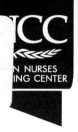

MW01041378

REVIEW AND RESOURCE MANUAL

Cardiac Vasular Nursing

Published by American Nurses Credentialing Center
Author: Linda Baas, PhD, MSN, RN, ACNP, FAHA

CONTINUING EDUCATION SOURCE
NURSING CERTIFICATION REVIEW MANUAL
CLINICAL PRACTICE RESOURCE

3RD EDITION

Library of Congress Cataloging-in-Publication Data

Baas, Linda S.
Cardiac vascular nursing review and resource manual / by Linda Baas. -- 3rd ed.
    p.; cm.
Rev. ed. of: Cardiac/vascular nursing review and resource manual. 2nd ed. c2006.
Includes bibliographical references and index.
ISBN 978-1-935213-36-9
1. Cardiovascular system-—Diseases—Nursing—Handbooks, manuals, etc. 2. Heart—-Diseases—
Handbooks, manuals, etc. 3. Heart—Nursing—Handbooks, manuals, etc. I. American Nurses
Credentialing Center. II. Cardiac/vascular nursing review and resource manual. III. Title.
    [DNLM: 1. Cardiovascular Diseases—nursing—Handbooks. 2. Cardiovascular Diseases—nursing-
Outlines. WY 18.2]
    RC674.C3744 2010
    616.1'0231--dc22
                                2010036962

The American Nurses Credentialing Center (ANCC), a subsidiary of the American Nurses Association
(ANA), provides individuals and organizations throughout the nursing profession with the resources they
need to achieve practice excellence. ANCC's internationally renowned credentialing programs certify
nurses in specialty practice areas; recognize healthcare organizations for promoting safe, positive work
environments through the Magnet Recognition Program® and the Pathway to Excellence ® Program;
and accredit providers of continuing nursing education. In addition, ANCC's Institute for Credentialing
Innovation provides leading-edge information and education services and products to support its core
credentialing programs.

Introduction to the Continuing Education (CE) Contact Hour Application Process for *Cardiac Vascular Nursing Review and Resource Manual*, 3rd Edition

The Institute for Credentialing Innovation now offers the continuing education contact hours for this manual online at www.NursingWorld.org, the American Nurses Association's Web site. This process involves answering approximately 25–30 questions that test knowledge of the information contained within this manual. The continuing education contact hours can be completed at any time and a certificate can be printed from the Web site immediately upon successful completion of the test.

After studying the manual and given an online multiple-choice test, the exam candidate will be able to:

1. Pass the posttest with at least 75% of the answers correct.
2. Select responses to test questions based on key principles, standards of practice, and theoretical basis of nursing practice.
3. Choose accepted therapeutic interventions in answering questions related to quality nursing practice.
4. Utilize direct and indirect professional role responsibilities and applications regarding nursing practice in answering test questions.

Upon completion of this manual and the online CE test, a nurse can receive up to a total of **30 continuing education contact hours** at a price of $60, only $2 per CE. (ANA members receive a discount on CEs.) The entire process—online test and evaluation form—must be completed by December 31, 2012 in order to receive credit. **To begin the process, please e-mail revmanuals@ana.org.** Your patience with this process is greatly appreciated.

Inquiries or Comments

If you have any questions about the CE contact hours, please e-mail The Institute at revmanuals@ana.org. You may also mail any comments to Editor/Project Manager at the address listed below.

Duplicate CE Certificates

Once you have successfully passed the CE test on NursingWorld, you may go back and re-print your certificate as often as you wish.

Conflicts of Interest

A conflict of interest occurs when an individual has an opportunity to affect educational content about health-care products or services of a commercial company with which she/he has a financial relationship.

The planners and presenters of this CNE activity have disclosed no relevant financial relationships with any commercial companies pertaining to this activity.

The Institute for Credentialing Innovation
American Nurses Credentialing Center, Attn: Editor/Project Manager
8515 Georgia Avenue, Suite 400
Silver Spring, MD 20910-3492
Fax: (301) 628-5342

A maximum of 30 contact hours may be earned by learners who successfully complete this continuing nursing education activity.

The American Nurses Association Center for Continuing Education and Professional Development is accredited as a provider of continuing nursing education by the American Nurses Credentialing Center's Commission on Accreditation.

ANCC Provider Number 0023

ANA is approved by the California Board of Registered Nursing, Provider Number 6178.

The ANA Center for Continuing Education and Professional Development includes ANCC's Institute for Credentialing Innovation.

Contents

Inflammation
Atherosclerosis
Thrombosis and Embolism
Altered Vascular Function
Altered Cardiac Function

Basic Principles
Subjective Information (History)
Physical Examination
Diagnostic Tests
Laboratory Tests Using Blood
Noninvasive Diagnostic Testing
Diagnostic Ultrasonography
Diagnostic Testing Using Radionuclides
Invasive Diagnostic Testing

Angina Pectoris
Myocardial Infarction
Valvular Heart Disease
Mitral Stenosis
Mitral Regurgitation
Aortic Stenosis
Aortic Regurgitation
Infective Endocarditis
Acute Pericarditis
Dilated Congestive Cardiomyopathy
Hypertrophic Cardiomyopathy
Restrictive Cardiomyopathy
Heart Failure
Atrial Fibrillation
Atrial Flutter
First-Degree Atrioventricular Block
Second-Degree Atrioventricular Block Type I
Second-Degree Atrioventricular Block Type II
Third-Degree Atrioventricular Block, Complete Heart Block
Ventricular Tachycardia
Ventricular Fibrillation
Sudden Cardiac Death
Pulmonary Artery Hypertension
Carotid Artery Occlusive Disease
Acute Management of Thrombotic CVA
Abdominal Aortic Aneurysm
Upper Extremity Arterial Occlusive Disease
Lower Extremity Arterial Occlusive Disease
Deep Vein Thrombosis
Chronic Venous Insufficiency

Cardiac Vascular Nursing
Review and Resource Manual

Taking the Certification Examination

When you sign up to take a national certification exam, you will be instructed to go online and review the testing and review handbook. (www.nursecredentialing.org/documents/certification/applicarion/generaltestingandreviewhandbook.aspx). Review it carefully and be sure to bookmark the site so you can refer to it frequently. It contains information on test content and sample questions. This is critical information; it will give you insight into the nature of the test. The agency will send you information about the test site; keep this in a safe place until needed.

GENERAL SUGGESTIONS FOR PREPARING FOR THE EXAM

Step One: Control Your Anxiety

Everyone experiences anxiety when faced with the certification exam.

- Remember, your program was designed to prepare you to take this exam.
- Your instructors took a similar exam, and have probably talked to students who took exams more recently, so they know how to help you prepare.
- Taking a review course or setting up your own study plan will help you feel more confident about taking the exam.

Step Two: Do Not Listen to Gossip About the Exam

A large volume of information exists about the tests based on reports from people who have taken the exams in the past. Because information from the testing facilities is limited, it is hard not to listen to this gossip.

- Remember that gossip about the exam that you hear from others is not verifiable.
- Because this gossip is based on the imperfect memory of people in a very stressful situation, it may not be very accurate.
- People tend to remember those items testing content with which they are less comfortable; for instance, those with a limited background in women's health may say that the exam was "all women's health." In fact, the exam blueprint ensures that the exam covers multiple content areas without overemphasizing any one.

Step Three: Set Reasonable Expectations for Yourself

- Do not expect to know everything.
- Do not try to know everything in great detail.
- You do not need a perfect score to pass the exam.
- The exam is designed for a beginner level—it is testing readiness for entry-level practice.
- Learn the general rules, not the exceptions.
- The most likely diagnoses will be on the exam, not questions on rare diseases or atypical cases.
- Think about the most likely presentation and most common therapy.

Step Four: Prepare Mentally and Physically

- While you are getting ready to take the exam, take good physical care of yourself.
- Get plenty of sleep, exercise, and eat well while preparing for the exam.
- These things are especially important while you are studying and immediately before you take the exam.

Step Five: Access Current Knowledge

General Content

You will be given a list of general topics that will be on the exam when you register to take the exam. In addition, examine the table of contents of this book and the test content outline, available at www.nursecredentialing.org/cert/TCOs.html.

- What content do you need to know?
- How well do you know these subjects?

Take a Review Course

- Taking a review course is an excellent method of assessing your knowledge of the content that will be included in the exam.
- If you plan to take a review course, take it well before the exam so you will have plenty of time to master any areas of weakness the course uncovers.
- If you are prepared for the exam, you will not hear anything new in the course. You will be familiar with everything that is taught.
- If some topics in the review course are new to you, concentrate on these in your studies.
- People have a tendency to study what they know; it is rewarding to study something and feel a mastery of it! Unfortunately, this will not help you master unfamiliar content. Be sure to use a review course to identify your areas of strength and weakness, then concentrate on the weaknesses.

Depth of Knowledge

How much do you need to know about a subject?

- You cannot know everything about a topic.
- Remember that the depth of knowledge required to pass the exam is for entry-level performance.
- Study the information sent to you from the testing agency, what you were taught in school, what is covered in this text, and the general guidelines given in this chapter.
- Look at practice tests designed for the exam. Practice tests for other exams will not be helpful.
- Consult your class notes or clinical diagnosis and management textbook for the major points about a disease. Additional reference books can be found online at www.nursecredentialing.org/cert/refs.html.
- For example, with regard to medications, know the drug categories and the major medications in each. Assume all drugs in a category are generally alike, and then focus on the differences among common drugs. Know the most important indications, contraindications, and side effects. Emphasize safety. The questions usually do not require you to know the exact dosage of a drug.

Step Six: Institute a Systematic Study Plan

Develop Your Study Plan

- Write a formal plan of study.
  - Include topics for study, timetable, resources, and methods of study that work for you.
  - Decide whether you want to organize a study group or work alone.
  - Schedule regular times to study.
  - Avoid cramming; it is counterproductive. Try to schedule your study periods in 1-hour increments.
- Identify resources to use for studying. To prepare for the examination, on your shelf you should have:
  - A good pathophysiology text.
  - This review book.
  - A physical assessment text.
  - Your class notes.
  - Other important sources, including information from the testing facility, a clinical diagnosis textbook, favorite journal articles, notes from a review course, and practice tests.
  - Know the important national standards of care for major illnesses.
  - Consult the bibliography on the test blueprint. When studying less familiar material, it is helpful to study using the same references that the testing center uses.
- Study the body systems from head to toe.
- The exam emphasizes health promotion, assessment, differential diagnosis, and plan of care for common problems.
- You will need to know facts and be able to interpret and analyze this information using critical thinking.

Personalize Your Study Plan
- How do you learn best?
  - If you learn best by listening or talking, attend a review course or discuss topics with a colleague.
- Read everything the test facility sends you as soon as you receive it and several times during your preparation period. It will give you valuable information to help guide your study.
- Have a specific place with good lighting set aside for studying. Find a place with no noise or distractions. Assemble your study materials.

Implement Your Study Plan
You must have basic content knowledge. In addition, you must be able to use this information to think critically and make decisions based on facts.
- Refer to your study plan regularly.
- Stick to your schedule.
- Take breaks when you get tired.
- If you start procrastinating, get help from a friend or reorganize your study plan.
- It is not necessary to follow your plan rigidly. Adjust as you learn where you need to spend more time.
- Memorize the basics of the content areas you will be required to know.

Focus on General Material
- Most of what you need to know is basic material that does not require constant updating.
- You do not need to worry about the latest information being published as you are studying for the exam. Remember, it can take 6 to 12 months for new information to be incorporated into test questions.

Pace Your Studying
- Stop studying for the examination when you are starting to feel overwhelmed and look at what is bothering you. Then make changes.
- Break overwhelming tasks into smaller tasks that you know you can do.
- Stop and take breaks while studying.

Work With Others
- Talk with classmates about your preparation for the exam.
- Keep in touch with classmates, and help each other stick to your study plans.
- If your classmates start having anxiety attacks, do not let their anxiety affect you. Walk away if you need to.
- Do not believe bad stories you hear about other people's experiences with previous exams.
- Remember, you know as much as anyone about what will be on the next exam!

Consider a Study Group
- Study groups can provide practice in analyzing cases, interpreting questions, and critical thinking.
  - You can discuss a topic and take turns presenting cases for the group to analyze.
  - Study groups also can provide moral support and help you keep studying.

Step Seven: Strategies Immediately Before the Exam

Final Preparation Suggestions
- Use practice exams when studying to get accustomed to the exam format and time restrictions.
  - Many books that are labeled as review books are simply a collection of examination questions.
  - If you have test anxiety, such practice tests may help alleviate the anxiety.
  - Practice tests can help you learn to judge the time you should take during an exam.
  - Practice tests are useful for gaining experience in analyzing questions.
  - Books of questions may not uncover the gaps in your knowledge that a more systematic content review text will reveal.
  - If you feel that you don't know enough about a topic, refer to a text to learn more. After you feel that you have learned the topic, practice questions are a wonderful tool to help improve your test-taking skill.
- Know your test-taking style.
  - Do you rush through the exam without reading the questions thoroughly?
  - Do you get stuck and dwell on a question for a long time?
  - You should spend about 45 to 60 seconds per question and finish with time to review the questions you were not sure about.
  - Be sure to read the question completely, including all four answer choices. Choice "a" may be good, but "d" may be best.

The Night Before the Exam
- Be prepared to get to the exam on time.
  - Know the test site location and how long it takes to get there.
  - Take a "dry run" beforehand to make sure you know how to get to the testing site, if necessary.
  - Get good night's sleep.
  - Eat sensibly.
  - Avoid alcohol the night before.
  - Assemble the required material—two forms of identification, admission card, pencil, and watch. Both IDs must match the name on the application, and one photo ID is preferred.
  - Know the exam room rules.
  - You will be given scratch paper, which will be collected at the end of the exam.
  - Nothing else is allowed in the exam room.
  - You will be required to put papers, backpacks, etc., in a corner of the room, or in a locker.
  - No water or food will be allowed.
  - You will be allowed to walk to a water fountain and go to the bathroom one at a time.

The Day of the Exam
- Get there early. If you are late, you may not be admitted.
- Think positively. You have studied hard and are well-prepared.
- Remember your anxiety reduction strategies.

SPECIFIC TIPS FOR DEALING WITH ANXIETY
- Test anxiety is a specific type of anxiety. Symptoms include upset stomach, sweaty palms, tachycardia, trouble concentrating, and a feeling of dread. But there are ways to cope with test anxiety.
- There is no substitute for being well-prepared.
- Practice relaxation techniques.
- Avoid alcohol, excess coffee, caffeine, and any new medications that might sedate you, dull your senses, or make you feel agitated.
- Take a few deep breaths and concentrate on the task at hand.

FOCUS ON SPECIFIC TEST-TAKING SKILLS
- To do well on the exam, you need good test-taking skills in addition to knowledge of the content and ability to use critical thinking.

ALL CERTIFICATION EXAMS ARE MULTIPLE CHOICE
- Multiple choice tests have specific rules for test construction.
- A multiple choice question consists of three parts: the information (or stem), the question, and the four possible answers (one correct and three distracters).
- Careful analysis of each part is necessary. Read the entire question before answering.
- Practice your test-taking skills by analyzing the practice questions in this book and on the ANCC Web site.

ANALYZE THE INFORMATION GIVEN
- Do not assume you have more information than is given.
- Do not overanalyze.
- Remember, the writer of the question assumes this is all of the information needed to answer the question.
- If information is not given, it is not relevant and will not affect the answer.
- Do not make the question more complicated than it is.

WHAT KIND OF QUESTION IS ASKED?
- Are you supposed to recall a fact, apply facts to a situation, or understand and differentiate between options?
- Read the question thinking about what the writer is asking.
- Look for key words or phrases that lead you (see Box 1–1). These help determine what kind of answer the question requires.

READ ALL OF THE ANSWERS
- If you are absolutely certain that answer "a" is correct as you read it, mark it, but read the rest of the question so you do not trick yourself into missing a better answer.
- If you are absolutely sure answer "a" is wrong, cross it off or make a note on your scratch paper and continue reading the question.
- After reading the entire question, go back, analyze the question, and select the best answer.
- Do not jump ahead.
- If the question asks you for an assessment, the best answer will be an assessment. Do not be distracted by an intervention that sounds appropriate.

Box 1–1. Examples of Key Words and Phrases

avoid	first	likely
best	contributing to	of the following
except	appropriate	most consistent with
not	most	
initial	significant	

- If the question asks you for an intervention, do not answer with an assessment.
- When two answer choices sound very good, the best one is usually the least expensive, least invasive way to achieve the goal. For example, if your answer choices include a physical exam maneuver or imaging, the physical exam maneuver is probably the better choice provided it will give the information needed.
- If the answers include two options that are the opposite of each other, one of the two is probably the correct answer.
- When numeric answers cover a wide range, a number in the middle is more likely to be correct.
- Watch out for distracters that are correct but do not answer the question, combine true and false information, or contain a word or phrase that is similar to the correct answer.
- Err on the side of caution.

ONLY ONE ANSWER CAN BE CORRECT
- When more than one suggested answer is correct, you must identify the one that best answers the question asked.
- If you cannot choose between two answers, you have a 50% chance of getting it right if you guess.

AVOID CHANGING ANSWERS
- Change an answer only if you have a compelling reason, such as you remembered something additional, or you understand the question better after rereading it.
- People change to a wrong answer more often than to a right answer.

TIME YOURSELF TO COMPLETE THE WHOLE EXAM
- Do not spend a large amount of time on one question.
- If you cannot answer a question quickly, mark it and continue the exam.
- If time is left at the end, return to the difficult questions.
- Make educated guesses by eliminating the obviously wrong answers and choosing a likely answer even if you are not certain.
- Trust your instinct.
- Answer every question. There is no penalty for a wrong answer.
- Occasionally a question will remind you of something that helps you with a question earlier in the test. Look back at that question to see if what you are remembering affects how you would answer that question.

ABOUT THE CERTIFICATION EXAMS

The American Nurses Credentialing Center Computerized Exam

The ANCC examination is given only as a computer exam, and each exam is different. The order of the questions is scrambled for every test, so even if two people are taking the same exam, the questions will be in a different order. The exam consists of 175 multiple-choice questions.

- 150 of the 175 questions are part of the test and how you answer will count toward your score; 25 are included to refine questions and will not be scored. You will not know which ones count, so treat all questions the same.
- You will need to know how to use a mouse, scroll by either clicking arrows on the scroll bar or using the up and down arrow keys, and perform other basic computer tasks.
- The exam does not require computer expertise.
- However, if you are not comfortable using a computer, you should practice using a mouse and computer beforehand so you do not waste time on the mechanics of using the computer.
- Know what to expect during the test.
- Each ANCC test question is independent of the other questions.
  - For each case study, there is only one question. This means that a correct answer on any question does not depend on the correct answer to any other question.
  - Each question has four possible answers. There are no questions asking for combinations of correct answers (such as "a and c") or multiple-multiples.
- You can skip a question and go back to it at the end of the exam.
- You cannot mark key words in the question or right or wrong answers. If you want to do this, use the scratch paper.
- You will get your results immediately, and a grade report will be provided upon leaving the testing site.

INTERNET RESOURCES

ANCC Web site: www.nursecredentialing.org

ANA Web site: www.nursesbooks.org; catalog of ANA nursing scope and standards publications and other titles that may be listed on your test content outline

National Guideline Clearinghouse: www.ngc.gov

2

Ethical and Legal Issues

Nurses are required to provide ethical and legal patient care that demonstrates respect for others. This chapter reviews the application of ethical theories and principles in clinical practice. The professional and legal regulation of practice also is discussed.

ETHICS

- Ethics is the systematic study of moral conduct and provides the framework for studying and examining moral dilemmas.
- Bioethics, also called biomedical ethics or medical ethics, is the study of moral conduct within the context of health care.
- Morality refers to norms about right and wrong human conduct that form a social consensus.
  - Moral virtues are socially valued character traits.
  - Five moral virtues for health professionals:
    1. Compassion combines active regard for another's welfare with an emotional response of sympathy, tenderness, and discomfort at another's misfortune or suffering.
    2. Discernment involves the ability to make judgments and decisions without being unduly influenced by extraneous considerations (e.g., fears, personal attachments).
    3. Trustworthiness involves ability and strength of character, dependability, and reliability.
    4. Integrity involves firm adherence to moral and ethical principles.
    5. Conscientiousness involves careful, dependable, competent practice.

ETHICAL PRINCIPLES

- *Beneficence* means to do good.
  - Promote the well-being of the patient
  - Prevent harm
- *Nonmaleficence* means to refrain from harm.
  - Obligates the clinician to avoid inflicting harm directly or intentionally
  - Balanced with beneficence—maximize benefits while minimizing harm
- *Autonomy* refers to the human right to make one's own decisions. Clinicians show respect for autonomy when they engage in the following behaviors:
  - Tell the truth
  - Respect the privacy of others
  - Protect confidential information
  - Obtain consent for interventions with patients
  - When asked, help others make important decisions
- *Justice* is the principle of fairness.
  - To treat others equally
  - To refrain from discrimination

Code of Ethics for Nurses

Box 2–1 lists the nine provisions of the Code. The full document includes interpretative statements related to each provision.

Selected Issues in Clinical Practice

Informed consent is based on respect for autonomy. There are five elements of informed consent related to treatments and procedures. Chapter 5 details specifics of informed consent related to research participation.

- Decisional capacity includes the ability to understand and make decisions.
  - Decisional capacity is specific, not global. It depends on the match between the patient's abilities and the specific decision-making task.
  - Decisional capacity may vary over time and be intermittent.
    - Physiological (e.g., illness, hypoxia) and situational factors (e.g., medically naive person admitted to the emergency department) may affect decision-making capacity.
    - If the patient's decisional capacity cannot be established initially, it is appropriate to assess his or her understanding, deliberative capacity, and coherence over time, and to consult with an expert when necessary.
    - Surrogate decision-makers are authorized to make decisions for patients when decisional capacity is impaired.
      - If possible, the surrogate decision-maker is required to make the decision that the incompetent patient would have made if competent. This is the "substituted judgment" standard. Surrogates may have written evidence of a person's wishes (e.g., a living will or letter), verbal evidence (i.e., conversations), or they may make inferences based on the person's history of relevant choices.

Box 2-1. Code of Ethics for Nurses

1. The nurse, in all professional relationships, practices with compassion and respect for the inherent dignity, worth, and uniqueness of every person, unrestricted by consideration of social or economic status, personal attributes, or the nature of health problems.
2. The nurse's primary commitment is to the patient, whether a person, family, group, or community.
3. The nurse promotes, advocates for, and strives to protect the health, safety, and rights of the patient.
4. The nurse is responsible and accountable for individual nursing practice and determines the appropriate delegation of tasks consistent with the nurse's obligation to provide optimum patient care.
5. The nurse owes the same duties to self as to others, including the responsibility to preserve integrity and safety, to maintain competence, and to continue personal and professional growth.
6. The nurse participates in establishing, maintaining, and improving healthcare environments and conditions of employment conducive to the provision of quality health care and consistent with the values of the profession through individual and collective action.
7. The nurse participates in the advancement of the profession through contributions to practice, education, administration, and knowledge development.
8. The nurse collaborates with other health professionals and the public in promoting community, national, and international efforts to meet health needs.
9. The profession of nursing, as represented by associations and their members, is responsible for articulating nursing values, for maintaining the integrity of the profession and its practice, and for shaping social policy.

From *Code of Ethics for Nurses With Interpretive Statements* (p. 4), by the American Nurses Association, 2001, Silver Spring, MD: American Nurses Association. Copyright 2001 by the American Nurses Association. Reprinted with permission.

- If the surrogate has no way of knowing what choice a person would have made, then the "best interests" standard should be used. That is, the surrogate should choose the option that appears to be in the best interests of the patient. Hence, surrogates are held to a higher standard of decision-making than competent persons. Competent persons may make healthcare choices that are eccentric, poorly reasoned, biased, and so on, but, unless evidence exists to support such a choice, a surrogate is compelled ethically and legally to act in the patient's best interests.
- The order of surrogate authority varies slightly by state but generally specifies the following list in descending order of priority:
  - Court-appointed guardian
  - Durable power of attorney
  - Spouse
  - Adult children (usually requires consensus)
  - Parents (usually requires consensus)
  - Adult siblings (usually requires consensus)

- Disclosure includes a core set of information about the treatment or research procedure, including the following:
  - Facts or descriptions that patients usually consider relevant when making a decision to refuse or consent.
  - Information the clinician believes to be relevant (e.g., alternative treatments).
  - The clinician's recommendation
  - The purpose of seeking consent
  - The nature and limits of consent (e.g., research studies include the right to withdraw from study without penalty).
  - Patients have the right to refuse to be informed regarding their healthcare decisions, however. In that situation, the clinician should document the refusal in the medical record.
- Understanding is difficult to assess. Patients and research subjects should understand at least what the clinician or researcher believes the patient needs to understand to authorize the procedure.
- Voluntariness implies that the patient agrees to the intervention without undue influence.
- Consent is the acceptance or refusal of the treatment or research study after the patient is adequately informed.
  - Consent can be withdrawn at any time.
  - A written form documenting that consent has occurred is required for some healthcare decisions such as sterilization, injection of a radioactive substance, surgery, etc. Which procedures and decisions require written evidence of consent is mandated occasionally by law and usually by institutional policies.
  - Regardless of whether written consent is required, all health care should be delivered using the model of informed consent including nursing-controlled activities such as ambulation following surgery, preoperative teaching, and so on. Written evidence of consent for such noninvasive activities is not required.

Advance Directives

A person while competent can complete a directive documenting his or her healthcare wishes or values or selecting a surrogate to make decisions during periods of incapacity.

- Living wills are directives that specify preferred treatment during periods of incapacity. They represent written evidence of a patient's wishes.
- Durable power of attorney for health care (DPAHC) is a legal document in which one person assigns authority to another to act as his or her surrogate if he or she is unable to make healthcare decisions.
  - In general, only the DPAHC includes healthcare decision-making authority.
- The Patient Self-Determination Act of 1990 requires healthcare facilities to develop programs to inform patients and staff about advance directives.

Access to Care

Access to care is a major ethical and political issue confronting the United States and is based on the principle of justice.

- Access is limited, in part, by economic considerations. Different insurance plans provide different reimbursement for, and therefore different access to, care.
  - Approximately 17% of the non-older adult U.S. population lacks health insurance of any kind.
  - Approximately 25% of the U.S. population has publicly supported care (e.g., Medicare, Medicaid) or insurance unconnected to employment.
  - Approximately 58% of the U.S. population has employer-based insurance.
- Principle of justice—fair distribution of resources; all are treated equally—implies a right to health care.
- The dilemma confronting the United States is how to fund and distribute health care fairly.

Nurse/Healthcare Team/Patient Relationships

- Veracity obligates the nurse to be truthful with patients and members of the healthcare team. A current example is the increased emphasis on the need to disclose healthcare errors to colleagues, the institution, the patient, and in some cases to government agencies.
- Privacy obligates the clinician to appropriately restrict access to the patient and to the health record. A current privacy issue is the need to restrict clinicians' access to the electronic medical record of any patients with whom they are not directly involved in care. This includes hospitalized colleagues, employees, public figures, and family or friends.
- Confidentiality requires clinicians to share information about the patient only with the patient and those health professionals who are involved in caring for the patient.
- Fidelity refers to faithfulness in keeping a promise. The nurse makes an implied promise to care for a patient based on the social contract the profession of nursing has established with the public. Fidelity requires that the nurse put the patient's interests above other interests, such as financial, personal, or other people involved in the patient's care or life.

Withholding and Withdrawing Treatment

Questions about withholding and withdrawing treatment derive from the principles of beneficence and nonmaleficence.

- Medical futility is a controversial concept.
  - Quantitative medical futility describes a situation where research and practice would suggest that there is less than a 1% chance that the treatment will have the intended effect, for example, CPR in a cachectic patient with metastasized cancer. Quantitatively futile treatments are not obligatory.
  - Qualitative futility describes situations where the treatment will have the intended effect but will not achieve a desired benefit (e.g., tube-feeding a patient who has suffered a severe stroke will provide nutrition but will not restore neurological function).

- Ordinary versus extraordinary treatments
  - The traditional rule is that extraordinary treatment can be withheld but ordinary treatment cannot.
  - The distinction between ordinary and extraordinary treatments is not clear and of uncertain moral and ethical meaning.
- Double effect: A single act may have two effects, one beneficial and one harmful. For example, a patient requiring high doses of a narcotic analgesic for pain control (intended, beneficial effect) may be at risk for respiratory depression (unintended, harmful effect). Questions to consider:
  - Is there an alternative treatment that provides the intended effect (pain control) without the unintended effect (respiratory depression)?
  - Is the treatment provided for its intended effect (pain control, not respiratory depression)?
  - Does the intended effect (pain control) outweigh the unintended effect (respiratory depression)?

Ethical Reasoning

Application of a systematic way of thinking about an ethical dilemma will help to reach a conclusion. Steps in the reasoning process include:
- Review facts and assumptions about the case or situation.
  - Clinical data and treatment options
  - Relevant law
  - Patient preferences and beliefs
  - Goal of treatment
- Define the ethical dilemma in specific terms.
  - An ethical dilemma requires a choice between courses of action that involves fundamental concepts of right and wrong.
  - Ethical dilemmas usually involve concepts of rights, duties, and responsibilities.
  - An ethical dilemma is not a difference of opinion about treatment or different appraisals of clinical facts.
- List possible courses of action.
- Choose a course of action, considering:
  - Patient preferences
  - Professional standards
  - Relevant law
  - Personal values and principles
- Evaluate the choice.
  - Consistent with ethical principles?
  - Consistent with decisions made in similar cases?
  - Consistent with values and principles of those affected (e.g., culturally sensitive)?
  - Consequences of the decision?

Ethical Decision-Making Resources

- Ethics committees are multidisciplinary groups that review ethical dilemmas and advise clinicians.
- Ethics consultation services provide "on-call" assistance to patients, families, and clinicians when confronted by ethical dilemmas.

- Formal educational programs in ethics provide clinicians with an understanding and a framework for decision-making.
- Policies related to ethical issues (e.g., do not attempt resuscitation policy) guide institutional practice.

Patients' Rights
- Patients' rights are derived from the ethical theory of Liberal Individualism.
- In 1990, the American Hospital Association codified the following in the Patients' Bill of Rights.
    - Right to considerate and respectful care
    - Right to information about diagnosis, treatment, and prognosis
    - Right to make decisions about the plan of care
    - Right to have advance directives
    - Right to privacy
    - Right to confidentiality
    - Right to review clinical records
    - Right to responsible care and services, including the right to transfer
    - Right to information about business relationships among the hospital, educational institutions, and payors that might influence care and treatment
    - Right to reasonable continuity of care
    - Right to be informed of hospital policies and procedures that regulate patient care, treatment, and responsibilities; includes the right to grievance and dispute resolution

REGULATION OF NURSING PRACTICE

Professional Regulation
- Professional practice standards are authoritative statements by which the nursing profession describes the responsibilities of nurses.
    - Standards of care describe a competent level of nursing care as demonstrated by the nursing process (includes assessment, diagnosis, outcome identification, planning, implementation, and evaluation).
    - Standards of professional performance describe a competent level of behavior in the professional role (includes activities related to quality of care, performance appraisal, education, collegiality, ethics, collaboration, research, and resource utilization).
- Nursing's social policy statement describes the discipline of nursing, its scope, and the profession's responsibility to society.
    - The 1980 Social Policy Statement defined nursing as "the diagnosis and treatment of human responses to actual or potential health problems."
    - Since that time, definitions of nursing acknowledge four essential features:
        - Attention to the full range of human experiences and responses to health and illness (i.e., not limited to actual or potential health problems)
        - Integration of objective data with understanding of the patient's subjective experience
        - Use of scientific knowledge in the process of diagnosis and treatment
        - Provision of a caring relationship that facilitates healing

– Scope of basic nursing practice involves promoting, supporting, and restoring health; preventing illness; and assisting with activities that contribute to a peaceful death.
  • Nurses in basic practice coordinate care, prepare patients for tests and procedures, and monitor the patient's response to various treatments.
  • Nurses in basic practice provide care in a variety of settings including hospitals, homes, schools, places of employment, correctional facilities, nursing homes, and community-based healthcare facilities.

Professional Certification

• Private (not governmental) agencies sponsor programs to certify that people meet certain criteria and are prepared to practice in that discipline or clinical area.
• Certification recognizes specialized knowledge and skills beyond that which is required for safe, basic practice. This differs from licensure, which is a legal recognition that enables one to practice in a profession such as nursing.

Legal Regulation of Nursing Practice

• Protects the public health, safety, and welfare
  – All states require licensure for nursing practice (e.g., registered nurse, licensed practical nurse).
  – Most states have additional requirements for advanced clinical nursing practice (i.e., nurse practitioner, clinical nurse specialist, nurse anesthetist, nurse midwife).
• Nurse practice acts are state laws that grant the right to practice nursing to people who meet predetermined standards (e.g., education).
  – Regulatory boards (e.g., Board of Nursing [BON]) are created under the nurse practice act and govern nursing practice in the state.
  – The BON is responsible for
    • Determining eligibility for licensing and relicensing
    • Approving and supervising educational programs
    • Enforcing the statute (i.e., the nurse practice act and the BON regulations)
    • Writing rules and regulations governing the practice of nursing
  – Basic grounds for disciplinary action
    • Fraud in obtaining a license
    • Unprofessional, illegal, dishonorable, or immoral conduct
    • Performance of specific actions prohibited by the act
    • Conviction of a felony or crime of moral turpitude
    • Drug or alcohol addiction rendering the person incapable of performing duties
  – Possible sanctions if found guilty of the above include
    • Revocation of license
    • Suspension of license for a specified period of time
    • Suspension of license for an unspecified period of time with the opportunity to reapply after a specified program of study or treatment
    • Prohibition of work in specified settings

LEGAL ASPECTS

Personal Accountability
- The individual is personally responsible for his or her own actions.
- The person who actually causes the harm has the primary responsibility.
- Duty to communicate may be the most important duty of the nurse.
  - Communicate change in the patient's condition to the physician.
  - Communicate concern about impaired practice to the nurse manager or supervisor.
  - Communicate concerns about short staffing to the appropriate person every time the situation occurs.

Employer and Supervisor Accountability
- An employer is liable for the actions of its employees within their scope of employment.
  - The employer may not be responsible if the employee is acting beyond his or her scope of employment.
  - Employer and supervisor responsibility does not eliminate personal responsibility.
- A supervisor may be liable for harm caused by an incompetent nurse, if the supervisor failed to assess the nurse's ability, if the employee has a known problem that can affect performance (e.g., alcoholism), or if the supervisor failed to provide adequate supervision.
- A healthcare facility is obligated to carefully monitor the credentials and competence of employees and independent contractors.

Independent Contractor Accountability
- The independent contractor is responsible for his or her own actions.
- The healthcare facility or organization may be liable also if it has reason to know that the independent contractor was incompetent and failed to act.

Torts
- A tort is a civil action for financial damages for injury to a person, property, or reputation.
- Negligence, an unintentional tort, is the most common cause of cases involving nurses.
  - Failure to adhere to the standard of nursing care (negligent practice) results in harm to the patient.
  - Four elements must be proved to establish a claim of negligence.
    - Duty:
      - It must be proved that the nurse had a duty (responsibility) to care for the patient.
      - The scope or limits of that duty must be proved. Published standards of care and the actions of a "reasonably prudent nurse" (expert witness) are used to establish scope of duty.
    - Breach of duty: It must be proved that the nurse deviated in some manner from the standard of care.
    - Injury or harm to the patient must result. Harm may be physical, emotional, or financial.
    - Causation: The breach of duty must be proved to be the proximate cause of injury.

- Protect yourself against negligent practice.
  - Know your practice area and remain current.
  - Know your abilities and limitations.
  - Know and follow the standards of care in your area.
  - Know and follow your facility's policies and procedures.
  - Know your patients and their families; build good relationships.
- Statute of limitations specifies the time limit within which a suit must be filed.
  - Established under state law.
  - Varies by nature of the complaint. In most states, a complaint of negligence must be entered within 2 years of the time the patient (or patient's representative) becomes aware of the injury.

- Torts generally result in financial settlements. The BON may take action regarding licensure in addition to the financial settlements resulting from a successful civil tort (malpractice) claim. Crimes carry the possibility of jail sentences.
- In some states, Good Samaritan Laws extend a degree of immunity to people providing care gratuitously in an emergency situation.
- Intentional torts contain purposeful action and the intent to do an act. The intent does not have to be hostile or malicious. There must be an understanding that the harmful outcome is highly likely or that the act was done with reckless disregard for the interest of the patient.
  - Assault and battery
    - An assault is a credible threat that causes another to become apprehensive of being touched in a manner that is offensive, insulting, provoking, or physically injurious.
    - If the threat (assault) is carried out, the act is battery.
  - Defamation is the wrongful injury to the reputation of another person.
    - Oral defamation is slander.
    - Written defamation is libel.
    - Statement must be made to a third person; statements made directly to the person are not defamatory.
    - Best protection against defamation: truth and privilege.
      - True statements are not a basis for legal action.
      - A privileged statement is one that could be considered defamatory in other situations, but is not because of a legally recognized higher duty that the person making the communication must honor.
  - Invasion of privacy occurs when an unauthorized person has access to confidential information.
    - Information about a patient is confidential and should not be released without permission of the patient.
    - Mandatory reporting of communicable diseases, suspicion of child or elder abuse, and other matters to the appropriate officials as required by law is not invasion of privacy.
      - Disclosure to the general public, media, or other interested parties is invasion of privacy.
      - Clinicians who access information about patients for whom they do not have direct responsibility are invading the privacy of those patients and may be subject to institutional or civil penalty.

– Fraud and misrepresentation are false or misleading statements that the patient relies on to his or her detriment.
– False imprisonment is the unlawful restriction of the freedom of a person, including physical restraint.

SUMMARY

As you prepare for the cardiovascular certification exam, remember that the basics of legal and ethical practice are part of the test content outline. Be sure to be able to apply concepts from the *Code of Ethics for Nurses* to a clinical situation, demonstrating knowledge of ethical theories and sound ethical decision-making. Know the difference between certification and licensure, what constitutes malpractice, and major tenets of the HIPAA legislation.

REFERENCES

Aiken, T. D. (2004). *Legal, ethical, and political issues in nursing.* Philadelphia: F. A. Davis.

American Hospital Association. (1990). *A patient's bill of rights.* Chicago, IL: Author.

American Nurses Association. (2001). *Code of ethics for nurses with interpretive statements.* Washington, DC: American Nurses Publishing.

American Nurses Association. (2003). *Nursing's social policy statement* (2nd ed.). Silver Spring, MD: American Nurses Publishing.

American Nurses Association. (2004). *Nursing: Scope and standards of practice.* Silver Spring, MD: American Nurses Publishing.

American Nurses Association. (2008). *Cardiovascular nursing: Scope and standards of practice.* Silver Spring, MD: American Nurses Publishing.

Beauchamp, T. L., & Childress, J. F. (2001). *Principles of biomedical ethics* (5th ed.). New York: Oxford University Press.

Butts, J. B., & Rich, K. L. (2005). *Nursing ethics across the curriculum.* Sudbury, MA: Jones & Bartlett

Fry, S., & Johnstone, M. J. (2008). *Ethics in nursing practice.* Oxford, UK: Wiley Blackwell.

Griffith, R., & Tengnah, C. (2008). *Law and professional issues in nursing: Transforming nursing practice.* Exeter, UK: Learning Matters.

Westrick, S., & McCormack-Dempski, K. (2009). *Essentials of nursing law and ethics.* Sudbury, MA: Jones & Bartlett.

3

Theory:
Nursing and Health

This chapter provides an overview of what constitutes a theory and why it is important, and an introduction to nursing theories, health-related theories, and pertinent theories from psychology and sociology. Theories from education are found in Chapter 6.

Theory is to nursing practice as a road map is to a cross-country car trip. Theory, like a road map, provides direction to facilitate successful outcomes. Theory, research, and practice are intertwined. Theory guides your specific approach to your practice. It is the rationale for doing things the way that you do them. Theory can arise from practice or be formulated from research findings. In addition, theory can guide the research. Some describe the relationship among theory, research, and practice as a three-legged stool. If you take any one of the three legs away, patient care is less effective.

GENERAL COMMENTS REGARDING THEORY

Theory and its components require a brief explanation.
- *Theory* is a set of concepts, definitions, and propositions that projects a systematic view of phenomena by defining specific interrelationships among the concepts for purposes of describing, explaining, and predicting phenomena.

- A *concept* is a word or phrase that describes an abstract idea or mental image of a phenomenon. Concepts are the building blocks of theory. For example, concepts with special relevance to nursing are "adherence, health, and cardiovascular fitness."
- A *proposition* is a statement about a concept or the relationship between two or more concepts. For example, a descriptive proposition related to health is "health is more than the absence of disease." A relational proposition is "cardiovascular fitness is a component of health."
- The purpose of theory is to describe, explain, or predict phenomena. Theory serves the discipline of nursing in several ways:
  - As an organized source for knowledge and research findings
  - To explain observations and predict outcomes
  - To stimulate new directions in practice and research
  - To develop research questions for testing
- Theory improves nursing practice by increasing understanding of phenomena; understanding influences behavior. Learning to think differently about phenomena enables one to try different approaches.
- When theory is shared by peers or adopted by a clinical unit, there is a shared approach to the care of the patient. For instance, self-care or adaptation may be the focus of the approach taken for patient care interventions.

NURSING THEORY

Often, Florence Nightingale is cited as the first nursing theorist. She proposed that nursing put the patient in the best possible condition (environment) for healing. The text by George provides an overview of many of the nursing theories.

- Nursing theory development really began in the 1960s as nurse educators tried to explain practice. Henderson and Johnson developed lists of activities that nurses did to support patients.
- In the 1970s, there was an informal agreement that nursing theory should address four concepts: patient, nursing, environment, and health. Theories differed in the way in which they viewed these four components (often called the metaparadigm of nursing) and the assumptions and propositions among the concepts.
- Early theories (Roy, Orem, Rogers) tried to explain all of nursing and these are grand theories. Some refer to grand theories as conceptual models that are more abstract than theories.
- More recent theories try to be more specific and explain a narrower focus of nursing, such as symptom management or health promotion.
- Examples of nurse theorists and their focus are provided in Table 3–1.

Table 3–1. Major Foci of Nursing Theories

Theorist	Major Focus	Brief Explanation of Key Points
Myra Levine	Conservation	Nurses provide therapeutic interventions to conserve patient energy to preserve structural integrity, personal integrity, and social integrity.
Dorothea Orem	Self-Care	Nursing provides care when the patient has a deficit. The form of care can be wholly compensatory, partially compensatory, or supportive-educative depending on the patient's needs. Goal is self-care.
Sister Callista Roy	Adaptation	Nursing helps in adaptation in four modes: physiologic, self-concept, role function, and interdependence. Adaptation occurs through the regulator (physiologic) and cognator (cognitive) functions.
Betty Neuman	Systems Model	Nursing assists the person to build strong lines of defense against stressors.
Martha Rogers	Unitary Man	People are open energy systems in constant interaction with others and the environment. Nurses assist the person to move forward and evolve to reach maximum human potential.
Helen Erickson, Evelyn Tomlin, Mary Ann Swain	Modeling and Role Modeling	Nurses model the client's world and then intervene to remodel the world to reach higher levels of health. Nurses practice five aims of interventions to use patient self-care knowledge, adaptive potential, and developmental residual to facilitate health.
Jean Watson	Transpersonal Caring	Nurses provide human caring that is holistic for the purpose of preserving dignity and wholeness.
Margaret Newman	Expanding Consciousness	People are energy fields that can expand consciousness. Nursing assists in this process.
Madeleine Leininger	Cultural Caring— Sunrise Model	All nursing care must be placed in a cultural context as health behaviors and beliefs are filtered through social systems, norms of behavior, and societal values.

Health and Illness

Health and illness are key concepts in nursing theory, research, and practice. In 1974, the World Health Organization (WHO) defined health as follows: "Health is a state of complete physical, mental, and social well-being and not merely the absence of disease and infirmity."

- This definition changed the conceptualization of health from an illness model to a competence model. Health became a positive condition to be attained.
- Four general conceptualizations of health are found in the nursing literature.
    - Clinical: Health is the absence of disease or injury.
    - Role: Health is the ability to perform role functions.
    - Adaptive: Health is adaptation or adjustment to life's demands.
    - Eudaimonistic: Health is the expression of the maximum potential of the person. The WHO definition is an example of eudaimonistic definition.
- Holistic theorists define health as a state or process in which the person experiences a sense of well-being and the integration of body, mind, and spirit interacting harmoniously with the environment. The American Holistic Nursing Association has identified specific nursing theories as holistic for certification of holistic nursing (*Modeling and Role-Modeling* by Helen Erickson, Evelyn Tomlin, and Mary Ann Swain; *Human Caring* by Jean Watson) focuses on what the person believes caused the health problem and the self-care knowledge of what will help the person regain health.
- Illness and disease are different concepts. Illness is the subjective experience of the symptoms and suffering to which the person assigns meaning. Disease is a discrete entity causing specific symptoms.
    - Some scholars conceptualize health and illness as existing on a single continuum, from optimum health to terminal illness.
    - Others conceptualize health and illness on two distinct, but interacting, continua. One continuum is anchored by no illness and terminal illness; the other by optimum health and poor health.

HUMAN BEHAVIOR

Theories of human behavior have been used to describe, explain, or predict health-related behavior. Theories and models that focus on individuals describe, explain, or predict the choices that individuals make about health-related behavior.

Maslow's Hierarchy of Needs

Abraham Maslow's hierarchy depicts human need as a pyramid with survival needs at the base and the most sophisticated needs at the apex of the pyramid. As needs are met at each level, the next higher level provides motivation for behavior. The first two steps often are described as basic needs while the next two steps are growth needs. Basic needs must be met before one can meet growth needs. Layers of the pyramid, from most basic to most sophisticated, are:

- Physiological survival needs—food, air, sleep, and shelter
- Safety needs—freedom from fear of threat to survival
- Belonging needs—affiliation and love
- Self-actualization needs—maximizing one's potential and achieving personal fulfillment

Human Development

Human development proceeds in a sequence of stages that are generally age-related. Each stage poses a challenge that the person must overcome. While Erik Erikson described the challenges for each stage across the life span, he also identified that if not successfully resolved earlier in life, this challenge may resurface later in life when a person is stressed. This helps explain that trust or autonomy may be a major concern for a person during the stress of an illness. The nurse must consider this and approach the patient in a way to help deal with the developmental challenge. The stages and challenges are:

- Trust versus mistrust
- Autonomy versus shame and doubt
- Initiative versus guilt
- Industry versus inferiority
- Identity versus role diffusion
- Intimacy versus isolation
- Generativity versus absorption
- Integrity versus despair

Social Cognitive Theory

Social cognitive theory (SCT) examines the mental processes through which thoughts, beliefs, and attitudes are converted into behavior. Perceived self-efficacy is a significant determinant of behavior.

- Perceived self-efficacy is a person's assessment of his or her ability to perform the actions necessary to achieve a desired outcome.
- Perceived self-efficacy is a thought or belief that is unrelated to actual skill level.
- Perceived self-efficacy is behavior-specific; a person's perceived self-efficacy for engaging in exercise may differ from his perceived self-efficacy for dietary change.
- Efficacy information is obtained from four sources.
  - Mastery experience is the most powerful source and comes from engaging in the behavior and evaluating personal performance.
  - Vicarious experience comes from watching others perform a task and hearing their self-evaluation and feedback.
  - Physiological cues provide information to the person through his or her level of autonomic arousal. People use physiological cues related to anxiety, fear, and tranquility to judge their competence.
  - Verbal or social persuasion is information presented by others to convince the person that he or she possesses the capacity to carry out a specific course of action. Verbal or social persuasion is the least powerful source of efficacy information.
- SCT and perceived self-efficacy have been used in several studies on the resumption of activity after an acute cardiac event. In general, perceived self-efficacy for a specific behavior is moderately to highly correlated with achievement of the behavior.

Health Belief Model

The Health Belief Model (HBM) explains why healthy people use health-protecting and disease-preventing services. The HBM has been refined and extended to explain individual responses to preventive services and illness treatment.

- In the HBM, three sets of variables interact and determine individual response.
  - Individual perceptions
    - Perceived vulnerability of the person
    - Perceived seriousness of the disease
    - Perceived benefits of preventive action
    - Perceived barriers to preventive action
  - Modifying factors
    - Demographics: age, gender, and ethnicity
    - Psychosocial characteristics: personality, social class, and peer group pressure
    - Structural characteristics: knowledge about the disease and prior contact with disease
  - Cues to action
    - Media campaigns
    - Advice from others
    - Postcard reminders
- The interaction of individual perceptions, modifying factors, and cues to action determines whether a person engages in a health-promoting behavior.
- The HBM has been used to explain health-related behavior and to guide program development to increase the likelihood of success.
- Across studies, perceived barriers to preventive action have been most consistently associated with health-promoting behaviors. When perceived barriers are high, the likelihood of adopting the preventive behavior is low.
- The HBM has been criticized for several reasons:
  - It places responsibility for action exclusively on the person;
  - It focuses on avoiding negative behavior, as opposed to embracing positive health behaviors; and
  - The motivation for behavior change comes from perceived threat or fear of illness.

Health Promotion Model

The Health Promotion Model (HPM) described by Nola Pender focuses on health-seeking rather than disease-preventing behaviors.

- In the HPM, two sets of variables interact and determine personal commitment to action:
  - Individual characteristics and experiences (including expectations); and
  - Behavior-specific thoughts and feelings.
    - Perceived benefits of action
    - Perceived barriers to action
    - Perceived self-efficacy
    - Activity-related effect
- The commitment to action may be modified or broken by competing demands and preferences.
- In general, studies that used the HPM produced evidence that supports the relationships between perceived self-efficacy, benefits of and barriers to action, and health-related behavior.

Transtheoretical Model

The Transtheoretical Model (TTM) describes a six-stage process of behavior change that was derived from a review of theories and research related to behavioral change conducted by Prochaska and DiClemente. The motivation to change and effective interventions to promote change differ by stage. Progression through the stages is not always linear. The average person recycles through the stages several times before behavior change is achieved. TTM is the theoretical model that is the basis of the Smoking Cessation Model from the National Institutes of Health and it is the rationale for asking all hospitalized patients about smoking status.

- In the precontemplation stage, the client has no intention of changing.
  - The client may deny that change is needed, blame others for the problem, or feel overwhelmed and demoralized.
  - Clinicians are most effective if they are empathetic and patient while offering hope for change.
- In the contemplation stage, the client acknowledges the need to change but is ambivalent and anxious about the change.
  - Clinicians can provide information, acknowledge ambivalence, help clarify goals, and eliminate barriers to change.
- In the preparation stage, the client begins to explore different options or ways to change the behavior. He or she is actively planning to change within the next month.
  - Clinicians can assist the client to make realistic plans about how to handle relapse while focusing on the future and the benefits of change.
- In the action stage, the client changes the behavior.
  - Clinicians assist the client to substitute alternative behaviors. Affirmation and support are helpful at this stage.
- In the maintenance stage, the client continues the change. If a lapse occurs it may result in fear and decreased self-efficacy.
  - Clinicians assist the client to view a lapse as a learning opportunity without imposing guilt. A lapse is not a defeat.
- In the termination stage, the client revises his or her self-image and the former behavior is no longer a threat.
  - Clinicians remain alert to risks for old behavior and continue to promote the client's self-efficacy for the behavior.
- The TTM developed through studying the process of smoking cessation with adults. Subsequent studies have shown its applicability to exercise and other behavior changes.

COMMUNITY-LEVEL BEHAVIOR CHANGE

Social Ecology Theory

Social Ecology Theory (SET) examines the way people influence and are influenced by their environment and pays particular attention to the interface between person and environment.

- Responsibility for health is shared between individuals and community systems.
- Health-promoting strategies are developed through community action and public policy. Programs based on SET focus on creating healthier communities to produce healthier people.
  - The role of the clinician is consultant and supporter of the change process.
  - The Minnesota Heart Health Program is an example of a community-based behavior change program. Strategies employed included community-level health education programs related to smoking cessation, exercise, and nutrition.

ORGANIZATIONAL CHANGE

Lewin's Planned Change

Kurt Lewin's process of planned change is the classic theory of organizational change.
- Successful change involves unfreezing existing structures, introducing the change and moving to a new level, and refreezing the structures to incorporate the change.
- Successful change requires identifying forces driving the change and those restraining the change. Change is accomplished by strengthening driving forces and reducing restraining forces.

Strategies for Organizational Change

Strategies for organizational change reflect individual change theories.
- Empirical–rational strategies for organizational change reflect the Theory of Reasoned Action.
  - The logic is as follows: Organizations are composed of people. People are rational. To create change, provide education and disseminate knowledge. Once the people see the benefit, they will adopt the change.
- Normative–reeducative strategies of organizational change reflect social cognitive theory.
- Power–coercive strategies of organizational change reflect motivational theories. The impetus for change is authority or organizational power. Change occurs because it reduces pain or harm as opposed to increasing pleasure or benefit.

Barriers to Organizational Change

Forces restraining acceptance of organizational change include:
- Threat to self-interest: the change will be harmful in some way
- Inaccurate perceptions of the effect the change will have
- Disagreement about the value of the change
- Low tolerance for change and uncertainty, which may be related to lack of self-confidence
- Time; a system that has been stable for a long time is resistant to change

Drivers for Organizational Change

Forces facilitating acceptance of organizational change include:
- People believe that the change is their idea or agrees with their ideas.
- People are part of the change process.
- Other people who are important to the person support the change.
- The change reduces burden or work.
- The change is introduced as a pilot with evaluation.
- The change is implemented using skillful, enthusiastic leadership that emphasizes communication and participation.

Rogers's Theory of Adoption of Innovation

Everett Rogers built upon Lewin's work and described a process of adopting innovation.
- A new change must undergo a process of diffusion in an organization that uses defined communication channels.
- People fall into five categories related to their response to change: innovators, early adopters, early majority, late majority, and laggards.
- Strategies for change should consider mobilizing early adopters and early majority.

FAMILY DYNAMICS

- Families are important in nursing practice. Families are conceptualized as the context within which the person exists and as the client for therapeutic intervention.
- Family may be defined as a small group of intimates related biologically, legally, or emotionally; a family is as it defines itself.
- Cardiovascular and other health risk factors cluster within families. The Framingham Heart Study found a higher than expected concordance between spouses for blood pressure, cholesterol, triglyceride, blood sugar, smoking, and pulmonary function.

Family Systems Theory
- Members of the family interact as a functional whole. Change in one element of the family system affects the whole system.
    - The family as a whole is greater than (and different from) the sum of its parts.
    - People are best understood within the family context.
- The family system is in contact with the environment, with input and output across its boundaries.
    - Families function to transmit culture.
    - Family members occupy a variety of roles and functions that may assume varying importance at different familial developmental stages.
    - Family members, especially the spouse, are the most important source of social support.
        - Social support has a direct effect on health.
        - The quality of family relationships has an indirect effect on health by buffering stress.
- Problems and symptoms occurring within family members reflect the family's adaptation to its total structure and environment at a given time.
- Adaptive efforts of family members affect the biological, interpersonal, and intrapsychic connections with the family (nuclear and extended) and the society.
    - Concurrent events in different parts of the family are connected in some way.
- There are normative expectations related to timing of major transitions within the family, such as leaving home, marriage, and childbirth.
    - "On time" events create less strain within the family than "off time" events.

Family Life Cycle
- As with individuals, family development follows a predictable course.
    - Unattached young adult
    - Newly married couple
    - Family with young children
    - Family with adolescent children
    - Family launching children and moving on
    - Later life family
- Families oscillate between periods of closeness (centripetal) and periods of distance (centrifugal). These periods reflect the needs of the family within its developmental stage. For example, a family with young children requires high cohesion (centripetal) while a family that is launching children requires more distance (centrifugal).

Family Response to Serious Illness

Family response to serious illness depends on when the illness occurs within the family life cycle, which family member falls ill, and the family's usual coping style. For example, a myocardial infarction may have different meaning to a family with young children versus a later life family. Family stress related to role change may differ depending on whether it is the husband or the wife who becomes ill.

CRISIS THEORY

Crisis is a response to hazardous events and is experienced as a painful state. A situation becomes a crisis because the person perceives it as threatening in a highly significant way. Clinicians describe crisis as a clinical syndrome involving emotional upset, increased tension, unpleasant affect, ineffective coping strategies, and impaired functioning.

- Life events associated with loss and threat can precipitate situational crisis.
  - Examples include death, divorce, major illness, job loss, rape, and trauma.
  - Positive events such as marriage and childbirth can create conflicts (for example, differences in values related to family or religion) that can lead to crisis. The arrival of the first child creates major change in the couple's relationship, which can cause conflict and stress related to loss.
- Developmental crises occur at predictable points at which new behavior must be learned for the person to move to the next level. Erickson identified three developmental tasks with potential for crisis that occur in adulthood:
  - Intimacy versus isolation in young adults
  - Generativity versus self-absorption in middle-aged adults
  - Integrity versus despair in older adults
- Crisis occurs when the usual coping strategies are unable to control effectively or resolve the tension generated by the situation. Each person usually functions within a specific range of effectiveness and personal satisfaction. In a crisis, there is overwhelming emotional distress that interferes with effective problem-solving.
  - A crisis is self-limited and some resolution occurs in 4 to 10 weeks.
  - All of the person's energy and resources focus on resolution of the crisis and reduction of the pain.
- The person in crisis is generally more open to accepting help. Minimal help may produce meaningful results.

Crisis Intervention

- Crisis intervention consists of short-term psychotherapy with specific goals.
  - To keep the person safe—prevent harm to self or others.
  - To return the person to the precrisis level of functioning or higher.
  - To enhance the coping repertoire and self-esteem.
- Crisis intervention techniques include reassurance, suggestion, support, environmental manipulation, and psychotropic medications.

SUMMARY

This chapter reviewed commonly applied nursing and psychosocial theories that guide nursing interventions. Be able to apply these theories to clinical practice of assisting patients to accept their disease, make lifestyle changes, and enhance coping and quality of life.

REFERENCES

Aguilera, D. C. (1998). *Crisis intervention: Theory and methodology* (8th ed.). St. Louis, MO: Mosby.

Bandura, A. (1986). *Social foundations of thought and action: A social cognitive theory.* Englewood Cliffs, NJ: Prentice-Hall.

Bowen, M. (1978). *Family therapy in clinical practice.* New York: Jason Aronson.

Bridges, W. (1991). *Managing transitions: Making the most of change.* Reading, MA: Addison-Wesley.

Burr, W. R., Leigh, G. K., Day, R. D., & Constantine, J. (1979). Symbolic interaction and the family. In W. R. Burr, R. Hill, F. I. Nye, & I. L. Reiss (Eds.), *Contemporary theories about the family* (pp.128–141). New York: Free Press.

Chinn, P. L., & Jacobs, M. K. (1987). *Theory and nursing: A systematic approach* (2nd ed.). St. Louis, MO: Mosby.

Dossey, B. M., Keegan, L., & Guzzetta, C. (2005). *Holistic nursing: A handbook for practice* (4th ed.). Boston: Jones & Bartlett.

Erickson, H. C., Tomlin, E., & Swain, M. A. (1988). *Modeling and role-modeling: A theory and paradigm for nursing.* Lexington, SC: Pine Press of Lexington.

Erikson, E. H. (1955). Growth and crises of the healthy personality. In C. Kluckhorn, H. A. Murray, & D. M. Scheider (Eds.), *Personality in nature, society and culture* (pp. 78–102). New York: Knopf.

Fawcett, J., & Downs, F. S. (1992). *The relationship of theory and research* (2nd ed.). Philadelphia: F. A. Davis.

Fishbein, M., & Azjen, I. (1975). *Belief, attitude, intention and behavior: An introduction to theory and research.* Reading, MA: Addison-Wesley.

George J. (2002). *Nursing theories: A base for professional practice.* Upper Saddle River, NJ: Prentice Hall.

Huber, D. (1996). *Leadership and nursing care management.* Philadelphia: W. B. Saunders.

King, K. M., Humen, D. P., Smith, H. L., Phan, C. L., & Teo, K. K. (2001). Psychosocial components of cardiac recovery and rehabilitation attendance. *Heart, 85*(3), 290–294.

Lenz, E. R., & Shortridge-Baggett, L. (2002). *Self-efficacy in nursing: Research and measurement perspectives.* New York: Springer.

Lewin, K. (1951). *Field theory in social science.* New York: Harper & Row.

Parker, M. (2005). *Nursing theories and nursing practice.* Philadelphia: F. A. Davis.

Pender, N. J. (1996). *Health promotion in nursing practice* (3rd ed.). Norwalk, CT: Appleton & Lange.

Peterson, S. J., & Bredow, T. S. (2004). *Middle range theories: Application to nursing research.* Philadelphia: Lippincott William & Wilkins.

Prochaska, J. O., & DiClemente, C. C. (1984). *The transtheoretical approach: Crossing traditional boundaries of change.* Homewood, IL: Dow-Jones-Irwin.

Rosenstock, I. M. (1974). Historical origins of the Health Belief Model. In M. H. Becker (Ed.), *The Health Belief Model and personal health behavior* (pp. 158–178). Thorofare, NJ: Slack.

Roy, C., & Roberts, S. L. (1981). *Theory construction in nursing: An adaptation model.* Englewood Cliffs, NJ: Prentice-Hall.

Smith, J. (1983). *The idea of health: Implications for the nursing profession.* New York: Teachers College.

Smith, M. J., & Liehr, P. R. (2008). *Middle range theory for nursing* (2nd ed.). New York: Springer.

Sullivan, M. D., LaCroix, A. Z., Russo, J., & Katon, W. J. (1998). Self-efficacy and self-reported functional status in coronary heart disease: A six-month study. *Psychosomatic Medicine, 60*(4), 473–478.

Tiffany, C. R., & Lutjens, L. R. J. (1998). *Planned change theories for nursing.* Thousand Oaks, CA: Sage.

4

Leadership

This chapter provides an overview of leadership principles and team building that apply to the role of the certified nurse. Case management goals appropriate for cardiovascular nursing are presented. An overview of quality management, performance improvement, and outcomes evaluation also are reviewed.

LEADERSHIP

Leadership is the personal characteristics or qualities that the leader uses to influence others to achieve an identified goal. Key attributes of a leader that promote the achievement of the identified goal are:

- The leader works effectively with members of the group or team.
- The leader facilitates communication among members of the group or team.
- The leader motivates the members of the group or team.

Leadership Styles

- Autocratic leadership uses power to influence group members. The leader makes the decision and gives minimal consideration to the ideas or suggestions of members.
- Participative leadership uses the democratic process for decision-making with group members. The leader encourages the participation of members and provides consistent feedback.
- Laissez-faire leadership uses minimal guidance and provides little feedback to group members. The leader is unwilling to make decisions and consequently does not initiate change.
- Transactional leadership focuses on daily activities and is comfortable with the status quo. The leader rewards group members for work completed and deals with problems after they have occurred.
- Transformational leadership articulates a vision and commitment to the organization's goals. The leader empowers members to achieve the goals and vision.

Leadership in Cardiovascular Care

Cardiovascular (CV) nurses assume a leadership role as they coordinate care. The complexity of cardiac and vascular care is increasing and there is a great need for interdisciplinary collaboration to meet patient care needs. Participative and transformational leadership styles facilitate group or team processes to achieve desired outcomes in patient care.

TEAM BUILDING

Team building involves many factors that promote good working relationships among team members. Teams collaborate to promote the efficiency of the organization and to optimize patient outcomes. Teams develop the highest potential of its members so that they contribute in significant ways, accept more responsibility, and share a commitment to the organizational goals and structure.

Team

- A team is a group of people committed to an identified, shared purpose, with common goals, complementary or shared skills, and a similar approach to completing the work. Each member is accountable to the team for the completion of assigned tasks.
- Attributes of a successful team include the ability to self-regulate, awareness of team member roles including strengths and weaknesses, adaptability to changing events, accountability for evaluating actions, and responsibility for revising the plan as necessary.

Team-Building Models

- The Traditional Model of Team Effectiveness views the team as a series of components that include team building, team processes, and team effectiveness. This model examines the symptoms of team effectiveness but does not look at the actual reasons such as motivation or cognitive processes that drive the team towards attainment of its goals.
  - Assumptions are that the team is passive, stable, and a behavioral entity.
  - Team building is geared towards redesigning behavioral processes by examining the signs of team effectiveness rather than the causes.
  - Team processes include communication, social integration, role clarification, and goal setting.
  - Process, attitudinal, and perceptual indicators measure team effectiveness.

- Cognitive Motivational Model of Team Effectiveness (CoMMTE) is based on the premise that each of the variables (i.e., assumptions, team causes, team processes, team effectiveness, team building) are interdependent and can be used to evaluate and redesign team-developed interventions.
  - CoMMTE assumes that the team is an active, dynamic, fluid, and cognitive–motivational entity.
  - Team causes or purposes include shared goals and actions as well as the ability to evaluate its actions and to redesign its interventions.
  - Team processes are self-regulated and have diagnostic prerogatives.
  - Team effectiveness is measured by the achievement of results.
  - Team building focuses on redesigning cognitive functioning by analyzing team effectiveness.

Benefits of Team Building in Health Care
- Nursing, medicine, and other healthcare professionals must provide integrated care that supports optimal use of healthcare resources to improve patient outcomes.
- Collaboration among nurses provides continuity of care by focusing on a plan that promotes teamwork to enhance positive patient outcomes and to coordinate care delivery.
- Interdisciplinary collaboration involves the joint contributions of professionals from other disciplines (such as medicine) working towards the common goals of improving quality of care and outcomes for patients.
- Teams can streamline healthcare services for patients while avoiding duplication or gaps in their care.

Team Building and Teamwork
- Clear expectations about the roles, skills, and goals of the team and its members enhance teamwork, reduce conflict, and promote success.
- Participative learning experiences foster collaboration among the members of the team.
- Effective communication among team members promotes team effectiveness.
- Support, encouragement, respect, and commitment among members facilitate teamwork.
- Recognition of one member of the team as the leader by other members enhances group processes.

Barriers to Team Building and Teamwork
- Healthcare professionals have not been taught about teamwork or team building.
- Sex role stereotyping and gender hierarchy have a negative effect on interdisciplinary groups.
- Role status of team members has the potential to impede communication within the group.
- Team members with traditional views of organizational roles may have difficulty with teamwork.
- Situations that promote lack of communication, support, and respect for team members impair teamwork.

Team Building for CV Care

- The formation of teams and subsequent team building are beneficial for the management of acute and chronically ill patients with cardiac and vascular health problems.
- Decreased length of stay for cardiac surgical patients mandates that healthcare services are coordinated within the hospital among nursing, cardiology, cardiac surgery, anesthesia, physical therapy, dietary, and respiratory therapy. The development of fast-track protocols for early extubation and discharge of these patients require interdisciplinary collaboration.
- The formation of teams to address the needs of hospitalized CV "outliers" also has been effective. Nurses use primary nursing to manage the nursing care needs while interdisciplinary teams develop clinical pathways. For example, the development of ventilator weaning and extubation protocols has decreased the duration of mechanical ventilation and hospitalization for patients after cardiac surgery.
- Teamwork has also been effective in coordinating the care of patients with chronic CV diseases (such as heart failure). The goal is to prevent readmissions because of symptom exacerbations. Intra- and interdisciplinary team efforts provide continuity in the transition from hospital to home with home-based case management systems to continue education efforts and assist in self-management.

CASE MANAGEMENT

Definitions

Nursing uses case management to coordinate the care of patients. Case management is defined differently by different professional organizations.

- The Case Management Society of America states that case management is "a collective process which assesses, plans, implements, coordinates, monitors, and evaluates the options and services required to meet an individual's health needs using communications and available resources to promote quality, cost-effective outcomes." This definition, while broad enough to encompass the different disciplines involved in case management, does not address nursing's unique role.
- The American Nurses Credentialing Center defines nursing case management as "a dynamic and systematic collaborative approach to providing and coordinating healthcare services to a defined population. It is a participative process to identify and facilitate options and services for meeting individuals' health needs, while decreasing fragmentation and duplication of care and enhancing quality, cost-effective clinical outcomes."

Case Management Models

- Nursing case management models evolved from primary nursing and were used traditionally in acute care settings.
  - Nurse case managers coordinate each patient's care throughout hospitalization as the patient moves to different locations in the institution.
  - Nursing case management plans use diagnosis-related group length of stay, critical pathway reports, and variance analysis, along with interdisciplinary collaborative group practice arrangements, to provide healthcare services to these patients.
- Community-based case management models use case managers to coordinate the care of patients from the hospital to the community and to long-term care settings, if indicated. These patients have chronic health conditions and need long-term healthcare services. Community-based models provide care and resources to high-risk patients across the continuum of care.
- Case management models have been modified to accommodate the needs of patients in a variety of community settings.
  - Long-term healthcare models are used for prior authorization screening to permit a service.
  - Rehabilitation case management targets chronic medical or psychosocial health problems that have a longer recovery or treatment time than acute health problems.
  - Occupational healthcare models focus on employee health, with return to work and wellness as the major goals.
  - Private case management involves subcontracting with individuals or groups for the coordination of services, advocacy, and counseling.
  - Insurance case management emphasizes the linkage of resources for patient care but is not involved with direct care.
  - Managed care and HMO case management models monitor access to services and advocate cost-effective alternatives to services. In some cases, permission for costly services is required but reimbursement is not necessarily granted.

Role of Case Managers

- Establish a professional case management relationship with the patient and family.
- Assist the patient and family in adapting to the health problem.
- Advocate for the patient and family.
- Ensure that patient and family education needs associated with the health problem are met.
- Manage, coordinate, and facilitate the healthcare services that the patient and family need.
- Make sure that healthcare services are appropriate, delivered within the required time frames, and coordinated across the continuum of care.
- Evaluate the quality and cost-effectiveness of healthcare services delivered to patients and their families.

TOTAL QUALITY MANAGEMENT

- Total quality management (TQM) is a way to run complex organizations to achieve the aims or mission of the organization.
- TQM emphasizes empowerment of employees.
  - An underlying principle is that most people are trying quite hard to do their best work, further the mission of the organization, and meet the needs of the customers.
- TQM recognizes that an organization or department has multiple customers who may have competing needs.
  - A customer is anyone who depends on a department to provide a service. Customers of nursing service include patients and families (external), but also physicians and other clinicians (internal).
  TQM focuses on meeting the needs of both internal and external customers.
- Quality problems occur when good people get caught in broken processes or systems that don't work.
  - The people doing the work have the most information about how the work gets done
  - Quality is cost-effective. Fewer resources are required to do the job right the first time than are required to do it multiple times until it is right.
- A key strategy of TQM is to involve the worker in improving the work processes through continuous quality improvement.

CONTINUOUS QUALITY IMPROVEMENT

- Continuous quality improvement (CQI) is an approach to improve quality that focuses on how the work gets done (process) rather than on who is doing the work (people).
- A process is a sequence of actions leading to an outcome that is important to customers (i.e., patients) who depend on the process.
- It often happens with complex processes that no one person or department understands the whole process. Therefore, CQI requires an interdepartmental team.
  - Suppose, for example, that it took too long for a patient who was experiencing a stroke to get from the emergency department (ED) to the CT scan needed to determine eligibility for a thrombolytic agent. A CQI team formed to address this quality problem might require representation from the ED, business office (patient registration), nursing (triage), medicine, transportation, and radiology.
- CQI empowers healthcare workers to reduce the cost and improve the quality of their work.
- The term Performance Improvement is another term for CQI. Performance Improvement may include conducting small studies of the operation or changed process to evaluate outcomes.

Shewhart Cycle
- Shewhart Cycle (also known as the Deming Cycle) is the planning and improvement process in widest use in U.S. healthcare organizations today. The cycle has four steps: plan, do, check, act (PDCA).
- The CQI team plans change by studying the process, deciding what could improve it, and identifying data to be used in monitoring the process.

- The team tests the proposed change by doing a small-scale trial or data simulation exercise. The team checks the effects of the trial by studying the results and modifies the planned change if necessary.
- The team acts to improve the process by implementing the change.
- The cycle repeats continuously. Small changes are implemented and evaluated until the process is as efficient as can be achieved. In the example of time from ED to angiography suite:
  - Plan: The team measured the average time from ED check-in to thrombolytic injection. They studied the process and determined that time waiting for transport was a critical factor.
  - Do: The team assigned a transporter to the ED for 1 month and continued to monitor time to thrombolytic injection.
  - Check: Pre- and post-intervention data were analyzed and the team found that time to thrombolytic injection was reduced by 25 minutes. The team consensus was that further reduction was possible.
  - Act: The 1-month trial of the transporter was extended another month and preprinted physician orders also were implemented. Time-to-thrombolytic-injection data were gathered continually.
  - Repeat: The data showed further reduction in time; the team continued to examine the process to identify further potential improvement.

CQI Relies on Data
- Quality issues are identified from data.
- Local and national data are used to establish benchmarks for quality care.
- Data are collected and analyzed to determine the effect of the change on the process of care.

Barriers to Implementing CQI Programs
- Organizational barriers include:
  - Resistance to change
  - Culture is so deeply ingrained that the behavioral change is in conflict with the organization's philosophy
  - Limited time for the change to take place
  - Lack of organizational support for CQI
- Management barriers include:
  - Management not accepting of role change associated with CQI
  - Organization's goals not clearly communicated to management
  - Lack of managerial support
- Process barriers include:
  - Data not available
  - National or local benchmarks not defined
- CQI team barriers include:
  - Inadequate team building
  - Key departments not represented
  - Lack of understanding by team members of the CQI process
  - Personal agendas

OUTCOME EVALUATION

Outcome evaluation is important for patients, healthcare providers, and the healthcare system. It can be used to evaluate the effect of care on the patient's recovery from cardiac and vascular procedures. This process also can be used to enhance the knowledge of healthcare providers, establish the criteria for clinical decision-making, evaluate the effectiveness of interventions, and identify areas for performance improvement.

An outcome is a change in status between two points in time. The change may be positive or negative.
- Frequently used patient outcomes include:
  - Morbidity or incidence of complications
  - Mortality
  - Hemodynamic parameters (e.g., pulmonary artery pressures, central venous pressures)
  - Laboratory values (e.g., blood sugar, prothrombin time, INR)
  - Symptoms (nausea, vomiting, pain, fatigue, angina, anxiety, depression)
  - Functional status (e.g., activities of daily living, sexuality, family function, employment)
- Frequently used healthcare provider outcomes include:
  - Change in knowledge or skill level
  - Compliance with practice standards
- Frequently used system outcomes include:
  - Service utilization
  - Length of hospital stay or duration of services
  - Cost of care or services
- Many organizations set standards for outcomes that hospitals now monitor. Some examples are
  - National Database of Nursing Quality Indicators (NDNQI) includes overall outcomes such as falls, nosocomial infections, nosocomial pressure ulcers, and hospital-related infections.
  - Joint Commission (formerly Joint Commission on Accreditation of Health Care Organizations or JCAHO) requires institutions to monitor a set of outcomes from a larger list that includes many of the NDNQI indicators but also 30-day readmissions for heart failure and smoking assessment and intervention.
  - Specialty medical organizations, for example, American Heart Association (AHA) outcomes that include discharge medication of ACE-inhibitors after admission for myocardial infarction (MI) or heart failure (HF), obtaining lipids on all cardiac patients within 24 hours of admission, beta blocker use in HF patients.

PROGRAM CERTIFICATION

A growing number of specialty organizations offer program certification in an effort to ensure that standards for patient care are in place and outcomes are monitored. Some examples of program certification include American Association of Cardiovascular and Pulmonary Rehabilitation, Chest Pain Center Certification, and Heart Failure Program Certification from the Joint Commission.

MAGNET RECOGNITION PROGRAM®

The American Nurse Credentialing Center is responsible for administration of the Magnet Recognition Program. This program is based on five Model Components that have been related to best outcomes of nursing care and enhanced staff professionalism. The program of self-study and review is an intense process that involves the support of administration and staff.

SUMMARY

This chapter provided a brief overview of the role of the cardiovascular nurse in case management, quality improvement, and performance improvement. As more national organizations set outcome measures that are linked to program certification and payment, all members of the staff are responsible for ensuring that these outcomes are monitored and programs put in place to continuously improve nursing and healthcare performance.

REFERENCES

Case Management Society of America. (2001). *Definition of case management.* Retrieved from www.cmsa.org.

Drummond, M. F., Sculpher, M. J., Torrance, G. W., & O'Brien, B. J. (2005). *Methods for the economic evaluation of health care programmes.* Oxford, UK: Oxford University Press.

Dunton, N., & Montalvo, I. (2009). *Sustained improvement in nursing quality: Hospital performance on NDNQI indicators, 2007–2008.* Silver Spring, MD: American Nurses Association.

Finkelman, A., & Kenner, C. (2009). *Professional nursing concepts: Competencies for quality leadership.* Sudbury, NJ: Jones & Bartlett.

Idvall, E., Rooke, L., & Hamrin, E. (1997). Quality indicators in clinical nursing: A review of the literature. *Journal of Advanced Nursing, 25*(1), 6–17.

Klainberg M & Dirschel . (2009). *Today's nursing leader: Managing, succeeding, excelling.* Sudbury, NJ: Jones & Bartlett.

Marquis, B. L., & Huston, C. J. (2009). *Leadership roles and management function in nursing: Theory and application* (6th ed.). Philadelphia: Lippincott Williams & Wilkins.

McCallin, A. (2001). Interdisciplinary practice—a matter of teamwork: An integrated literature review. *Journal of Clinical Nursing, 10*(4), 419–428.

McClure, M. L., & Hinshaw, A. S. (2002). *Magnet hospitals revisited: Attraction and retention of professional nurses.* Washington, DC: American Nurses Publishing.

Newell, M. (2008). *Using nursing case management to improve health outcomes.* Philadelphia: Lippincott Williams & Wilkins

Sullivan, E. J. (2008). *Effective leadership and management in nursing* (7th ed.). Englewood Cliffs, NJ: Prentice Hall.

Tomey, A. M. (2008). *Guide to nursing management and leadership.* St. Louis, MO: Mosby.

5

Research

Nursing research provides the scientific basis for practice and begins by asking pertinent questions regarding the best way to provide care. Cardiovascular nurses may contribute to nursing research in many ways, including identifying research questions, consulting with researchers on designs, collecting data, analyzing results, and reporting findings. The scope of the research can range from small performance improvement studies done on a single nursing unit to multicenter studies. If not conducting studies, nurses must be aware of the literature. So all nurses need basic knowledge of research in order to read, critique, and apply results of published nursing studies. Nurses with advanced education in research methods are expected to conduct research, but all nurses can collaborate with a nurse researcher to answer practice-related questions. This chapter reviews basic understanding of statistics, quantitative research designs, and qualitative research methods.

PROBLEM IDENTIFICATION

Sources of Ideas for Research Problems
- Clinical practice
  - The idea emerges: For example, how can the nurse relieve patient and family anxiety about early hospital discharge?
  - Brainstorm with colleagues: Do others perceive anxiety about early discharge to be a problem? Why is it a problem? Does it have bad outcomes?

- Review the literature: Has the question been answered? Is the answer definitive? Are observable variables suggested or supported by the literature?
- Identify variables: What concepts contained in the questions have the ability to vary?
  - Possible patient-related variables: Age, gender, procedure, and prehospitalization anxiety.
  - Possible nurse-related variables: Age, gender, education, and experience.
  - Possible system-related variables: Discharge planning procedure, length of hospital stay, and referral to home care.
- Continuous quality improvement trends
- Theory
  - Some scholars believe that the purpose of nursing research is to generate and test theory, and research that is unrelated to theory is trivial.
- Literature
- Priorities set by professional organizations and funding agencies
- Conferences and colleagues

Problem Evaluation

- Does the problem occur frequently? Does it occur infrequently but have a significant effect on outcome?
- Can the problem or question be answered by collecting observable data?
- Will answering the question result in better care?
- Are the resources necessary to answer the question available? Is it feasible, practical?
- Is the question ethical? Will some good come to the participant or society? Are the risks outweighed by the benefits of participation?
- Is the nurse's level of interest in the question sufficient to sustain the effort?

Stating the Question or Problem

- A research question is a concise statement, worded in the present tense that includes one or more variables (or concepts).
- Kinds of research questions
  - Descriptive: For example, "How is anxiety related to early discharge manifested in patients and families?"
  - Exploratory or relational: For example, "What is the relationship between predischarge anxiety and postdischarge behavior?"
  - Predictive: For example, "Does self-efficacy, predischarge anxiety, or family structure best predict postdischarge behavior?"
  - Experimental or quasi-experimental: If one can predict the outcome, the next step would be to modify the outcome. If one knew, for example, that self-efficacy predicted postdischarge behavior, then one could prescribe a self-efficacy enhancement intervention to influence postdischarge behavior.

RESEARCH METHOD

The research question and the existing knowledge about the phenomena of interest determine the research method used.

- Qualitative methods are inductive; quantitative methods are deductive.
- Qualitative methods are used in the following situations.
  - When the question is broad and little is known about the subject. For example, "How do midlife women decide to begin an aerobic exercise program?"
  - To achieve a deep, rich understanding of the phenomena—discovery, exploration, and description of the phenomena. For example, "What factors contribute to women's delay in seeking emergency care when experiencing symptoms of myocardial infarction?"
  - In combination with quantitative methods—for triangulation or as a complement
  - For instrument development
  - To generate hypotheses about relationships for subsequent testing
- Quantitative methods are used to
  - Explain and predict phenomena;
  - Generate evidence of cause and effect;
  - Test theory or instruments; and
  - Evaluate the effectiveness of interventions.

QUALITATIVE METHODS

General Characteristics
- Qualitative methods allow the researcher to gain insight through discovering meaning.
- Qualitative methods are a way to explore the richness and complexity of phenomena.
- Qualitative data are expressed in words rather than numbers.
- Data collection and analysis occur concurrently.
- Theoretical or purposive sampling is used. Using insights from the data, the researcher selects informants with particular characteristics to increase theoretical understanding of the phenomenon.
- Researchers are concerned with the trustworthiness of qualitative studies.

ENSURING TRUSTWORTHINESS

- Credibility is the truth-value of the study. It has been compared to the internal validity of a study using quantitative methods. When assessing the credibility of the study, the reviewer considers the period of engagement with the study, the use of multiple data sources (triangulation), and whether the researcher checked with the informants and included their responses before publishing the study.
- Transferability of a study has been compared to the external validity of a study using quantitative methods. In general, the result of a qualitative study is deep, rich description of a phenomenon or process. Results are not directly transferable to other settings or populations. The understanding gained may be used to inform other studies or practices.

- Dependability of a study has been compared to the reliability of a quantitative study. The researcher maintains scrupulous records about methods and decisions that can be reviewed and verified in a process audit.
- Confirmability of a study has been compared to the objectivity of a quantitative study. The issue here is the extent to which the meanings assigned to the data are grounded in the events and the culture rather than in the researcher's experience. "Would another analyst find similar meaning in the data?"

Phenomenological Research

Phenomenological research is used to describe experiences as they are lived from the perspective of the study participant.

- Phenomenology is not just a research method but also a philosophy that guides the research process.
- The first step in conducting a phenomenological study is to identify the phenomenon of interest.
- The research question asks, "What is the human experience and meaning of this phenomenon?"
- Sampling requires locating and identifying people living with the phenomenon who are willing to share their thoughts, feelings, and experiences with the researcher.
- Data are generated and collected through observation, interview, videotape, and descriptions written by participants.
- Analysis consists of attaching meaning to statements and the outcome is a theoretical statement responding to the research question.
  - Excerpts from the data are used to support the theoretical statement.
  - Many nurses are familiar with Benner's phenomenological study of nursing knowledge acquisition, *From Novice to Expert* (1984).

Grounded Theory

Grounded theory is a research method used to understand basic social processes. It has its roots in sociology.

- The first step is to identify the social process of interest.
- Data are generated and collected through participant observation and intensive interviewing.
- Data are coded and categorized.
  - Constant comparative analysis compares each piece of data with every other piece.
  - The categories are found within the data, not preconceived.
  - Data are collected until all of the characteristics of the category are revealed.
- The outcome is a theory grounded in the data from which it was derived explaining the social process of interest.

Ethnography

Ethnography is a research method used to understand a culture (or subculture) from its own perspective. Ethnography has its roots in anthropology.

- The first step with ethnography is to identify the culture to be studied.
- Literature review provides a background for the study.
  - The researcher seeks a general understanding of the phenomena to be examined specifically within the culture.
  - Studies of health behavior and experiences of homeless people may use ethnographic methods, for example.

- Data generation and collection require access to the culture and key informants.
  - Key informants are members of the culture who are willing to share their knowledge of the culture and the phenomena.
  - The researcher becomes immersed in the culture through active participation.
- Data are collected through observation and interview.
- Analysis involves identifying meaning attached to the data and events by the informants. Members of the culture validate meaning before the results are final.
- The outcome is a detailed description of the phenomena as experienced within the culture.

Historiography

Historiography examines past events.
- The first step is to select the topic and questions to be examined.
- Next the researcher must identify sources of data and obtain access to these sources.
  - Data may include letters, memos, and mementos.
- Analysis involves synthesis of the data collected.
- The outcome is a cogent retelling of historical events and their meaning.
  - Examples of historical studies include reports of nurses imprisoned during World War II, founding of early schools of nursing, biographies of nursing leaders, and nursing during the flu epidemic of 1918.

Content Analysis

Content analysis is a method used to classify words in text by their theoretical importance.
- Content analysis differs from other qualitative methods because it uses numbers to represent frequency; order; or intensity of words, phrases, or sentences.
- Content analysis is sometimes used in historical research.
- Theoretically significant categories are identified. Data are classified into categories and the number of data bits assigned to the category is determined.
- Descriptive statistics may be used to count and summarize data.

QUANTITATIVE METHODS

General Concerns and Issues

- Variables
  - An independent variable is the stimulus or activity that is manipulated by the researcher to create an effect on the dependent variable.
    - Control is very important in experimental and quasi-experimental designs. It can refer to the use of a control group or efforts to maintain consistency of methods.
    - The greater the amount of control the researcher has, the stronger the evidence from the study.
  - A dependent variable is the response, behavior, or outcome that the researcher wants to predict or explain.
  - Extraneous variables are all of the other factors that can vary and may influence the dependent variable.
    - The researcher uses research design and statistical methods to reduce the effect of extraneous variables.
  - Demographic variables are characteristics of the subjects that are collected for descriptive purposes.

- Causality—support for causal relationships
    - Correlation or association alone does not prove causality.
    - Three conditions must be met to establish causality.
        1. Strong relationship between the proposed cause and effect
        2. Proposed cause must precede the effect in time
        3. Proposed cause must be present every time the effect occurs
    - Multicausality—multiple factors contribute to the effect or outcome.
    - Probability addresses relative, rather than absolute, causality. It describes the likelihood that one factor caused another.
- Validity of a study is a measure of the truth or accuracy of the study. There are multiple aspects of validity that contribute to strength of the evidence provided by a study.
    - Statistical conclusion validity is concerned with whether the conclusions made through statistical analyses accurately reflect the real world.
        - Type I error occurs when the researcher concludes that there is a difference between two groups when in reality there is no difference.
            - The risk of Type I error increases when the researcher conducts multiple statistical analyses of relationships or differences.
            - Some relationships or differences that do not reflect true population relationships or differences may be found within the sample by chance.
        - Type II error occurs when the researcher concludes that there is no difference between two samples when there is a true difference.
            - Low statistical power is the most common cause of Type II error. This is usually because of a small sample size.
    - Internal validity is the extent to which the effect detected in a study results from the relationship between the independent and dependent variable and not from some extraneous factor.
    - Construct validity is the goodness of the fit between the definition of a concept of interest and its method of measurement.
    - External validity describes the extent to which study findings can be generalized beyond the sample used in the study.

Quantitative Designs
- Descriptive designs are used when the purpose is to delineate characteristics of a sample or setting. The purpose is not to generalize to a larger population.
- Correlational designs study a population by systematically examining a representative sample. Findings may be generalized to the population represented by the sample.
    - Cross-sectional designs collect data at one point in time.
    - Longitudinal designs collect data at more than one point in time.
    - Correlational designs may be used also to describe relationships between or among factors when the intent is not to make inferences about a larger population.
- Quasi-experimental and experimental designs are used to test hypotheses about causal relationships.
    - Control is a basic characteristic of experimental and quasi-experimental designs. Control is the ability of the researcher to manipulate the independent variable and to eliminate, hold constant, or measure the effect of extraneous variables.

- Elements of a true experimental design include:
  - At least two groups—experimental and control
  - Random assignment of the sample to the experimental and control groups
  - Pretests before the manipulation of the independent variable (often included but not mandatory)
  - Posttests following manipulation of the independent variable
- When random assignment cannot be met, the design is quasi-experimental.

Sampling

Sampling involves selecting a group of people or elements to participate in a study.

- Population refers to the entire set of people or elements that meet the sampling criteria. Accessible population refers to the set of people or elements that meet the sampling criteria and to which the researcher can gain access.
- Sampling criteria are the characteristics essential for inclusion in the target population.
  - Inclusion criteria are characteristics that must be present for a subject to be included in the population.
  - Exclusion criteria are characteristics that when present cause a subject to be excluded from the population.
- Representativeness is the extent to which the sample is like the population.
- Adequate sample size for a study is determined by the anticipated effect size, power of the statistical tests, and significance level.
  - Effect size is the amount of an impact or the strength of the relationship between the independent and dependent variables.
  - Power is the capacity of the statistical test to detect significant differences or relationships that exist between groups in the sample. The minimal acceptable power for a study is .80, meaning there is an 80% probability of correctly discerning a difference between two groups.
  - Understanding the research literature requires understanding the importance of statistical significance. Statistical significance relies on the concepts of error and sampling and is applied in statistical analyses.

Sampling Error

Parameters describe population characteristics or attributes; statistics describe sample characteristics.

- Sampling error is the difference between a sample statistic and a population parameter.
  - If the sample does not reflect the population, sampling error will be large.
  - Random variation is the expected difference that occurs when one measures a variable in different subjects from the same sample.
  - Systematic variation occurs when subjects vary in some specific way from the population as a whole.
- Random sampling is a way to ensure that every individual in the population has an equal chance to be selected into the sample.
  - Random sampling assures that the sample represents the population and minimizes systematic variation.
  - Random samples include simple random samples, stratified random samples, and cluster samples.

Box 5–1. Understanding the *p* Value

The *p* value reported in research is something that many readers find intimidating. It should not be so difficult to understand. Keep the following in mind when reading research.

- The significance level is set by the researcher and determines the probability of making a Type I error (concluding that there is a difference between two groups when in reality there is no difference).
- In general, researchers use a probability of .05 or less when analyzing data.
- When a test of difference is significant at the .05 levels, the researcher may conclude that there is a 95% probability that the two groups are different. Thus, the differences found were likely because of the intervention and not chance.
- If the study involves more serious outcomes, like those found in a drug or device study, the researcher may try to achieve a $p < .01$ or $p < .001$. This would ensure that there is even less risk that the results were due to chance.

- In nonprobability sampling, every individual in the population does not have an equal chance to be selected.
  - Nonprobability sampling reduces the likelihood that the sample represents the population, increasing the risk of systematic variation.
  - Nonprobability samples include convenience and quota samples.
    - Random assignment to group is used in an attempt to control systematic bias within convenience samples.

Epidemiology

Epidemiology is the study of events occurring in large samples or the population.

- Population studies are often done to determine the natural progression of the disease or treatment and to assess the effect of risk factors on disease manifestation and outcomes.
  - The Framingham Heart Study has resulted in the largest database on risk factors for cardiovascular disease.
    - It began as a study of approximately 5,000 residents of Framingham, MA (a suburb of Boston), and has continued for 6 decades, studying the offspring of original participants.
    - Results can be used to determine a risk score for 10-year probability of cardiovascular event (myocardial infarction [MI] or death). Risk stratification is discussed further in Chapter 8.
- Epidemiological studies provide a mechanism for determining probability of events occurring.
- Analyses often are reported as incidence, prevalence, and relative risk.
  - Prevalence is the total number of cases of the disease in the population at a given time.
  - Incidence is the number of new cases of the disease in the population during a given period of time.
  - Relative risk is the risk of an event relative to the exposure (see Box 5–2).

Box 5–2. Understanding Relative Risk Ratios

Relative risk (RR) is the probability of an event occurring. It helps the clinician see the relative importance of controlling for or eliminating a factor.
- Relative risk of 1 means that there is no difference in the occurrence of an event in two groups of people (e.g., 20-year-old men and 20-year-old women).
- An RR > 1 means that the event is more likely to occur in the group with the specific factor (e.g., CAD in smokers vs. nonsmokers).
- An RR < 1 means the event is less likely to occur in the group getting the treatment than those not receiving it (e.g., cardiac rehabilitation after MI vs. those not in rehab).
- An RR of 2 means the risk is twice that of the group without the factor.
- A risk factor with an RR of 2.5 is more of a concern than another risk factor with an RR of 1.8.
- Knowing the RR helps prioritize the importance of modifying risk factors.

Measurement

Measurement is the process of assigning numbers to objects, events, or situations according to a rule.
- Levels of measurement
  - Nominal scale is the lowest level of measurement. Numbers function as labels or categories and cannot be used for calculation. For example, the numbers on baseball players' shirts are labels only. When the variable gender is measured using 1 for female and 2 for male, the numbers represent categories only.
    - The categories are mutually exclusive.
    - All of the data fit in one of the categories (exhaustive).
  - Ordinal scale represents sequence or order; members of a set are ordered from most to least with respect to some characteristic. For example, a graduating student may be first or tenth in a class. The number is significant in terms of relative position.
    - Categories are mutually exclusive and exhaustive.
    - Categories can be ordered, but intervals are not equal.
  - Interval scale has order and equal numerical distance between intervals. For example, temperature is measured on an interval scale. The difference between 70° and 80° is the same as the difference between 50° and 60°. A temperature of 0° does not indicate the absence of temperature, however.
    - Categories are mutually exclusive and exhaustive.
    - Categories can be ordered.
    - Intervals are equal, but the scale does not contain absolute zero.
  - Ratio scale is the highest form of measurement and exists on a continuum. Weight, length, and volume are examples of ratio-level measurements. Zero represents the absence of weight, length, or volume. Because absolute zero is contained in the scale, one can say that 10 pounds is twice as heavy as 5 pounds.
    - Categories are mutually exclusive and exhaustive.
    - Categories can be ordered.
    - Intervals are equal.
    - Scale contains absolute zero.

Measurement Issues

- It is not possible to measure a concept perfectly. Measurement error is the difference between the concept in reality and as measured by an instrument.
- There are three components to a measured score: the true score, the observed score, and the error score. The observed score equals the true score plus the error score.
- There are two components to the error score: random error and systematic error.
- Random error causes the observed score to vary around the true score.
  - According to measurement theory, the sum of random errors is zero. Some observed scores will be higher than the true scores and some will be lower, but taken together the errors will add to zero.
  - Random error is not correlated with the true score. Random error will not cause the mean score to be higher or lower than the true mean but will increase the amount of unexplained variance around the true mean. Random error cannot be eliminated.
- Systematic error causes the observed score to vary from the true score in a consistent (systematic) way. For example, a scale that consistently weighs subjects as 2 pounds heavier than their true weight adds systematic error. Systematic error affects mean scores.
  - The goal in measurement is to reduce systematic error as much as possible.
- Reliability of a measure reflects the consistency or reproducibility of scores obtained with the measure.
  - Reliability testing provides an indication of the amount of random error inherent in the measurement of the concept within the sample.
  - Reliability of a measure is expressed as a correlation coefficient with 1.00 representing perfect reliability and 0.00 representing no reliability.
  - Estimates of reliability are specific to the sample being tested.
    - Reliability testing is performed on each instrument used in a study before other statistical analyses are done.
    - Internal consistency is measured by the Cronbach alpha statistic. It is a method of examining a survey to see if the items are somewhat similar or consistent in measuring a concept. A reliability coefficient of 0.80 is the minimal acceptable level for established instruments. For newly developed instruments, a reliability coefficient of 0.70 may be accepted.
- Validity of a measure reflects the extent to which an instrument represents the concept being measured within the specific situation. Validity of a measure determines the appropriateness, meaningfulness, and usefulness of inferences made from scores on the measure.
  - Systematic error reduces the validity of measures.
  - Evidence for the validity of an instrument develops through repeated use over time in a variety of situations. Traditionally, the various means of accumulating evidence have been grouped into categories. The use of category labels does not indicate different kinds of validity, but different types of evidence.
    - Content-related evidence examines the extent to which the method of measurement includes representative elements from a domain of content.
      - Content-related evidence often relies on expert judgment to identify appropriate elements for inclusion.
      - Factor analysis is a statistical method that examines clusters of relationships among items. Once the clusters are identified mathematically, the analyst explains theoretically why the items grouped as they did.

- Criterion-related evidence examines the performance of an instrument in comparison with other measures, preferably a "gold standard."
- Evidence of validity accrues from differential prediction of future or concurrent events.
  · The ability to predict future performance.
  · The ability to differentiate between groups known to be high and low in the concept of interest.
- Sensitivity is the ability of a measure to detect relevant change in the concept.

DATA COLLECTION STRATEGIES

- Observation
  – Answers questions about overt human behavior (e.g., actions, facial expressions, body language)
  – Allows phenomena to be studied in their natural environment
- Self-report—interviews, questionnaires, and surveys
  – Answers questions about facts, beliefs, feelings, and attitudes
  – People may be unwilling or unable to answer the questions. Questions may not be answered truthfully.
- Existing data—public records, medical records, national databases
  – Existing data may be used to answer a new question. For example, an investigator might use census data to explore a health-related question.
  – Personal health (medical) records often are used in case series. Health records may contain biases of the healthcare clinician.
- Physiological measures (e.g., blood pressure, heart rate, blood tests)

PROTECTION OF HUMAN RIGHTS

- Research studies are reviewed by an institutional review board (IRB) prior to starting data collection.
  – The purpose of the IRB is to protect human subjects. The IRB was created to protect the public from the abuses that occurred decades ago with the Tuskegee syphilis study, total body radiation studies, and prisoner drug and surgical studies.
  – The protection of human rights focuses on the provision of informed consent to participate in the study.
    • Informed consent assumes the subject voluntarily participates, has complete information to make the decision, and has the cognitive capacity to make the decision.
    • Vulnerable populations include children, pregnant women, elderly, prisoners, and those with mental handicaps.
- Consent can be obtained in two manners.
  – Consent can be documented by a witnessed signature on a consent form. In this case the subject is known to the researcher, who must maintain confidentiality of the individual subject's identity.

– Consent can be implied if a person given complete information about the study voluntarily completes a survey, but does not sign a consent form. In this instance the responses are completely anonymous and the identity of the subject is not known to the researcher or anyone else.

• Risks and benefits of participation in a study must be fully disclosed. Risks must not be unduly high and must be weighed against the potential benefits.

• Data safety monitoring boards (DSMB) are often created to provide an independent group that reviews the data to ensure that the study is being conducted as planned and that the intervention is not harmful. Studies may be stopped early at the advice of the DSMB if the results are so positive that everyone should get the intervention or so poor that no additional subjects should be put at risk by receiving the treatment.

DATA ANALYSIS

• The research question, methods used to obtain data, and characteristics of the data determine the appropriate statistical tests to be used.

• Descriptive statistics provide precise, standard ways to summarize and communicate complex information about a sample.
  – Measures of central tendency
    • The mode is the numerical value or score that occurs with the highest frequency.
    • The median is the score at the exact center of the distribution. Exactly 50% of scores are above the median and 50% of the scores are below the median.
    • The mean is the sum of scores divided by the number of scores included in the sum.
  – Shape of the distribution
    • Symmetry—left side of the curve is a mirror image of the right side of the curve. When a curve is symmetrical, all three measures of central tendency are equal. When a curve is not symmetrical, it is skewed.
      ▪ Positive skew—the largest portion of data falls below the mean; the curve has a tail extending to the right.
      ▪ Negative skew—the largest portion of data falls above the mean; the curve has an initiating tail.
    • Modality—a curve may be unimodal, bimodal, or multimodal. Symmetric curves are usually unimodal.
    • Kurtosis—describes the peakedness of the curve, which is related to the spread or variability of the scores.
  – Measures of dispersion
    • The range is the mathematical difference between the highest and lowest scores.
    • The standard deviation is the average amount by which scores vary around the mean.
    • The variance is the average of the squared standard deviations. It is frequently used in statistics but is difficult to interpret as a measure of dispersion.

- Measures of association
    - Contingency tables or cross tabulations allow visual comparison of summary data related to two variables within the sample.
        - Contingency tables are used to examine nominal or ordinal level data.
        - Chi-square is a statistic designed to test for differences between cells in contingency tables.
    - Correlation coefficients provide information about the direction, strength, and shape of relationships. Values range from –1.00 (a perfect and inverse correlation) to +1.00 (a perfect and positive correlation).
- Inferential statistics allow the investigator to go beyond description of the sample and make probabilistic inferences about the population.
    - Parametric statistics require assumptions about the distribution of data—normality and homogeneity of variance, for example.
    - Nonparametric statistics make no assumptions about the shape of the distribution.
        - Nonparametric statistics are particularly relevant when the distribution is not normal or the sample size is small.
        - Nonparametric statistics are commonly used to analyze nominal and ordinal-level data.
    - Hypothesis testing of differences and association between variables
        - Tests of difference
            - Parametric: t-test, ANOVA
            - Nonparametric: Mann-Whitney U test, sign test
        - Tests of association
            - Parametric: Pearson correlation coefficients
            - Nonparametric: Spearman and Kendall correlation coefficients
- Meta-analysis is a method used to pool the statistics from multiple studies and report overall outcomes.
    - A rigorous review of the literature is undertaken and each study is treated as a subject in the meta-analysis.
    - This method is particularly useful when some studies found positive results while others were negative.
    - It is also useful when the sample sizes of the studies were small and power was low.
    - Combining studies for a meta-analysis can help clarify the usefulness of an intervention and provide more evidence to change practice.

EVIDENCE-BASED PRACTICE

Evidence-based practice is the synthesis and use of scientific information (i.e., evidence) to direct practice.

Sources and Kinds of Evidence

- National guidelines may be research-based, represent the consensus of experts, or more commonly both.
  - The Agency for Healthcare Research and Quality serves as a clearinghouse for published practice guidelines that summarized evidence related to specific topics. (www.ahrq.gov or www.guideline.gov). Another major source of cardiovascular practice guidelines is the American Heart Association/American College of Cardiology (www.americanheart.org).
  - Evidence-based guidelines
    - Contain comprehensive review and summary of existing research
    - Rate the quality of the evidence; place highest value on evidence from randomized clinical trials (RCT)
      - Strongest evidence: rating A—results of two or more RCTs
      - Rating B—results of two or more controlled clinical trials
      - Rating C—results of one controlled trial, two case series or descriptive studies, or expert opinion
    - Expert panel makes practice recommendations based on evaluation of the evidence.
- Professional organizations publish research-based protocols (e.g., Nurses Improving Care for Healthsystem Elders [NICHE], sponsored by the Hartford Foundation at NYU); Cochrane also publishes large reviews.
- Research utilization: Before using research in practice, a comprehensive analysis should be performed.
  - Locate relevant clinical nursing research.
  - Critique the research to determine transferability, feasibility, and readiness for use in practice.
    - Assess quality of the research—the strength of the evidence and applicability to clinical practice.
    - Studies that have been replicated generate more confidence in outcomes.
- Local data—Continuous quality improvement (CQI)
  - Revise systems and processes on the basis of data about the process itself.
  - CQI measures the current status, locates comparative data, and establishes benchmarks.
  - Change in practice is initiated; data continue to be gathered and analyzed; additional change is implemented as indicated.
  - The improvement process is continuous and cyclical.

OUTCOMES EVALUATION

The growing expense of health care led to focus on outcomes—how to maximize the benefit associated with the resources used in health care. An outcome is a change in patient health status between two or more points in time.

- Health status encompasses physiologic, functional, cognitive, emotional, and behavioral health.
- Outcomes can be positive, negative, or neutral changes in health status. Outcome is a function of baseline condition of the person and treatment factors. Frequently used outcome measures
    - Patient satisfaction measures
    - Functional health status
    - Mortality rates

SUMMARY

This chapter provided an overview of research methods and basic statistics. For the certification exam, be sure that you understand the basics of reading research and applying results to practice. Review the test content outline for specifics to review.

REFERENCES

Benner, P. (1984). *From novice to expert: Excellence and power in clinical nursing practice*. Menlo Park, CA: Addison-Wesley.

Burns, N., & Gove, S. K. (2006). *Understanding nursing research: Building an evidence-based practice*. Philadelphia: Elsevier.

Burns, N., & Gove, S. K. (2008). *The practice of nursing research: Appraisal, synthesis and generation of evidence*. Philadelphia: Saunders Elsevier.

DiCenso, A., Guyatt, G., & Ciliska, D. (2005). *Evidence based nursing: A guide to clinical practice*. St. Louis, MO: Elsevier Mosby.

Fawcett, J., & Garity, J. (2009). *Evaluating research for evidence-based nursing practice*. Philadelphia: F. A. Davis.

Grove, S. K., & Burns, N. (2009). *The practice of nursing research: Appraisal, synthesis and generation of evidence*. St. Louis, MO: Saunders Elsevier.

Mateo, M. K., & Kirchoff, K. T. (Eds.). (1999). *Using and conducting nursing research in the clinical setting* (2nd ed.). Philadelphia: Saunders.

Polit, D. F., & Beck, C. T. (2007). *Nursing research: Generating and assessing evidence for nursing practice*. Philadelphia: Lippincott Williams & Wilkins.

6

Communication, Education, and Counseling

Communication is essential to education, counseling, assessment, and all other interactions with patients, family members, and other members of the interdisciplinary healthcare team. Thus, communication is an essential skill for all nurses. Therapeutic communication fosters ways to improve interactions so that optimal patient outcomes are reached. This chapter begins with an overview of communication and is followed by concepts essential in patient education. Theories of adult learning are presented along with the education process. Health literacy is a current concern related to patient education and so it will be discussed to help raise the awareness of this problem so that nurses can develop more appropriate educational materials. Finally, patient counseling techniques will be included. The focus of counseling is on the role of the nurse in helping patients make behavioral change for a healthier lifestyle.

COMMUNICATION

Communication is the core of all interactions in nursing. Therapeutic communication is the intentional use of communication techniques to enhance the patient-nurse relationship. This section provides an overview of interviewing skills including verbal and nonverbal communication, recognizing communication barriers and cultural influences on communication, protecting privacy in communication, and providing accurate and complete documentation of communication.

Essential Components of Therapeutic Communications

- The use of interpersonal skills to help patients is "therapeutic use of self." It helps build a trusting relationship in which patients are willing to share personal information about their physical and emotional health. Three important techniques enhance the nurse's ability to develop therapeutic communication.
  - Exhibiting empathy or the attempt to appreciate or understand the feelings or emotional responses of another. An example of this might be a response of "it sounds like that was very upsetting to you."
  - Demonstrating unconditional acceptance of the person as one who deserves care. There are times when this is challenging but the nurse must overcome aversion to behaviors and focus on the person as being worthy of care. Acceptance is shown in the response "I see." It does not mean agreement or disagreement but simply understanding what is expressed.
  - Recognizing the patient's worth as an individual can be as simple as sitting with the person and sharing a moment of silence. It also can entail reaffirming the patient's strengths. An example might be "In the past you made changes to promote health and you indicated that attending cardiac rehabilitation helped with that change. It sounds like making changes through group participation is one of your strengths."
- The nonverbal aspects of therapeutic communication are important considerations.
  - Prior to the encounter the nurse should be aware of troubling thoughts and try to clear the mind so that there is intent to concentrate on the interaction. This may involve centering exercises that also help to calm the body and mind through a quick meditation-type activity. This allows for a more mindful approach to the communication.
  - Provide a comfortable setting that is free of distractions for the communication.
  - Face the patient on the same level (e.g., both seated) and turn your body toward him or her.
  - If possible, do not allow interruptions in the interaction. This is most important when doing initial assessments.

Characteristics of Therapeutic Communications

- Allow the patient the opportunity to talk without jumping to conclusions before you have all of the data.
- Be sure to obtain complete data by repeating and clarifying what you think you heard.
- There are many positive communication techniques. Table 6–1 lists some of these techniques for you to review.
- Negative communication techniques should be avoided. Table 6–2 lists common mistakes made in communication in health care.

Barriers to Effective Communication

- Language is an obvious barrier for the person who does not speak English or for whom English is a second language.
  - Use only interpreters who are trained and competent to act in this capacity for healthcare discussions. Never rely on family members because they may hide or offer inaccurate information in what they perceive to be the best interest of the patient.
  - Picture boards can be used for common phrases or patient needs.

Table 6–1. Interviewing Techniques That Promote Positive Communications

Positive Interviewing Techniques	Rationale	Example
Offering leads	Gives permission to speak freely	What happened next? Please continue.
Restating	Clarifies information	So you take a blue pill in the morning and evening.
Reflecting	Gives opportunity to restate or add to a response	Does that include everything you wanted to tell me about the pain you experienced?
Focusing	Links a problem to a bigger health concern	Do you have more coughing after smoking?
Clarifying	Provides validation and aids in interpretation	Was the bruise as large as the palm of your hand?
Sequencing	Provides an order for events	Did the shortness of breath or dizziness happen first?
Encouraging participation	Affirms the person's value and permits free expression	What do you think about the plan of care?
Encouraging evaluation	Allows the patient to assess a situation	What do you think caused this to occur?
Making observations	Aids in interpreting nonverbal messages	You have been yawning frequently over the past few minutes. Do you feel like you have been getting a good night's sleep?
Summarizing	Clarifies important information	So your family has a strong history of early heart disease but not cancers. Is that correct?

- Vision and hearing deficits provide challenges and are discussed under patient education.
- Healthcare literacy may be low. This is discussed in more detail under patient education. Be clear in your communications and remove all jargon. For instance, in a recent survey people were asked what ambulatory care is and most people responded that it was care delivered in an ambulance.
- Culture can be a barrier to communication. Every culture has norms for verbal and nonverbal communication.
    - In many cultures, it is inappropriate to make eye contact or face the person.
    - There may be culturally specific communication norms based on gender, age, or social status.
    - Be sensitive to the potential for cultural norms. Customer service departments often can help with determining culturally relevant communication needs.

Table 6-2. Interviewing Techniques That Inhibit Communication

Negative Interviewing Techniques	Rationale	Example
Why questions	Often judgmental and makes one defensive	Why in the world would you do that?
Giving advice	Often unwanted	Let me tell you what I would do in that situation.
False reassurance	Devalues feelings and promotes false hope	Everything will be just fine.
Using clichés	Trite and does not demonstrate interest in the patient	Tomorrow is a new day. You will feel better in the morning.
Defensive response	Does not show empathy	I am sure the previous nurse did not forget your pain medication. She would not do that.
Leading questions	Makes it difficult to not agree	I am sure you never smoked, or did you?
Using jargon	Difficult for the patient to understand	Has your BP been well-controlled? For this angiogram you will be NPO.

- The common use of electronic medical records is a newly recognized barrier to effective communication. Often the nurse faces the computer instead of the patient when obtaining the health history. Nurses must be cognizant of this potential barrier and find ways to maintain effective communication and then document data. Also, patient room design should be done in a way to minimize this problem by considering where the computers are placed.
- Lack of privacy is a barrier that must be considered. Do obtain history and sensitive data in a setting that affords the highest level of privacy possible. As discussed in Chapter 2, HIPAA guidelines require the protection of personal and health information about patients.

Documentation of Communication
- The medical record is where all data collected during the initial history and subsequent patient interactions are documented.
    - All documentation should be clear, unbiased, and precise.
    - Documentation should be timely so that pertinent information is shared among healthcare providers.
    - Rely upon information in the past medical record to help guide the current plan of care.
    - Care plans should document any barrier to communication.
    - Any patient education, counseling, family teaching, or family care conference should be documented in the medical record.

PATIENT EDUCATION AND ADULT LEARNING

The purpose of patient education is to provide the patient (family) with the knowledge and skills needed for self-care. Many of our major chronic health problems today are the result of behaviors that are not health-promoting. While avoiding blaming the person for his or her disease, the clinician must provide information to support or facilitate behavior change. This section will present principles of adult learning, the process of patient education, and discharge planning. The nurse needs to keep in mind that adult learning is a persistent change in behavior based on experience.

Characteristics of Adult Learners
• Adult learners come with problems to solve and learn best when content is related to the immediate need, problem, or deficit.
  – Adult learners are self-directed.
  – Adult learners are motivated and have a need to know.
• Adult learners have life experience that can hinder or facilitate learning.
  – Learning is enhanced when new content builds on past experience and is related to something the learner knows.

Domains of Learning
• Cognitive learning deals with the intellectual or knowledge area and involves acquiring facts, reaching conclusions, or making decisions.
• Affective learning consists of changing the attitudes, feelings, and interests the person has toward an object or idea.
• Psychomotor learning involves mastering physical skills or motor activities.

Conditions for Learning
• Learning depends on three conditions: motivation to learn, ability to learn, and the learning environment.
• Motivation describes the effect of internal and external forces on the person that initiate, direct, and maintain behavior.
  – Motivation to learn is based on previous knowledge, attitudes, and sociocultural factors.
  – Motivation is the willingness of the person to learn.
  – Six theories of motivation offer insight about why people may learn or change.
    • A desired behavior is reinforced or rewarded.
    • A behavior change satisfies a need for food, shelter, love, or self-esteem.
    • Changing the behavior relieves cognitive dissonance.
      – Cognitive dissonance is the tension felt when a deeply held belief is challenged by an inconsistent behavior.
      – A change in behavior can reduce the dissonance or tension.
      – Specific motivational interviewing skills can help increase the tension and lead the person toward adopting a positive or healthy behavior.

- The causal explanations or attributions a person makes about the situation affect his or her motivation to change.
    - For example, patients who attribute their heart attack to a high-fat diet may be more likely to change their diet than those who attribute their heart attack to bad luck or genetics.
    - Locus of control is a key concept in attribution theory.
        * People with an internal locus of control attribute success or failure to their own efforts.
        * People with an external locus of control attribute success or failure to external factors, such as luck, fate, or difficulty of the task.
- Individual differences in personality may influence motivation to learn or change.
    - Optimism is a personality trait that has been positively associated with seeking information and changing behavior.
    - Learned helplessness causes a person to believe he or she will fail no matter what is tried, thus making the person less likely to learn or change.
    - Coping style may be a part of personality structure, although coping style also may be learned. Additional information about coping is in Chapter 17.
- The person's perceived ability to achieve the goal affects motivation.
    - Self-efficacy is correlated positively with activity level after a heart attack.
- Ability to learn reflects the learner's developmental level, physical wellness, and intellectual thought processes.
    - Developmental level refers to the stage of life of the person. Each stage is accompanied by developmental tasks and concerns. For example, a young adult is concerned with establishing intimacy and close personal relationships. An older adult understands his or her purpose in life and seeks to share accumulated wisdom.
        - Literacy level involves reading, comprehension, problem-solving, math calculation, and the application of these abilities.
            - Illiteracy is found among all ethnic groups and at all socioeconomic levels.
            - Cues to low literacy include the following behaviors:
                * Withdrawing or avoiding learning situations
                * Excuses when asked to review printed material—too tired, forgot my glasses, gave it to my partner to take home, for example
                * Listening and observing very carefully to memorize how things work
            - Health literacy is the level of literacy required to function in the health environment. Health literacy, which is discussed later in this chapter, cannot be predicted from educational level.
        - Language. Does the learner speak and understand English? If not, are the interpreter's skills sufficient to explain?
    - Physical wellness includes the required level of strength, coordination, and sensory acuity for learning.
        - Physical size and strength must match the task to be performed or the equipment to be used.
        - Coordination is the dexterity required for complex motor skills. Consider, for example, the dexterity required to prepare and administer insulin injections. If dexterity is inadequate an alternative method of administration must be found.

- The sensory acuity level needed to receive information and respond appropriately to teaching includes vision, hearing, touch, taste, and smell.
    - Instructor awareness can compensate for some reduced or impaired sensory acuity (see Table 6–3).
  - Multiple intellectual processes are necessary for learning to occur. For example, the ability to pay attention, to understand language, to manipulate symbols, to retrieve information from memory, and to transfer learning to novel situations.
    - Intellectual ability can be affected by health status (e.g., person with receptive aphasia because of a stroke), developmental stage (e.g., child vs. adult), and genetic factors (e.g., person with Down syndrome).
- The environment can have a significant impact on the ability to learn. Many factors may need to be addressed to facilitate learning and minimize barriers to learning.
  - Teacher/learner ratio
    - Some people may learn better in a group, but others may find a group too distracting.
    - Some may learn better in small, interactive groups while others learn better in large groups where there is more anonymity.
    - Groups provide the opportunity for adults to learn from one another's experiences and understand the material presented.
    - Much patient education is presented in a one-to-one—nurse-to-patient—session. One-to-one teaching is sometimes called counseling. It tends to be more responsive to individual concerns and approaches.

Table 6–3. Sensory Impairments With Implications for Patient Teaching

Sensory Impairment	Implications for Teaching
Reduced hearing acuity	• Get person's attention prior to speaking. • Use simple sentences. • Face the patient and stand no more than 6 feet away. • Refrain from standing in front of a window or bright light, which may cast a shadow across your face or glare in patient's eyes. • Request feedback frequently to ensure the patient heard and understood what you said. • If the patient has a hearing aid, be certain it is functioning, adjusted properly, and in use.
Reduced visual acuity	• Vision-enhancing devices: clean glasses, adequate light, or magnifying glasses • Adequate contrast: black ink on white paper • Adequate font size for written materials (minimum 14 point) • Avoid blue, blue-green, and violet hues in printed materials and posters. • Consider using audiotapes to enhance learning.

– Privacy and the assurance of confidentiality are necessary when addressing sensitive issues (e.g., HIV status, genetic counseling).
– Comfortable physical environment
  • Moderate temperature
  • Sufficient lighting that minimizes glare
  • Minimal extraneous noise
  • Adequate ventilation
  • Appropriate and comfortable furniture

Health Literacy

• Health literacy is a strong predictor of health status.
  – Those who understand healthcare instructions have higher levels of health. This result has been replicated in many studies.
  – It is estimated that 90 million Americans have low health literacy skills and are at risk for further health problems.
• Many organizations now make a concerted effort to address the gap between healthcare language and laypersons' skill in understanding those terms.
  – The REALM tool can be used to assess health literacy independent of educational level and reading ability. Learning depends on three conditions: motivation to learn, ability to learn, and the learning environment.
  – Use simple terms to explain concepts that healthcare providers commonly use. For example, "blockages in blood vessels" is a simple way to describe atherosclerosis.
  – The National Institute for Literacy proposes that healthcare workers follow the "4 Bs."
    • Be informed about health literacy and recognize it.
    • Be caring and sensitive in your approach to the patient.
    • Be realistic about resources available and the rate of learning.
    • Be there and be supportive of progress patients make.
• Boxes 6–1 and 6–2 provide further information about health literacy.

Box 6–1. Possible Signs of Low Health Literacy

• Difficulty locating needed healthcare providers and services
• Difficulty filling out complex health forms
• Inability to give a clear or accurate health history
• Lack of preventive health care
• Inadequate knowledge of the results of risky behaviors
• Inability to participate in self-care of chronic health conditions
• Difficulty following medication regimen or undergoing diagnostic testing
• Inability to report what they have been told in the past about their health condition
• Handing healthcare materials to someone else to read or take care of
• Misperceptions, mispronunciations, misuses of common healthcare terms or conditions
• Withdrawn or aloof during discussions of diagnosis or plans of care
• Limited proficiency in the English language

Box 6–2. Interventions for Persons With Low Health Literacy

- Identify patients with limited literacy levels.
- Use simple language and short sentences and define technical terms.
- Supplement instruction with appropriate materials (videos, models, pictures, etc.).
- Ask patients to explain your instructions (teach-back method) or demonstrate the procedure.
- Ask questions that begin with "how" and "what," rather than closed-ended yes/no questions.
- Organize information so that the most important points stand out, and repeat this information.
- Reflect the age, cultural, ethnic, and racial diversity of patients.
- For limited English proficiency (LEP) patients, provide information in their primary language.
- Improve the physical environment by using lots of universal symbols.
- Offer assistance with completing forms.

PATIENT EDUCATION PROCESS

The patient education process parallels the nursing process.

Assessment

Assessment data are used to define learning needs and develop a teaching plan to meet the needs of the person.

- Assessment of need to learn
  - What does the patient know, feel, and believe about his or her health condition?
  - What does he or she need to know?
- Assessment of motivation to learn
  - What motivates this person to learn or change?
    - The learner with an internal locus of control may be eager to change his or her health behavior because the change will enhance feelings of control.
    - The learner with an external locus of control may be difficult to involve in learning and behavior change. He or she does not believe that individual behavior affects health status.
    - The learner who believes someone else controls his or her health (e.g., the nurse or a family member) may expect "someone else" to correct the condition.
  - Are there health-related cultural beliefs that may affect learning? Who should be included in the teaching and decision-making processes?
- Assessment of readiness to learn
  - Are there attitudes or beliefs that may hinder the ability to learn?
    - Some people do not believe that health behaviors affect health status (e.g., people who continue to smoke with peripheral vascular disease). Others believe that it does not matter what they do; illness is going to happen.

- Perceived benefits of changing behaviors differ among learners. Some people may not want to devote the time and energy to change a behavior that they do not believe will improve their quality of life. Others may feel that any effort to change is good.
  - Teaching strategies and techniques used for affective learning (changing attitudes and beliefs) differ from those used for cognitive learning (attaining facts and information).
  - Does the learner have the necessary energy and endurance or will fatigue hinder learning?
    - Patient fatigue often limits the amount of information that can be presented in one session.
  - Is the learner comfortable?
    - Is pain controlled and the patient mentally alert?
    - Does the patient feel safe with the instructor and in the setting?
      - Privacy and confidentiality assured.
      - Patient perceives the instructor as knowledgeable.
  - Are there sensory impairments for which the instructor must compensate?
  - Does the patient have the physical maturity and coordination needed to learn psychomotor skills?

Diagnostic Statement and Objectives

- Nursing diagnoses provide broad diagnostic statements. The following NANDA-I diagnoses may require educational intervention:
  - Deficient knowledge (specify)
  - Ineffective coping
  - Ineffective health maintenance
  - Noncompliance
- Learning objectives are developed in the cognitive (facts and information), affective (attitudes and beliefs), and psychomotor (skills) domains.
- Learning objectives are developed in behavioral terms that specify performance, conditions, and outcome.
  - Performance: Action verbs describe what the learner will do. For example, make a list or solve a problem.
  - Conditions: Identify specific circumstances that will be included in the action. For example, place, time of day, or equipment and tools to be used for teaching should be clearly noted.
  - Criteria: Indicate how achievement of the objective will be evaluated or measured (e.g., test score, accuracy, or frequency).
- Although objectives are developed and written by the instructor, they must be relevant to the learner. Mutual objective-setting helps to assure relevance.

Intervention: Teaching–Learning

- The role of the instructor is to facilitate learning. The role of the student is to learn.
- Structured teaching has been shown to be more effective than unstructured teaching.
- The instructor selects teaching strategies that help the learner to achieve his or her objectives.

- Teaching strategies may be more or less effective depending upon the learning domain, learner characteristics, the learning environment, and the skill of the instructor.
  - Lecture is used commonly when teaching groups.
    - Lecture is an effective method for presenting facts (cognitive learning), but is less effective for affective or psychomotor learning.
    - Lecture combined with discussion is more effective than lecture alone.
      - Discussion allows the learner to express personal feelings and concerns, to ask questions, and to clarify misunderstandings.
  - Question and answer (Q & A) sessions focus the discussion on specific learner needs.
    - Q & A sessions can facilitate both cognitive and affective learning.
    - Q & A sessions are effective in teaching groups and in one-to-one teaching.
      - In groups, people may learn from others' questions.
    - Q & A sessions require active learner participation.
    - Q & A sessions are not effective unless the learner has prior knowledge about the subject. The learner must know enough to recognize and ask questions.
  - Demonstration with return demonstration is an effective strategy for teaching psychomotor skills.
    - Explanation while slowly demonstrating the skill transitions into offering cues to the learner while he or she practices the skill.
    - Repeated practice with praise reinforces the behavior and helps the learner to move toward independent functioning.
    - Supervised return demonstration assists with evaluation of learning.
    - Demonstration/return demonstration is effective with small groups and in one-to-one teaching.
  - Role-playing is an effective strategy for teaching in the affective domain (i.e., attitudes and beliefs).
    - The learner responds to a stimulus based on his or her experience while the teacher offers guidance and feedback.
    - The role-playing may need to be repeated several times before the learner is able to internalize the behavior.
    - In role-modeling, the instructor may take the role of the patient and demonstrate an appropriate response.
  - Oral or written tests may be used for evaluation of cognitive and psychomotor learning.
    - Tests can be used as a part of assessment (pretest) and as an evaluation method to check progress.
    - Oral may be better than written tests when literacy is a concern.
    - Some learners are intimidated by written tests.
  - Simulation or case study method can be used to teach and evaluate the application of material to different situations.
    - Simulation may be computer-based or may use actors to create the scenario.
    - The scenario is presented and the learner interacts with the computer or actor.
    - Solutions and recommendations offered by the learner in response to the scenarios allow instructors to evaluate the effectiveness of their teaching.
  - Teaching tools include books, pamphlets, pictures, films, slides, audio- and videotapes, models, programmed instruction, and computer-assisted learning modules.
    - Selection of effective teaching tools depends on the planned instructional method, learning needs assessed, and the learning ability of the student.

- The instructor must evaluate tools for content, format, reading level, and appropriateness of illustrations before use.
  - Content must match the patient's reading level and present the subject material clearly and logically.
    - Avoid technical language.
    - Standardized reading level assessment formulas can be used to establish readability (e.g., SMOG). These formulas are now included as tools in many word processing programs.
  - Content must be relevant to the situation and contain accurate, current information.
  - Format of the materials affects learning. In general, materials should
    - Be organized with important general points presented first;
    - Progress to specific information based on general points; and
    - Be logical and "user friendly" (e.g., Q & A format).
  - Illustrations enhance learning by emphasizing and reinforcing the written message. They increase motivation by attracting attention, adding variety, and providing breaks in the text.
    - Illustrations should focus on the crucial aspects of the content.
    - Effective illustrations
      - Are simple, uncluttered, and labeled legibly
      - Graphic symbols may help if there are language barriers
      - Colors should be accurate and portray a realistic image
    - Learner interpretation of illustrations may be influenced by literacy level, cultural beliefs, and prior experience.
  - Layout and design of printed material can greatly influence its effectiveness.
    - Font should be clear and easy to read.
    - Type size should be 12–14 point, especially for the older learner.
    - Maintain case contrast; avoid all capitals. Use bold for emphasis.
    - Ink color should offer sufficient contrast with the paper color.
    - Glossy paper may produce glare and make reading difficult.
    - Adequate spacing of text, illustrations, and "white space" makes the materials easier to read.

Evaluation and Reteaching

- Evaluation is used to measure learning and health-related outcomes, monitor performance, and determine competence. Information gathered during evaluation is used to redirect teaching with the goal of improving responses and outcomes.
- Direct and indirect measurements are used for evaluation.
  - Direct measurement involves observing the learner and recording behaviors. The observer may use tools to guide the observations and rate behavior, such as
    - Rating scales (e.g., Likert, numerical [1–10, 0–5, 1–100], or visual analog scales)
    - Checklists of required behaviors
    - Anecdotal notes (i.e., written observations of behavior)
  - Indirect measurement makes the assumption that learning has occurred when learners have achieved at a predetermined level. Indirect measurement does not measure behavior directly.

- Oral questioning is a flexible form of indirect measurement.
  - Oral questioning allows immediate feedback to the learner and the correction of areas of weakness by the instructor.
  - Oral questioning may be difficult for the learner if oral expression or language is a problem.
- Written tests are an indirect measure of cognitive learning. The most effective tests are well-written, based on identified learning objectives, and involve increasing levels of difficulty.

Documentation

- Document in the clinical record the content presented, written materials provided, and the patient's understanding of the information.
- Document a plan for reinforcement of information or referral to specialized educational programs.

PATIENT EDUCATION AND COUNSELING

- Knowledge is necessary, but not sufficient, to change health behavior.
- Patient education and counseling often occur in busy practice settings.

Strategies

- Several patient education and counseling strategies have been described that can be implemented in brief periods of time during routine health visits.
  - Frame the teaching to match the patient's perceptions.
  - Fully inform patients of the purposes and expected effects of interventions and when to expect these effects. For example, when a smoker quits smoking, risk for cardiac and vascular mortality drops significantly in the first year and then more gradually through ensuing years.
  - Suggest small changes rather than large ones. Loss of 3 to 4 pounds in 4 weeks is better than recommending loss of 25 pounds in 6 months.
  - Be specific. If a patient is walking a mile 3 days a week, recommend increasing frequency to 5 days a week.
  - It is sometimes easier to add new behaviors than to eliminate established behaviors. It may be easier to add moderate exercise than to reduce caloric intake.
  - Link new behaviors to established behaviors. For example, link riding an exercise bicycle for 30 minutes to watching the evening news.
  - Use the power of the profession. Direct, explicit, simple measures are powerful. For example, the message "You have smoked your last cigarette" may be effective if given by a trusted health professional.
  - Get explicit commitments from the patient.
  - Use a combination of strategies. Educational efforts that incorporate individual counseling, group classes, and written materials are more likely to be effective than single strategies.
  - Involve office staff. Patient education and counseling is a shared responsibility of physicians, nurses, health educators, dietitians, and allied health professionals. The provision of educational materials in the waiting area may stimulate interest and discussion of health-related topics.

- Refer; an increasing number of educational programs are available through community agencies, national voluntary organizations, and health facilities.
- Monitor progress through follow-up contact. Inquire at each visit about progress and challenges. Telephone calls initiated by the professional to the patient to assess progress may provide external motivation for change.

HEALTH SELF-MANAGEMENT

Health self-management issues include health maintenance, disease prevention, and health promotion.

Health Maintenance

Health maintenance activities are behaviors that maintain or improve health over time. Health maintenance depends on three characteristics: perception of health, motivation to change when needed, and adherence to prescribed interventions.
- Perception of health involves one's understanding of current health status and having the knowledge to manage positive health behaviors.
  - Health perceptions include the importance of health, the ability to control health, and the benefits of and barriers to healthy behavior.
  - Factors affecting health perception include age and developmental stage, personality characteristics, and physical wellness. These factors are discussed previously in this chapter.
- Motivation to change is determined by the responsibility that the learner assumes for health. Factors that may affect motivation to change were discussed previously in this chapter.
- Adherence to (or compliance with) prescribed intervention requires making the decision to change or comply, setting goals, and actually making the therapeutic lifestyle changes.
  - Making a decision and commitment to change may be difficult to achieve but are essential first steps.
  - Goals need to be realistic and achievable. Failure occurs when goals are unrealistic and too difficult to achieve.
  - Making and maintaining lifestyle changes over time is often difficult.
    - Negative life events (e.g., the death of a spouse, family member, or close friend) can weaken the patient's resolve and old behaviors may resurface.
    - The professional helps the patient view the reoccurrence of old behavior as a temporary lapse rather than as a failure.
  - A positive social support system helps the patient focus on the treatment goals.

Disease Prevention

Disease prevention is the organized effort to limit the development and progression of lifestyle-related illness. Three areas of disease prevention are primary, secondary, and tertiary.
- Primary prevention precedes the occurrence of disease and is used with healthy populations.
  - Primary prevention aims to decrease the probability of disease.
  - Primary prevention includes immunizations, health education programs, and activities such as eating a healthy diet, avoiding tobacco products, and exercising regularly.

- Secondary prevention involves screening to detect and treat disease in its earliest stages, before symptoms are present.
  - Early detection and treatment are associated with improved health outcomes and reduced morbidity and mortality.
  - Secondary prevention includes screening programs such as cholesterol screening, vision/hearing screening, and blood pressure screening.
- Tertiary prevention attempts to reduce complications and disability from established disease, thereby improving quality of life.
  - In rehabilitation, the goal is to minimize residual dysfunction and to maximize functional level.
  - An example of tertiary prevention is a cardiac rehabilitation program that includes lifestyle changes such as altering dietary and exercise habits, remodeling attitude, and modifying response to stress.

Health Promotion

Health promotion refers to risk-reduction strategies applied at the population level (macro level). Nurses have major roles as educators for the prevention of disease and enhancement of quality of life and as citizens to influence health policy.
- Passive health promotion requires no action by the person, for example
  - Fluoridation of municipal drinking water
  - Fortification of milk with vitamin D
  - Addition of iodine to table salt
- Active health promotion is the adoption of and participation in health programs by the person (micro level), for example
  - Achieving and maintaining an ideal weight
  - Eating a healthy diet
  - Not smoking or using tobacco
  - Exercising regularly
  - Reducing stress

DISCHARGE PLANNING

Discharge planning facilitates the patient's transition between settings along the continuum of care. Discharge planning usually begins with admission to an institutional setting (hospital or nursing home) and continues until full recovery occurs, or the patient's condition is stabilized at the highest possible functional level.

Key Elements

Key elements addressed in discharge planning include changes in the patient's condition, coordination and facilitation of care, and negotiation of roles and responsibilities.
- Transitions involve changes in patient condition. These changes may require adjustment by patients and their families.
  - Mobility may be altered because of disease, surgery, or trauma. For example, an independent elderly patient may require a walker after surgery for an injured hip.
  - Self-concept may change and need to be addressed. For example, a person may feel "damaged" and less confident after myocardial infarction (MI) or heart surgery.

- Role performance may be altered permanently or temporarily after a stroke or aneurysm repair. The person may be unable to return to his or her former occupation, and roles within the family and community may need to be renegotiated.
  - Similarly, short- or long-term self-care deficits may be present for the stroke patient.
- Coordination of care is the identification, implementation, and direction of treatment prior to discharge.
  - In the acute care setting, coordination of care is facilitated by the use of multidisciplinary care paths or critical pathways.
    - Care paths or critical pathways sequence interventions to achieve expected outcomes over a projected length of stay for specific case types.
    - If care is provided according to these guidelines and variance from the guidelines is addressed promptly, the patient will be discharged in a timely manner and in as healthy a condition as possible.
  - Home care and long-term-care agencies use similar case-specific clinical guidelines for care coordination.
- Facilitation of care and discharge requires the anticipation of discharge needs upon admission.
  - Initial assessment of potential discharge needs is done when the patient is admitted to the facility or service.
  - Initial assessment of family resources and caregiving ability must occur also.
- Negotiation is the process by which discharge goals and roles and responsibilities are determined or assigned.
  - Negotiation may be formal or informal.
  - Negotiation may be necessary in the following examples.
    - The patient who is unable to manage at home may need supportive care, such as a visiting nurse, temporary nursing home placement, or outpatient rehabilitation.
    - The patient's health problems may require more family involvement, such as 24-hour supervision. The family may select a responsible person or multiple family members may agree to be present for specified times.
- Medication reconciliation is a major focus of current patient safety and must be included in all discharge planning. This is particularly important because previous home medications must be compared against hospital medications. Instructions should clearly address which medications are added, stopped, continued at same dose, and continued at an adjusted dose.

Levels of Discharge Planning

Levels of discharge planning vary based on patient needs, family support, and financial resources. There are three levels of discharge planning currently used in hospitals: basic, simple, and complex.

- Basic discharge planning may require only patient teaching.
  - The clinical nurse may do the teaching (e.g., wound care or medication actions).
  - Specialists, (e.g., dietitians, enterostomal nurses, lactation nurses, diabetes educators) may be involved with the teaching.
- Simple discharge planning involves referring the patient to community resources. This usually involves giving the necessary information to the patient or family, such as
  - Sources for durable medical equipment
  - Private-pay, in-home service agencies
  - Sources for outpatient therapies (e.g., speech, physical or occupational therapy)

- Complex discharge planning involves interdisciplinary collaboration, coordination, and negotiation. The discharge planner, the patient (when possible), and the family work together with community-based, subacute, or long-term care services to formulate the most appropriate discharge plan.
  - Community-based care may be needed when the patient remains in the home environment but requires supervision or therapy on an intermittent basis, for example
    - Daycare programs for the cognitively impaired adults
    - Home care services may include nurses, aides, therapists, and durable medical equipment companies.
  - Subacute care is designed for patients who are too ill to be discharged from the hospital to a traditional extended care facility or home. There are four types of subacute care facilities.
    - Transitional units are an alternative to continued hospital stays for patients with complex nursing or medical care needs (e.g., deep wound management, complicated vascular or cardiac surgery).
    - General units are for stable patients who require a moderate level of care (e.g., long-term intravenous therapy).
    - Chronic units are for patients with little or no hope of recovery (e.g., ventilator-dependent patients).
    - Long-term transitional units are for patients with medically complex conditions when recovery is expected (e.g., acute ventilator support with difficulty weaning).
  - Nursing homes offer care to patients experiencing debilitating acute or chronic illnesses (e.g., multiple sclerosis, muscular dystrophy, surgery, trauma).
    - Skilled nursing facilities provide care that requires licensed healthcare professionals such as nurses or therapists (e.g., tube feedings, care of stage 3 and 4 wounds).
    - Nursing facilities care for patients who cannot independently perform activities of daily living.
    - Residential facilities such as assisted-living centers and group homes offer supervision of patients who are fairly independent and able to perform most or all self-care activities.

SUMMARY

This chapter covered key aspects of communication, patient education, health literacy, and counseling for lifestyle change. Much of the content of the certification exam focuses on these basic nursing skills. Be sure to review the test content outline and match your knowledge against that framework for the examination.

REFERENCES

Balzer-Riley, J. (2007). *Communication in nursing* (6th ed.). St. Louis, MO: Elsevier-Mosby.

Bandura, A. (1986). *Social foundations of thought & action: A social cognitive theory.* Englewood Cliffs, NJ: Prentice-Hall.

Burnard, P., & Gill, P. (2009). *Culture, communication and nursing.* Essex, UK: England Pearson Education.

Hernandez, L., for Institute of Medicine. (2009). *Health literacy, ehealth, and communication: Putting the consumer first: Workshop summary.* Washington DC: Institute of Medicine.

Jackson, M. (2009). *Pocket guide for patient education.* New York: McGraw Hill.

Kennedy Sheldon, L. (2008). *Communication for nurses: Talking with patients* (2nd ed.). Sudbury, MA: Jones & Bartlett.

Knowles, M. (2005). *The adult learner: The definitive classic in adult education and human resource development* (6th ed.). Burlington, MA: Elsevier.

Maville, J. A., & Huerta, C. G. (2008). *Health promotion in nursing* (2nd ed.). Albany, NY: Thompson Delmar.

Mayer, G. G. (2007). *Health literacy in primary care: A clinician's guide.* New York: Springer.

Munoz, C., & Luckmann, J. (2005). *Transcultural communication in nursing.* St. Louis, MO: Elsevier-Mosby.

NANDA International. (2009). *Nursing diagnoses: Definitions & classification 2009–2011.* Sudbury, MA: Jones & Bartlett.

Pender, N., Murdaugh, C., & Parsons M. A. (2005). *Health promotion in nursing practice* (5th ed.). Los Altos, CA: Appleton & Lange.

Rankin, S. H., Stallings, K. D., & London, F. (2005). *Patient education in health and illness.* Philadelphia: Lippincott Williams & Wilkins.

Redman, B. K. (2006). *The practice of patient education: A case study approach.* St. Louis, MO: Mosby.

Rollnick, S., Miller, W. R., & Butler, C. C. (2008). *Motivational interviewing in health care: Helping patients change behavior.* New York: Guilford Press.

Cardiac and Vascular Risk

The Framingham Heart Study has provided the richest source of data on predictors of heart and vascular disease. Much information can be found at the Web site http://www.framinghamheartstudy.org/. In 1948, the original cohort of 5,206 adults (two-thirds of the adult population of Framingham, MA) were recruited to participate in examinations every 2 years. The offspring study was started in 1971, recruiting 5,124 children of the original participants. In 2001, Generation 3 Study began with 4,095 adult grandchildren of the original participants. Over the decades these people have biennial complete histories, physical exams, and laboratory studies to look for the best predictors of developing coronary artery disease, stroke, atrial fibrillation, and many more cardiac disorders. From 1950 to 2008, various researchers have published 1,973 papers based on Framingham study data. Current emphasis is on biomarkers and genetics as risk factors for heart disease. Several decades ago, the Framingham studies were criticized for underrepresenting minorities, a reflection of the population of the town where recruitment began. Therefore, the Omni study was added in 1994 with 506 new subjects of Black, American, Hispanic, Asian, and Native American decent. In 2003, the Omni Second Generation Study recruited an additional 410 minority offspring. Over the years, the Framingham study has provided the best source for identifying risk factors for heart and vascular disease. The studies have resulted in scoring mechanisms for predicting the occurrence of future disease and are now widely used in clinical practice. In recent years the American Heart Association has issued guidelines, based on the current research findings, for evaluating potential risk factors that provide a basis for when population screening should be done. This information guides practice protocols and community education.

CORONARY HEART DISEASE (CHD)

Risk Identification

- The term "cardiac risk factor" describes the characteristics found in healthy people that are independently related to the subsequent development of CHD. These characteristics are termed modifiable and nonmodifiable.
- Modifiable cardiac risk factors include hypertension, hypercholesterolemia, low high-density lipoprotein cholesterol (HDL-C) level, diabetes mellitus, tobacco use, and obesity.
- Nonmodifiable cardiac risk factors include age, gender, and family history of premature CHD in a first-degree relative (males < 55 years, females < 65 years).
- Patients having experienced a CHD event have the highest risk of experiencing another event. This risk is greater than 20% over 10 years, based on the results of the Framingham studies.
- Patients with a CHD risk equivalent have the same level of CHD risk (> 20% in 10 years), but have not yet experienced a CHD event.
- There are three CHD risk equivalent groups.
  - Patients with two or more cardiac risk factors
  - Patients with other forms of atherosclerotic vascular disease: peripheral vascular disease, abdominal aortic aneurysm, and symptomatic carotid artery disease
  - Patients with type 2 diabetes
- Patients with a 20% or greater 10-year risk of a coronary event should be treated as aggressively as people who already have CHD, regardless of symptom profile.
- Calculating the CHD risk score is the first part of the approach to lipid management of all adults.
- The Framingham Risk Calculators can be downloaded or used online at the Framingham Study Web site (http://www.framinghamheartstudy.org/) or the National Institute of Health Web site (http://hp2010.nhlbihin.net/atpiii/riskcalc.htm) for downloadable program, (http://hp2010.nhlbihin.net/atpiii/calculator.asp?usertype=prof for online calculator).

Core Risk Factors

- Modifiable
  - Hypertension
    - There is a 27% increase in risk for every 7 mm Hg increase in diastolic blood pressure (BP).
    - Isolated systolic hypertension (systolic BP > 160 mm Hg) markedly increases the risk for nonfatal myocardial infarction (MI) and cardiovascular death among general population samples and low-risk groups.
    - Pulse pressure, a potential surrogate for vascular wall stiffness, predicts first and recurrent myocardial infarction. Higher pulse pressure, especially after age 60, was as strong a predictor of CHD as systolic blood pressure.
    - With effective antihypertensive therapy, CHD risk is reduced but remains higher than in someone without hypertension. Hypertension treatment is detailed in Chapter 9.
    - BP goal should be lower in people with diabetes and those with renal disease (i.e., < 130/85 mm Hg).
    - The Joint National Committee (JNC) sets the standards for hypertension treatment. JNC7 was issued in 2004 and JNC8 is scheduled for release in 2010.

- Dyslipidemia
    - Estimates suggest that 45% of American adults have total cholesterol levels greater than 200 mg/dL and that 20% of American adults have total cholesterol levels of 240 mg/dL or greater.
    - A 10% increase in serum cholesterol is associated with a 20% to 30% increase in risk for CHD.
    - LDL-C is the primary target for lipid lowering because of the strength of this independent risk for CHD. Non-LDL-C (HDL and triglycerides) is a secondary target for intervention.
    - The lower the concentration of HDL-C, the greater the risk of CHD.
        - HDL-C below 40 mg/dL is classified as low.
        - HDL-C above 60 mg/dL is classified as high and is associated with lower CHD risk.
    - Evidence supports elevated triglyceride (TG) level as an independent predictor of CHD risk.
        - TG levels in the borderline high and high range (150 mg/dL to 500 mg/dL) are associated with increased CHD risk.
    - Saturated fatty acids increase low-density lipoprotein cholesterol (LDL-C) levels. Monounsaturated fatty acids lower LDL-C and do not affect HDL-C.
    - The Advisory Treatment Panel 3 (ATP3) was released by the National Cholesterol Education Panel in 2003. The ATP4 will be published in 2010.
- Diabetes mellitus
    - Type 2 diabetes accounts for about 90% of all diabetes cases. Underlying causes of type 2 diabetes are obesity, physical inactivity, and genetics.
    - Diabetes is associated with an accelerated atheromatous process resulting in increased risk for atherosclerotic disease. This risk qualifies diabetes as a CHD risk equivalent (10-year risk of CHD event > 20%).
    - Age-adjusted rates for CHD are two to three times higher among men with diabetes and three to seven times higher among women with diabetes than among their counterparts without diabetes.
    - Three-fourths of all deaths among people with diabetes result from CHD. By age 40, CHD is the leading cause of death in both men and women with diabetes.
        - There is a twofold increase in mortality in those who have diabetes at the time of MI, as well as increased risk for heart failure.
    - Metabolic syndrome is a constellation of lipid and nonlipid risk factors of metabolic origin. Metabolic syndrome is a generalized disorder closely linked to insulin resistance, implicating impaired insulin action.
        - Excess body fat (particularly abdominal obesity) and physical inactivity promote the development of insulin resistance.
        - The diagnosis of metabolic syndrome is made when three or more of the risk determinants are present.
            - Waist circumference (at the iliac crest) > 40 inches for men or > 35 inches for women.
            - Triglyceride > 150 mg/dL
            - HDL-C < 40 mg/dL for men and < 50 mg/dL for women
            - BP > 135 mm Hg systolic or > 85 mm Hg diastolic
            - Fasting blood glucose 110 mg/dL

Table 7-1. Gender and Race/Ethnicity Prevalence of CHD in the United States

	Males	Females
White (Caucasian)	8.8%	6.6%
Black	9.6%	9.0%
Hispanic and Mexican-American	5.4%	6.3%

- Nonmodifiable risk factors include:
  - Age
    - 85% of people who die of CHD are age 65 years and older.
    - About 80% of CHD mortality in people below age 65 occurs during the first MI.
    - Lifetime risk of developing CHD after age 40 is 49% for men and 32% for women.
    - In general, men (ages 35–65) have a higher risk for CHD than women. In women, the onset of CHD generally is delayed by 10 to 15 years (ages 45–75).
  - Gender
    - The incidence of CHD in women lags behind men by 10 years for total CHD and by 20 years for more serious clinical events such as MI and sudden death.
    - In men, the three major presentations of CHD (angina, sudden death, and MI) are equally distributed. Women with CHD more frequently present with angina symptoms.
    - CHD kills more women than all cancers combined.
    - In 50% of men and 63% of women who died suddenly of CHD, there were no previous symptoms of this disease.
    - Within one year after their first recognized MI, 25% of men and 38% of women will die.
    - Within 6 years after a recognized heart attack, 18% of men and 35% of women will have another heart attack.
    - Women in the United States are more likely to die of CHD than any other cause.
      - CHD rates in women after menopause are two to three times those of women before menopause.
      - Women taking oral contraceptives who also smoke have an increased risk of CHD.
  - Ethnicity
    - According to the Centers for Disease Control and Prevention, in 2007 the overall heart disease crude death rates per 100,000 population for the five largest U.S. racial/ethnic groups were
      - Hispanics, 69.2;
      - Asians and Pacific Islanders, 73.0;
      - Native Americans and Alaska Natives, 82.5;
      - Blacks (non-Hispanics), 189.8; and
      - Whites (non-Hispanics), 235.5.
    - Among Native Americans and Alaska Natives ages 65 through 74, the rates (per 1,000 population) of new and recurrent heart attacks are 25.1 for men and 9.1 for women.

- Family history
  - Family history is considered positive when CHD events are confirmed in first-degree male relatives before age 55 or first-degree female relatives before age 65.
  - Typically, the presence of premature CHD in the family history is accompanied by a family history of other cardiac risk factors.
- Socioeconomic
  - In developed countries, CHD is a disease concentrated in the lower socioeconomic, less educated sector of the population.
  - In developing countries, CHD is a disease of urban middle and upper classes and is virtually unknown in the traditional country villages.
  - Among the cardiovascular diseases, CHD is the leading cause of death in urban areas in rapidly industrializing countries (e.g., China).

Life Habit Risk Factors (Modifiable)

- Smoking
  - Smoking is the most important modifiable risk factor for CHD, accounting for 400,000 deaths annually.
  - Compared to nonsmokers, those who consume more than 20 cigarettes per day have a two- to threefold increase in CHD risk.
  - Smoking acts synergistically with oral contraceptives to increase CHD risk.
  - Smoking may enhance oxidation of LDL-C, as well as decrease HDL-C, impair coronary vasodilation, increase C-reactive protein and fibrinogen, and enhance monocyte adhesion to endothelial cells.
  - Smoking increases risk for coronary spasm and for ventricular ectopic activity.
  - Smoking cessation decreases the risk of first MI by 65%.
- Obesity
  - Obesity adversely influences other vascular risk factors, causing hypertension, dyslipidemia, glucose intolerance, and insulin resistance.
  - Obesity is independently associated with left ventricular hypertrophy (LVH), while weight loss can reduce left ventricular mass.
  - Waist-to-hip ratio, a surrogate for abdominal obesity, is an independent marker of vascular risk for women and older men.
  - Waist circumference measurements indicating increased risk are > 40" in men and > 35" in women.
- Physical Inactivity
  - Mortality data suggests that more than 200,000 deaths result from inactivity annually.
  - Physical inactivity is associated with other CHD risk factors including decreased HDL-C, insulin resistance, and hypertension.
  - Physically fit but overweight people have a CHD risk similar to that of people without CHD risk factors.
- Diet and nutrition
  - The effect of diet on risk is mediated through lipids, BP, and obesity.
  - There is growing interest in the Mediterranean diet, which is rich in monounsaturated fats as well as fruits and vegetables.

- Alcohol abuse
  - The relative risk of death from cardiovascular disease (CVD) in moderate drinkers compared to nondrinkers was 0.7 in men and 0.6 in women.
  - The protective effect of moderate alcohol intake on CVD may be mediated through increased HDL-C, decreased platelet aggregation, and fibrinolysis.
  - Alcohol abuse leads to hypertension, hemorrhagic stroke, and sudden cardiac death.
- Mental stress
  - Mental stress can cause coronary vasoconstriction, particularly in atherosclerotic arteries, reducing myocardial oxygen supply.
  - Catecholamines promote alterations in thrombosis and coagulation, favoring clot formation.
  - Increases in coronary deaths during missile attacks and earthquakes have been documented.

Emerging Risk Factors

- Hyperhomocysteinemia
  - Elevated homocysteine levels are independently associated with CVD.
  - Mechanisms include endothelial toxicity, accelerated oxidation of LDL-C, impaired endothelial-derived relaxation factor, and decreased flow-mediated arterial vasodilation.
  - Deficiencies in folate and vitamins B-12 and B-6 lead to elevated serum levels of homocysteine, while supplementation decreases levels.
- Hypercoagulability
  - Fibrinogen is positively associated with age, obesity, smoking, diabetes, and LDL-C, and inversely associated with HDL-C, alcohol abuse, physical activity, and exercise level.
  - The relative risk of CV events is 1.8 times higher for people in the top as compared with the bottom third of baseline fibrinogen concentration.
  - Factor VII levels, plasminogen activator inhibition, and platelet aggregation have been associated with CVD risk.
- Estrogen status
  - In premenopausal women, the age-adjusted incidence and mortality for CHD is lower than in men; however, the rates converge after menopause.
  - Aside from lipid benefits (deceased LDL-C with increased HDL-C, Apo A1, and triglycerides), estrogen decreases LDL oxidation, promotes endothelial vasodilation, decreases fibrinolytic capacity, and enhances glucose metabolism.
  - Postmenopausal hormone replacement therapy (HRT) is no longer recommended for cardioprotection. The Women's Health Initiative (WHI), a prospective study, found that HRT increased the incidence of MI, stroke, and blood clots.
- Lipoprotein (a) [Lp(a)]
  - Studies suggest a positive association between Lp(a) and vascular risk, although levels are elevated after acute ischemia, making measurement unreliable.
  - Limitations on the utility of Lp(a) screening include lack of testing standardization, variability of levels among racial groups, and unclear predictive value.
  - LDL reduction markedly reduces any adverse hazard associated with Lp(a).
- Triglyceride (TG)
  - Elevated levels of TG are related to decreased HDL-C, elevated levels of small dense LDL particles, and procoagulant state.

- Lowering triglyceride results in a significant reduction in CVD events.
- Oxidative stress
  - Vitamin E, beta carotene, and other natural antioxidants have failed to show a beneficial effect on CHD risk or disease progression.
  - American Heart Association discourages the use of antioxidant vitamin supplements and recommends dietary modifications.
- Left ventricular hypertrophy (LVH)
  - The incidence of LVH increases with age, BP, and obesity.
  - LVH is independently associated with increased incidence of CVD.
  - There are no conclusive data to support the theory that a reduction in LV mass can improve CV outcome independent of a decrease in BP.
- Inflammatory processes
  - Evidence linking inflammation to atherosclerosis stems from studies focusing on acute and chronic phases of CHD.
  - Acute phase reactants such as high-sensitivity C-reactive protein (hs-CRP), ICAM–1 (adhesion molecules), and IL–6 and tumor necrosis factor (cytokines) are inflammatory markers measured in the plasma.
  - hs-CRP and serum amyloid A have been shown in several studies to be markers of risk.
    - People with elevated hs-CRP levels had a relative risk of future vascular events three to four times higher than people with lower levels, an effect independent of other risk factors.
    - A recent study found that treating elevated CRP with statins (a known anti-inflammatory) in people with normal lipids reduced cardiovascular events.
    - At this time routine screening of hs-CRP is not recommended by the AHA; however, this may change in the future.
  - Numerous infectious agents are being considered as possible causes of vascular injury and inflammation (e.g., cytomegalovirus, *Chlamydia pneumoniae*, *Helicobacter pylori*, herpes simplex virus).
  - Extravascular foci of chronic infection might include gingiva, the bronchi, the urinary tract (including the prostate), or diverticular disease.

Risk Stratification

As mentioned near the beginning of this chapter, the Framingham Heart Study has developed and updated mathematical health risk appraisal models that relate risk factors to the probability of developing CHD.

- The new gender-specific models incorporate primary and secondary, or subsequent, risk appraisal.
- Primary models assess CHD risk in persons free of CV disease, including MI, coronary insufficiency, angina pectoris, stroke, TIA, heart failure, and intermittent claudication.
  - Risk factors included in the Framingham model are triglyceride level, alcohol use, and menopausal status.
- Subsequent CHD models are applicable for people with a history of CHD or ischemic stroke who have survived the acute period after the event.
  - Risk factors include age, blood lipid levels (total cholesterol and HDL-C), diabetes, systolic blood pressure (SBP), and smoking.

- The probability of developing CHD within a 10-year period is calculated by assigning points to each risk factor. Points are summed and probability of CHD read from a Framingham Risk Table.
  - Example of a 55-year-old male smoker with elevated cholesterol and high blood pressure
    Age: 6 points
    Total cholesterol/triglyceride: 10 points
    No diabetes: 0 points
    Smoker: 4 points
    SBP: 140 mm Hg on medication, 4 points
    Total points = 24, which indicates a 9% probability of a CHD event within 10 years.
- The risk tables are included in the appendix of the ATP-III Guidelines.

STROKE

Risk Identification
- Stroke is the third leading cause of death in the United States.
- There are 700,000 incident strokes annually.
- 4.4 million people are stroke survivors.
- The most common varieties of complete strokes are atherothrombotic brain infarcts (61% excluding TIAs), followed by cerebral embolus (24%).
  - 83% were ischemic
  - 10% were intracerebral hemorrhage
  - 7% were subarachnoid hemorrhage
  - 7.6% of ischemic strokes and 37.5% of hemorrhagic strokes result in death within 30 days.

Core Risk Factors
- Nonmodifiable
  - Age
    - The risk of stroke doubles in each successive decade after 55 years of age.
    - 28% of stroke victims are < 65 years of age.
  - Gender
    - Stroke prevalence is higher in men than women, with the exception of those 35 to 44 years old and those > 85 years, among whom women have slightly greater age-specific incidence than men.
    - Fatality rates are higher in women than men; one in six women who suffer a stroke will die of it.
  - Race/ethnicity
    - Blacks and some Hispanic Americans have an almost twofold increased incidence of stroke in comparison with whites.
    - The increased incidence of stroke in Blacks is because of higher prevalence of hypertension (HTN), obesity (in women), diabetes, increased LP(a) levels, smoking (in men), and low socioeconomic levels.
    - Black men and women were more likely to die of stroke than White men and women.

- Chinese and Japanese men and women have a high incidence of stroke.
  - Family history
    - Paternal or maternal history of stroke may be associated with increased stroke risk.
    - Mechanisms include genetic heritability of stroke risk factors, inheritance of susceptibility to effects of risk factors, and familial sharing of cultural, environmental, and lifestyle factors.
    - There is a fivefold increase in stroke prevalence among monozygotic (identical) twins in comparison with dizygotic (fraternal) twins.
  - Socioeconomic factors
    - In one study, women living in economically deprived areas had an increased risk of stroke.
- Modifiable
  - HTN
    - Major risk factor for both cerebral infarct and intracerebral hemorrhage
    - The incidence of stroke increases in proportion to both systolic and diastolic BP.
    - Two-thirds of people who experience a first stroke have BP > 160/95 mm Hg.
    - Isolated systolic hypertension (ISH) is an important risk factor for older adults.
    - ISH is defined by JNC VII as systolic BP > 160 mm Hg and diastolic BP < 90 mm Hg.
    - The SHEP (Systolic Hypertension in the Elderly Program) trial showed a 36% reduction in incidence of stroke with antihypertensive therapy.
  - Diabetes, hyperinsulinemia, and insulin resistance
    - People with insulin-dependent diabetes have an increased susceptibility to atherosclerosis and risk factors (e.g., HTN, obesity, abnormal blood lipids).
    - Metabolic risk factors known as the metabolic syndrome, which includes hyperinsulinemia and insulin resistance and results in hyperglycemia, increased VLDL, decreased HDL, and HTN, have been identified in some people with type 2 diabetes.
    - The relative risk of ischemic stroke in people with diabetes ranges from 1.8 to 8.0.
    - People with glucose intolerance have double the risk of brain infarction compared to those with normal glucose tolerance.
    - Tight control of HTN in people with diabetes significantly reduces stroke incidence.
  - Asymptomatic carotid stenosis
    - Cerebral ischemic events occurred more frequently among patients with severe (> 75%) carotid artery stenosis, progressing carotid artery stenosis, or heart disease, and in men.
    - The annual risk of stroke was 3.2% over 5 years with 60% to 99% carotid artery stenosis.
    - Some studies suggest that the rate of stroke may be higher for patients with progressing stenosis and those with more severe stenosis than in those with stable disease.
    - As with asymptomatic carotid bruit, asymptomatic carotid artery stenosis is an important indicator of concomitant ischemic cardiac disease.
  - Atrial fibrillation (A fib)
    - The annual risk of stroke for patients with nonvalvular A fib is 3% to 5%, with the condition being responsible for 50% of thromboembolic strokes.
    - Two-thirds of strokes in A fib patients are cardioembolic.

- The Framingham Heart Study showed a dramatic increase in stroke risk with A fib in advancing age: in 50- to 59-year-olds, the increase risk was 1.5% over those without A fib and in 80- to 89-year-olds, the risk increased to 23.5% over those in the same age group without A fib.
- Predictors of high risk for stroke were advanced age, prior TIA or stroke, systolic HTN, history of HTN, impaired LV function, diabetes, and women > 75 years of age.
- Other cardiac diseases
  - 20% of ischemic strokes are because of cardiogenic embolism from other cardiac diseases (e.g., ischemic cardiomyopathy, valvular heart disease, and intracardiac congenital defects).
  - MI
    - 8% of men and 11% of women will have a stroke within 6 years after MI.
    - Post-MI development of A fib is a common source of cardiogenic emboli.
    - Overall occurrence of stroke in acute MI is 0.8%, with 0.6% being ischemic.
    - Risk factors for stroke post-MI demonstrated preexisting factors such as previous stroke, A fib, old age, heart failure, and heart rate > 100 bpm were more important than treatment with thrombolysis, which was a borderline significant risk factor.
- Cardiac surgical procedures
  - Perioperative stroke occurs in 1% to 7% of patients having coronary artery bypass grafting.
  - History of prior neurologic events, advanced age, female gender, diabetes, and A fib accompanied by low cardiac output syndrome were identified as risk factors for early and delayed stroke.
  - Other factors include the duration of cardiopulmonary bypass and the presence of aortic atherosclerosis and macroemboli.
- Hyperlipidemia
  - One study showed a continuous and progressive increase in thromboembolic stroke rates with rising levels of cholesterol.
  - An inverse relationship exists between HDL-C level and stroke risk. (High HDL-C is associated with lower stroke risk.)
  - In the 4S trial (Simvastatin Survival Study), the simvastatin-treated group experienced a 51% reduction in ischemic nonembolic stroke.
- Sleep apnea
  - Sleep-related breathing disorder appears to be a risk factor for stroke.
  - Pathogenic mechanisms are decreased cerebral perfusion, increased coagulability, and diurnal HTN.
- Sickle cell disease (SCD)
  - The prevalence of stroke by age 20 in patients with SCD is at least 11%.

Life Habit Risk Factors

- Smoking
  - Effects of smoking are multifactorial, affecting both systemic vasculature and blood function.
  - Some effects include increased arterial wall stiffness, increased fibrinogen levels, increased platelet aggregation, decreased HDL, and increased hematocrit.
  - Smokers have twice the relative risk of cerebral infarct of nonsmokers.

- – The relative risk of stroke among former smokers was 1.34 in the Nurses' Health Study and 1.26 in the Physicians' Health Study.
  - – Stroke risk declined to the level of nonsmokers at 5 years from cessation.
  - – Exposure to environmental tobacco smoke caused a 20% to 70% increased risk of coronary events.
- Obesity
  - – Obesity increases the risk of stroke because of the association with HTN, hyperglycemia, and abnormal blood lipids.
  - – Abdominal obesity in men is an independent risk factor for stroke.
  - – Weight gain in women is an independent risk factor for stroke.
- Physical inactivity
  - – Several studies have demonstrated an inverse association between levels of physical activity and stroke incidence.
  - – Protective effects of physical activity may be mediated through its role in controlling HTN, cardiovascular disease, diabetes, and body weight. Other mechanisms include decreasing fibrinogen and platelet activity and increasing tissue plasminogen activator activity and HDL concentration.
- Diet and nutrition
  - – Data regarding the effects of general nutritional status on stroke are limited.
  - – An increment of one serving of fruit and vegetables per day was associated with a 6% decreased risk of stroke.
- Alcohol abuse
  - – There is a protective effect against stroke with two drinks per day (one drink = 12 oz beer, 4 oz wine, 1.5 oz 80-proof spirits, or 1 oz 100-proof spirits).
  - – Risk for stroke increases for those drinking more than five drinks per day compared to nondrinkers.
  - – There is a direct dose-dependent effect of alcohol consumption on hemorrhagic stroke.
- Drug abuse
  - – Studies examining the effects of illicit drug abuse on stroke risk have been neutral.
  - – Pathogenesis of stroke in this subset of patients is likely multifactorial (e.g., sudden increases in BP, vasculitis).

Emerging Risk Factors

- Hyperhomocysteinemia
  - – Homocysteine concentrations increase with age, with men having higher levels than women, especially at younger ages.
  - – Homocysteine is toxic to the vascular wall and this may include cerebral arteries.
  - – Case-controlled studies have shown an association between hyperhomocysteinemia and stroke. However, no randomized trials have been done to determine whether lowering levels decreases the risk of stroke.
- Hypercoagulability
  - – Limited data exist on the association between antiphospholipid antibodies and cerebrovascular arterial thrombosis.
  - – In one study, elevated anticardiolipin antibody was demonstrated to be an independent stroke risk factor across three ethnic groups, conferring a fourfold increased risk of ischemic stroke.
  - – Studies examining other coagulation abnormalities (factor V Leiden, protein C deficiency, protein S deficiency, antithrombin III deficiency) have been poorly adjusted for other stroke risks.

- Hormone replacement therapy (HRT)
  - The impact of postmenopausal HRT on stroke risk appears to be negative. There was an increase in stroke in the WHI in those on HRT and the Framingham Heart Study that found a 2.6-fold increase in the relative risk of atherothrombotic stroke among women receiving HRT compared to nonusers.
- Oral contraceptive use
  - The risk of ischemic stroke is increased in oral contraceptive users, but the absolute increase in risk is small because of the low stroke incidence in this population. The greatest risk is women over 35 who also smoke and take oral contraceptives.
- Lipoprotein (a) [Lp(a)]
  - Lp(a) is an independent risk factor for ischemic stroke, especially in young adults.
  - The ratio of apolipoprotein B to apolipoprotein A1 was associated with carotid atheroma.
- Inflammatory processes
  - Atherosclerosis, the most common cause of stroke, is now believed to be a disease of chronic inflammation.
  - *Chlamydia pneumoniae* has been identified in atherosclerotic carotid plaques and localizes to regions of altered plaque morphology.
    - The relationship between serum antibody titers to *C. pneumoniae* and stroke is likely because of its role in plaque progression and destabilization.
    - The benefit of antibiotic therapy for *C. pneumoniae* is unclear.
  - High-sensitivity C-reactive protein (hs-CRP) and serum amyloid A, markers of acute infection, may be associated with stroke.
    - Levels are elevated in smokers and in healthy men with vascular risk factors.
    - There is a significant and positive association between plasma hs-CRP levels and risk for stroke.

Risk Stratification

The Framingham Heart Study has developed a health risk appraisal for the purpose of predicting the risk of stroke.
- Risk factors measured include age, systolic BP, use of antihypertensive therapy, diabetes, smoking, prior CVD (coronary heart disease, cardiac failure, intermittent claudication), atrial fibrillation, and LVH measured by electrocardiogram.
- The 10-year probability of stroke is determined according to a point system. Points associated with each risk factor are summed. Risk associated with number of points is determined from a Framingham Stroke Risk Profile.
  - Example of a 70-year-old male, smoker with hypertension and diabetes:
    70 y.o. male: 5 points
    SBP 180 mm Hg: 7 points
    On HTN therapy: 2 points
    Diabetes: 2 points
    Smoker: 3 points
    Total = 19 points = 32.9% probability
    - This patient has a 32.9% 10-year probability of stroke, equating to a stroke risk 2.4 times higher than average.

PERIPHERAL VASCULAR DISEASE

Risk Identification

Peripheral vascular disease (PVD) is a manifestation of the atherosclerotic process that affects 12% to 14% of the general population.

- Approximately one half of the 8.4 million Americans with PVD are symptomatic.
    - An estimated 840,000 present with critical leg ischemia.
    - Approximately 3.4 million present with symptoms of intermittent claudication (IC).
- The prevalence of symptoms of IC increases with age.
    - 5% of men and 2.5% of women over age 60 experience symptoms of IC.
    - Three times as many have an abnormal ankle brachial index.
- Symptoms of IC are usually stable over a 5- to 10-year period.
    - 73% have no significant change in symptoms.
    - 16% experience deterioration in symptoms.
    - 7% require peripheral vascular bypass surgery.
    - 4% have a major amputation.

Core Risk Factors

- Diabetes
    - People with diabetes are three to four times more likely to develop PVD than those without diabetes.
    - The atheromatous process in people with diabetes particularly affects smaller, more distal vessels, making options for revascularization more difficult.
- HTN
    - Those with HTN are 1.5 to 2.5 times more likely to develop PVD than those without.
    - HTN is a significant risk factor for atherosclerosis when it coexists with other risk factors such as smoking and diabetes.
- Hyperlipidemia
    - Relative risk for developing PVD is 1.1 per 10 mg/dL increase in total cholesterol.
- Age
    - The prevalence of PVD in Americans increases with age.
        - 3% ages 40 through 59 (about 2.1 million people)
        - 8% ages 60 through 69 (about 1.6 million people)
        - 19% age 70 and older (4.7 million people)
    - In men, half of new cases of PVD present in the fifth decade.
    - In general, disease presentation is later in women. By the seventh decade, prevalence is similar.
- Ethnicity
    - Risks of developing PVD seem to be race-neutral and are similar in White, Black, and Japanese-American people.

Life Habit Risk Factor

- Tobacco use
    - Cigarette smoking is the most prominent high-risk behavior in developing PVD.
    - Smokers are 2.5 to 3 times more likely to have PVD than nonsmokers.

Emerging Risk Factor

- Hyperhomocysteinemia
  - Genetic and nutritional factors, such as deficiencies in folate, vitamin B12 and vitamin B6, are associated with increased levels of homocysteine (> 15 mmol/L). It is suggested that hyperhomocysteinemia is an independent risk factor associated with PVD.
  - The relative risk of developing PVD in those with hyperhomocysteinemia is 1.7 to 2.6.

Risk Stratification

- PVD is an independent predictor of increased risk of cardiac death.
  - Half of patients presenting with PVD have symptoms of CHD or electrocardiographic abnormality.
  - 90% of those with PVD have abnormalities on coronary angiography.
  - 40% have duplex evidence of carotid artery disease.
- All-cause mortality rates are two to three times higher for those with PVD than those without PVD.
- More than 30% of cardiovascular patients have peripheral arterial occlusive disease.
- Symptomatic PVD carries at least a 30% risk of death within 5 years and almost 50% within 10 years, due primarily to MI (60%) or stroke (12%).
  - Asymptomatic patients (ankle brachial index < 0.9) have a two- to fivefold increased risk of fatal or nonfatal cardiovascular events.

OVERALL CARDIAC AND VASCULAR RISK

- Gender and race/ethnicity differences are known across the various diagnoses. This information is important to educate the public and attempt to reduce or eliminate other factors that may increase risk.
- Table 7–2 provides an overview of the prevalence of disease by race/ethnicity.

Table 7–2. Prevalence of Select Cardiovascular Disorders by Race and Ethnicity

	Heart Disease	Coronary Heart Disease	Hypertension	Stroke
White (not Hispanic)	11.4%	6.1%	22.2%	2.2%
Black (not Hispanic)	10.2%	6%	31.7%	3.7%
Hispanic	8.8%	5.7%	20.6%	3.7%
Asian American	6.9%	4.3%	19.5%	2.6%
Native American, Alaska Native	10.5%	5.6%	25.5%	NK
Pacific Islander, Native Hawaiian	NK	NK	28.5%	NK

NK = not known.

Note. Adapted from "Heart Disease and Stroke Statistics—2009 Update" by the American Heart Association, 2009, Dallas, TX: Author.

SUMMARY

This chapter provided an overview of the various risk factors for coronary heart disease, stroke, and peripheral vascular disease. The Framingham Heart Study also was explained to provide a framework for understanding the background on the topic as well as understanding the Framingham Risk Score. Nonmodifiable, modifiable, and lifestyle factors were discussed. The next chapter will provide background on risk factor reduction. After that, you will find a specific chapter devoted to hypertension and another chapter for hyperlipidemia.

REFERENCES

American Heart Association. (2009). *Heart disease and stroke statistic—2009 update.* Dallas, TX: Author. Available online at http://www.amhrt.org/downloadable/heart/1240250946756LS-1982%20Heart%20and%20Stroke%20Update.042009.pdf.

D'Agostino, R. B., Russell, M. W., Huse, D. M., Ellison, R. C., Silbershatz, H., Wilson, P. W. F., & Hartz, S. C. (2000). Primary and subsequent coronary risk appraisal: New results from the Framingham Study. *American Heart Journal, 139*(2), 272–281.

Elifaf, M. (2001). The treatment of coronary heart disease: An update: Part 1: An overview of the risk factors for cardiovascular disease. *Current Medical Research and Opinion, 17*(1), 18–26.

Expert Panel on Detection, Evaluation, and Treatment of High Blood Cholesterol in Adults. (2001). Executive summary of the Third Report of the National Cholesterol Education Program (NCEP). Expert Panel on Detection, Evaluation, and Treatment of High Blood Cholesterol in Adults (Adult Treatment Panel III). *Journal of the American Medical Association, 285,* 2486–2497.

Hlatky, M. A., Greenland, P., Arnett, D. K., Ballantyne, C. M., Criqui, M. H., Elkind, M. S. V., ... American Heart Association Expert Panel on Subclinical Atherosclerotic Diseases and Emerging Risk Factors and the Stroke Council. (2009). Criteria for evaluation of novel markers of cardiovascular risk: A scientific statement from the American Heart Association. *Circulation, 119,* 2408–2416.

Jones, D. W., Peterson, E. D., Bonow, R. O., Gibbons, R. J., Franklin, B. A., Sacco, R. L., ... American Heart Association. (2009). Partnering to reduce risks and improve cardiovascular outcomes: American Heart Association initiatives in action for consumers and patients. *Circulation, 119,* 340–350.

Pearson, T. A., Mensah, G. A., Alexander, R. W., Anderson, J. L., Cannon, R. O. 3rd, Criqui, M. ... American Heart Association. (2003). Markers of inflammation and cardiovascular disease: Application to clinical and public health practice: A statement for healthcare professionals from the Centers for Disease Control and Prevention and the American Heart Association. *Circulation, 107,* 499–511.

Ridker, P. M., Danielson, E., Fonseca, F. A., Genest, J., Gotto, A. M. Jr., Kastelein, J. J., ... JUPITER Study Group. (2008). Rosuvastatin to prevent vascular events in men and women with elevated C-reactive protein. *New England Journal of Medicine, 359,* 2195–2207.

The Writing Group for the WHI Investigators. (2002). Risks and benefits of estrogen plus progestin in healthy post-menopausal women: Principal results of the Women's Health Initiative randomized controlled trial. *JAMA, 288*(3), 321–333.

INTERNET RESOURCES

American Heart Association: http://americanheart.org/
Centers for Disease Control and Prevention: http://www.cdc.gov/
Framingham Heart Study http://www.framinghamheartstudy.org/
National Health and Nutrition Examination Survey (NHANES): http://www.cdc.gov/nchs/nhanes/
National Institutes of Health: http://www.nhlbi.nih.gov/guidelines/cholesterol/index.htm
Women's Health Initiative: http://www.whiscience.org/

8

Risk Reduction

The presence of cardiovascular disease (CVD) is associated with characteristic modifiable and nonmodifiable risk factors. There is general agreement, although not consensus, that modifying risk factors can reduce the likelihood of developing or slow the progression of CVD. This chapter provides guidelines for primary, secondary, and tertiary prevention strategies for risk reduction. General procedures for cardiac rehabilitation are included.

LEVELS OF PREVENTION

Primary, secondary, and tertiary levels of prevention constitute a three-tiered model of intervention that promotes optimum outcomes by promoting health, preventing disability, reducing disease progression, reducing morbidity and mortality, and preserving function and quality of life. The presence or absence of clinical disease, not the nature of the intervention, defines the level of prevention.

Primary Prevention

- Primary prevention concerns promoting health and delaying or preventing disease in the general population. Primary preventive interventions occur before clinical indications of disease develop.
- Primary prevention of CVD involves helping children make healthy lifestyle choices and avoid choices that increase risk (e.g., tobacco use, physical inactivity, excessive body weight, high-fat diet).
- Primary prevention strategies include education, public law and policy (e.g., no tobacco for people under 18 years of age), the reduction of environmental hazards (e.g., secondhand smoke), and chemoprophylaxis (e.g., aspirin use among people without known CVD).

Secondary Prevention

- Secondary prevention concerns the early detection of disease or health problems and intensive treatment while the outcome can be altered favorably.
- Secondary prevention of CVD involves detecting and treating risk factors such as hypertension (HTN) and dyslipidemia before a cardiac or vascular event (e.g., myocardial infarction [MI], stroke, arterial occlusion) occurs. Secondary prevention includes intensive management of risk after an acute event to prevent subsequent events and death.
- The goal of secondary prevention is to control risk factors and to achieve therapeutic protection of arteries from plaque rupture.

Tertiary Prevention

- Tertiary prevention is concerned with treatment of the disease or health problem to avoid negative sequelae and to return the person to the highest possible functional level.
- Tertiary prevention of CVD includes poststroke rehabilitation and programs that modify work responsibilities to enable people to return to work after an acute cardiac event. (Cardiac rehabilitation programs use both secondary and tertiary prevention strategies. The emphasis on adopting a healthy lifestyle to prevent future events is an example of secondary prevention. The emphasis on resuming role responsibilities after an acute cardiac event is an example of tertiary prevention.)
- The goals of tertiary prevention are to minimize disability and to preserve or restore function and quality of life.

CARDIOVASCULAR DISEASE PREVENTION

- Preventing CVD requires individual, community, and societal effort.
- Data support the benefits of preventing and treating CVD.
- CVD is present in almost 50 million Americans and is the leading cause of death for both men and women in the United States.
- CVD is a large source of the chronic disability and health costs encountered in the world, making prevention a cost-effective goal with far-reaching consequences.
- Lifestyle modifications can reduce the risk of developing CVD by approximately 50%.

- Mortality from CVD in all races has been reduced by about 50% since the 1960s. This reduction is believed to be the result of multidisciplinary prevention and management strategies including changes in dietary and smoking habits, physical activity, and lipid and HTN management.
- Future research should be multidisciplinary, aimed at prevention across the life span, and examine disease progression and precipitants of acute events among various ethnic, racial, and socioeconomic groups.

Risk Factor Modification
- Many of the risk factors of CVD are modifiable: physical inactivity, tobacco use, obesity, HTN, diabetes, and lipid management.
- Successfully applied preventive interventions can reduce mortality and morbidity, acute coronary event rate, and rehospitalization for disease progression, thereby reducing healthcare costs.
- An organized system to reduce risk through a variety of preventive strategies is more likely to be effective than single strategies applied unsystematically.
  - Health needs assessment can identify populations at risk and prioritize individual and environmental interventions.
- Healthcare professionals need to assess patients' need for information, ability to comply, and barriers to successful change before selecting strategies to promote change in lifestyles.
- Educating people about the benefits that can be obtained from risk factor reduction may motivate people to try and then to adhere to lifestyle changes.

Expressions of Relative Risk
- Relative risk is the ratio of the likelihood of coronary heart disease (CHD) developing with and without a given risk factor.
- Absolute risk is the probability of developing CHD in a specified finite period, meaning a high relative risk early in life may correspond to a high absolute risk later in life. The Framingham Risk Score is an example of absolute risk.

TOBACCO USE AND EXPOSURE

Health Risks
- Cigarette smoking is a powerful risk factor for developing CVD.
- Smoking accelerates the rate of coronary plaque development.
- The Framingham Heart Study indicates that smoking may destabilize coronary plaques, promoting plaque rupture, and therefore, myocardial infarction.
- Smoking is the major cause of peripheral arterial disease and doubles the risk of ischemic stroke.
- The longer and the more packs per day smoked, the greater the risk of developing CVD.
- Smoking is quantified in pack years, which is the number of years smoked by the number of packs per day.
- While smoking rates continue to decline in most regions, it is still between 20% and 30% of adults in various regions of the country. It is the most important factor targeted in risk reduction programs.

Table 8-1. Neuroreceptor Stimulation Associated With Nicotine

Receptor	Response
Dopamine	Pleasure, reward
Norepinephrine	Arousal, appetite suppression
Acetylcholine	Arousal, cognitive alertness
Glutamate	Learning, memory enhancement
Serotonin	Mood modulation, appetite suppression
Beta endorphin	Alleviates anxiety, reduces tension
GABA	Alleviates anxiety, reduces tension

Physiologic Effects

- Cigarette smoking contains many harmful substances in addition to nicotine and tar.
- Nicotine is the addictive agent in cigarettes and it reaches the brain within 11 seconds of inhaling the cigarette smoke.
  - Nicotine is readily absorbed by the lung surface but is poorly absorbed in the acidic stomach. It is metabolized to cotinine, which is excreted in the urine.
    - The half-life of nicotine is 2 hours. (See Chapter 15 for a discussion of half-life). By four to five half-lives, the drug is virtually eliminated from the blood.
    - The half-life of cotinine is 19 hours, so serum or urine testing can detect if the person has smoked in the last 3 to 5 days.
  - Nicotine stimulates many brain centers, resulting in physiological responses found in Table 8–1. These responses are pleasurable and what drives people to continue to smoke. Withdrawal from nicotine produces the opposite effects.
  - Cardiovascular effects of nicotine include increased heart rate and blood pressure (BP) through increased catecholamine release.
  - Smoking accelerates atherosclerosis by increasing low-density lipoprotein cholesterol (LDL-C) and reducing high-density lipoprotein cholesterol (HDL-C), increasing endothelial wall damage, increasing myocardial work and oxygen demand, and increasing inflammation as marked by higher levels of C-reactive protein (CRP).
  - The problems are further complicated by decreased oxygen-carrying capacity of the blood because of carbon monoxide attachment to hemoglobin.
  - Smoking mediates the development of thrombus by increasing coronary vasoconstriction, increasing fibrinogen levels, increasing platelet adhesion and aggregation, and increasing blood viscosity.

Cessation Techniques and Guidelines

- Smoking intervention systems increase the proportion of smokers who are identified, counseled about cessation, referred to cessation programs, and supported in their efforts to quit.
- Cessation of smoking may reduce mortality and reinfarction rates by 50%.
- Smoking behaviors involve nicotine addiction, pleasure attainment, and habit; therefore, all three factors should be assessed to plan the most appropriate interventions.
- Cessation techniques may include temptation management, cue extinction, contingency management, persuasive techniques, pharmacologic agents, and behavior modification.
- Pharmacologic approaches to cessation programs include nicotine replacement products and agents to block specific neuroreceptors. These products are discussed in more detail in Chapter 15.
- Begin with the five A's as defined in the Transtheoretical Model (discussed in Chapter 2). Ask if the person smokes, advise to quit, assess readiness to change, assist to set goals, and arrange for referral or treatment. Recall that the specifics of intervention are based on the stage of change (precontemplation, contemplation, preparation, action, maintenance, or termination).

NUTRITION

Skills

Required skills for patients to engage successfully in dietary modification include reading food labels before purchasing groceries, selecting appropriate foods from restaurant menus, using appropriate cooking styles, and taking medications, if indicated.

Lipid Management

Normalizing blood lipids may reduce the rates of coronary events and death from CVD.
- Diet, exercise, and drug therapy have been shown to be effective strategies in achieving optimum cholesterol levels.
    - LDL-C < 100 mg/dL
    - HDL-C > 40 mg/dL for men and > 50 for women
    - Triglyceride < 200 mg/dL
- Low-fat, low-cholesterol choices for a healthy diet include:
    - Five servings of a variety of fruits and vegetables daily
    - Six or more serving of whole grain daily
    - Fat-free or low-fat items
    - Balance daily caloric intake by calorie expenditure. A quick estimate of calories needed for a specific weight is to multiply weight in pounds by 15 (if active) or by 13 (if sedentary).
- People without CVD, diabetes, or high LDL-C should consume less than 30% of their total calories as fat; less than 10% as saturated fat, and less than 300 mg of cholesterol per day.
- People with CVD, diabetes, or high LDL-C should consume less than 30% of total calories as fat, less than 7% as saturated fat, and less than 200 mg of cholesterol per day.

Weight Management

- Body mass index (BMI) is used to define overweight and obesity.
    - BMI = weight in kilograms divided by height in meters squared or
    - Estimated BMI = (weight in pounds divided by height in inches squared) multiplied by 704.5
- The healthy range for BMI is 18.5 to 24.9 kg/m^2.
    - Overweight is defined as a BMI of 25 to 29.9 kg/m^2.
    - Obesity is defined as a BMI of 30 kg/m^2 or higher.
    - Morbid obesity is defined as a BMI of 35 kg/m^2 or higher.
- Treatment goals for cardiovascular health are
    - BMI below 25 throughout adult life. (BMI of 25 corresponds to 110% of ideal body weight).
    - If BMI is 25 through 30, diet and exercise management is recommended.
        - A caloric deficit of 500 calories per day should result in weight loss of 0.45 kg (1 lb) per week. The recommended weight loss rate is 1 lb per week.
        - Pharmacologic agents may be indicated for BMI above 30.
- A threshold level of BMI is not entirely appropriate because adipose tissue in the abdomen affects the risk of CHD more than distribution in the pelvic area.
    - BMI does not take into account distribution of body fat.
    - Research shows that increased waist circumference and waist-to-hip ratio predict comorbidities and mortality from obesity.
        - Desirable waist circumference is less than 35 inches (88 cm) for women and less than 40 inches (102 cm) for men.
        - Waist-to-hip ratio is the waist measurement divided by the hip measurement. Desirable waist-to-hip ratio is less than 0.8 for women and less than 1.0 for men.
- BMI or obesity independently predicts coronary atherosclerosis in Whites. The relationship between obesity and CVD morbidity and mortality is less clear for other groups.
    - Weight loss is associated with improved lipid levels, less insulin resistance, and lower blood pressure.
    - Cardiac rehabilitation may aim for a reduction of 5% to 10% of body weight to improve risk factors.
- Prevention of obesity by diet and regular physical activity is a high priority to reduce CVD risk.
- Obesity is associated with a number of comorbidities, including heart disease.
- Heredity may explain 30% to 70% of obesity, but environmental factors must be considered as contributors to the increasing prevalence of obesity.
- Weight loss is particularly important for patients with HTN, elevated triglycerides, or elevated blood glucose levels.
- Bariatric surgery may be the most appropriate weight loss approach that reduces mortality and controls cardiac risk factors for morbidly obese patients.

Metabolic Syndrome

- Metabolic syndrome is a clustering of several metabolic risk factors in one patient, which predisposes the person to premature CHD.
  - Metabolic syndrome is diagnosed when three or more of the following factors are present:
    - Abdominal obesity
    - Elevated triglycerides
    - Low HDL cholesterol
    - High blood pressure (> 130/> 85 mm Hg)
    - Fasting glucose above 110 mg/dL
- Metabolic abnormalities include defective glucose uptake by the skeletal muscle, increased release of free fatty acids by adipose tissue, over-production of glucose by the liver, and hypersecretion of insulin by pancreatic beta cells.
- The Framingham Risk Score does not contain all of the risk determinants used to diagnose the metabolic syndrome. The importance of metabolic syndrome as a risk factor may be underestimated.

Divalent Cations (Electrolytes)

- Sodium
  - For the general population, the American Heart Association (AHA) recommends eating less than 6 grams of salt or 2,400 mg of sodium per day. This is half to one-third of what the average American consumes daily.
  - Lower sodium guidelines may be recommended for patients with HTN and heart failure.
- Potassium, calcium, and magnesium
  - Low calcium consumption (300 to 600 mg per day) is associated with HTN.
  - High potassium consumption is associated with lower blood pressure in people with HTN.
- The DASH study (Dietary Approaches to Stop Hypertension) manipulated dietary intake of potassium, calcium, and magnesium while holding sodium intake constant.
  - A diet rich in fruits, vegetables, and low-fat dairy products significantly reduced systolic and diastolic pressure in comparison with a "normal" diet.
    The DASH diet has been shown to reduce homocysteine levels also.
  - Care should be taken when salt substitutes are used in the diet because such substitutes often are high in potassium.

Alcohol Use

- Urban residents tend to have more education beyond high school, higher alcohol use, smoke more cigarettes, and have higher medical specialist usage than rural populations.
- There is a U-shaped relationship between alcohol consumption and blood pressure. Light drinkers have lower BP than both those who abstain and those who drink more heavily.
- There is evidence from observational studies that red wine reduces risk of heart attack.
- AHA recommends moderate alcohol consumption in appropriate people.
  - Not more than one alcoholic beverage for women, and two for men, per day.
  - An alcoholic beverage is defined as 12 oz of beer, 4 oz of wine, 1½ oz of 80-proof liquor, or 1 oz of 100-proof liquor.

EXERCISE AND ACTIVITY

Physical activity can be cost-effective and flexibly scheduled, and need not require special equipment or location.

Activity Guidelines for Healthy People
- Physical activity is recommended for primary and secondary prevention of CVD.
  - An active lifestyle from childhood is important in the primary prevention of atherosclerosis.
  - School programs should include aerobic activities (such as running, swimming, walking, and dancing), flexibility (stretching), and resistance exercises (free weights or exercise machines).
  - Physical inactivity is associated with at least a twofold increase in risk for cardiac events.
- Exercise and activity reduce CVD risk through lowering blood pressure, reducing platelet aggregation, raising HDL-C, and improving glucose metabolism.
  - Physical activity also helps psychologically to improve mood (reduces feelings of depression and anxiety).
  - Personal satisfaction is an important consideration in selecting an activity that will become an almost daily choice.
  - Intensity, duration, and frequency of exercise as well as mode are the components of an exercise prescription. This will be described in more detail under the section on Cardiac Rehabilitation later in this chapter.
  - Exercise can be either isotonic or isometric.
    - Isotonic exercise is the movement of large muscles in a rhythmic fashion, using predominantly aerobic metabolism. Aerobic metabolism is more efficient than anaerobic (38 ATP produced vs. 2) but requires more oxygen and thus blood flow. Examples are running, walking, cycling, and swimming.
    - Isometric is muscle contraction without movement and is associated with anaerobic metabolism. Examples include weight lifting and resistance training.
    - Physiologic changes with exercise are detailed in Table 8–2.
    - Over time, exercise training improves ventilatory capacity, oxygen diffusing capability, and muscle mitochondria size and energy sources.
    - Initially most of cardiac output increase is because of increased heart rate, but with training, the stroke volume increases. This means that with training you can do more work with a lower heart rate and systolic blood pressure because the stroke volume is much greater at work and at rest.
    - While most of the physiologic benefits are derived from aerobic exercise, it is still recommended that every healthy person have some anaerobic exercise for muscle strength training and some degree of flexibility exercise for balance and coordination.
    - Oxygen consumption can be estimated by the rate-pressure-product (RPP). It is the heart rate multiplied by the systolic blood pressure. The linear increase in this is a representation of the increase in actual oxygen needed to perform the work.

Table 8-2. Physiologic Changes That Occur During an Episode of Exercise (Acute Changes)

Parameter	Aerobic Exercise	Anaerobic Exercise
Heart Rate	Increase corresponding to effort	No change
Systolic Blood Pressure	Increase corresponding to effort	Little increase
Diastolic Blood Pressure	Unchanged or 10 mm increase or decrease	Increase corresponding to effort
Stroke Volume	Increase corresponding to effort	No change
Cardiac Output	Increase corresponding to effort; may increase to 30 L/min in a trained athlete	No change or minimal increase
Oxygen Consumption	Increase corresponding to effort	No change

- Primary prevention
  - All children and adults should participate in at least 30 minutes of moderate aerobic physical activity most, if not all, days of the week.
    - Activities of moderate intensity include brisk walking, cycling, swimming, and yard work.
    - Children and adults who already meet this standard of activity will receive additional benefits from increased duration or intensity of activity.
  - The American Heart Association recommends vigorous (aerobic or isotonic) activity for at least 30 to 60 minutes, 3 to 4 days per week at 50% to 75% of maximum heart rate for most healthy people. A rough estimate of maximum heart rate is derived by subtracting age from the constant of 220. Actual maximum heart rate is determined on an exercise test.
  - Intensity also may be measured by the onset of breathlessness or fatigue. The Borg scale provides a rating of perceived exertion (scaled from 6 to 20) and is used in community exercise programs and outpatient cardiac rehabilitation programs.
  - People with acute illnesses such as influenza or upper-respiratory infections should decrease or stop physical activity for up to 2 to 3 weeks, while recovery occurs.
  - Exercise testing (measurement of functional capacity) is not routinely required for primary prevention without other existing risk factors.
  - It is most desirable to complete the recommended duration of physical activity in one set; however, it can be accumulated in intervals of 10 to 15 minutes throughout the day to total 30 to 60 minutes.
  - For those unable to maintain or increase intensity level, frequency and duration should be increased to compensate.
  - Table 8-3 provides a summary of the benefits of exercise training.

Table 8–3. Physiologic Benefits of a Training Program of Isotonic Exercise

	Resting State	Submaximal Exercise	Maximal Exercise
Heart Rate	Decreased	Decreased	No change
Blood Pressure	Decreased	Decreased	No change
Rate Pressure Product	Decreased	Decreased	No change
Stroke Volume	Increased	Increased	No change
VO$_2$ (Oxygen Consumption)	No change	No change	Increased

Note: Submaximal exercise refers to any activity that the person may do such as walking up steps or doing the laundry. Maximal exercise refers to the highest level of activity possible and this is usually measured by treadmill walking/running or stationary cycling.

- Secondary prevention
  - Secondary prevention is physical activity after a heart attack or stroke has occurred or for those at great risk of developing CVD. The goal is to prevent further cardiac and vascular events or disability from disease.
  - Walking has been shown to increase survival, decrease recurrent events, and may slow the progression of CVD.
  - Additional benefits of walking include improved quality of life, decreased incidence of hospitalization, and reduced need for repeat invasive percutaneous coronary interventions.
  - Walking for patients with intermittent claudication should be 60 minutes a day, with stops for rest if pain develops.
  - Regular light or moderate physical activity started in middle age or older age has been shown to reduce mortality from CVD.
- Tertiary prevention
  - Tertiary prevention minimizes disability, improves function, and improves quality of life.
  - Cardiac rehabilitation provides a multidisciplinary approach to tertiary prevention.
  - Exercise testing is recommended before starting an exercise program after an acute cardiac event.

Safety Considerations
- Risk should be assessed, preferably with an exercise test, prior to the initiation of an exercise prescription following a cardiac event or in a high-risk person.
- In the early recovery period following a cardiac event (i.e., during the second week), the goal is to walk 5 to 10 minutes and perform nonresistive range of motion.
- Later in recovery, activity is guided by the results of a symptom-limited exercise test and includes:
  - Exercise involving large muscle groups performed for a total of 20 to 30 minutes, plus warm-up and cool-down periods before and after, at least three to four times per week.

- Low-risk patients are characterized by the absence of ischemia and significant dysrhythmia.
  - The majority of patients requiring secondary prevention are classified as low risk and can implement an exercise prescription at home or in the community.
  - In low-risk patients, primary prevention guidelines apply.
  - Follow-up exercise testing is recommended on an annual basis.
- Activities progress as tolerated up to a moderate level of intensity.
- During early recovery from an acute event and in the initial stages of an exercise program, an increase of 20 beats per minute above resting heart rate may be used as a guideline for the progression of activity.
- Once a steady state of activity is tolerated without symptoms, dysrhythmia, or excessive tachycardia, the duration of exercise may be increased in 5-minute increments each week, while intensity can be increased at a frequency of three to six times weekly.
- High-risk patients are encouraged to attend medically supervised exercise sessions.
  - Moderate- to high-risk patients have ischemia and/or significant dysrhythmia on symptom-limited exercise testing.
    - Significant dysrhythmia includes ventricular tachycardia, symptom-producing dysrhythmia, and hemodynamic instability.
    - Signs of ischemia include the presence of chest pain, 2 mm ST-segment depression or elevation, or a decrease in systolic blood pressure more than 20 mm Hg from base line.
  - Exercise prescriptions for moderate- to high-risk patients require medical supervision, such as cardiac rehabilitation.
  - Exercise for older people may best be done initially under supervised conditions for a brief period of time.

CARDIAC REHABILITATION

First developed in the 1960s, cardiac rehabilitation programs are designed to take advantage of the benefits of walking during prolonged hospitalization and promote secondary prevention in a formal, structured program.

- Cardiac rehabilitation is a multidisciplinary approach to improve physical and psychosocial outcomes of people with cardiovascular conditions.
  - Cardiac rehabilitation includes exercise, education, and lifestyle change.
  - Cardiac rehabilitation generally consists of three phases.
    - Phase I is inpatient and the goal is prevent or reduce deconditioning effects, begin the education of patient and family, and prepare the patient for discharge. See Table 8–4 for deconditioning effects. Range of motion exercises and early ambulation reduce the effect of deconditioning.
    - Phase II is an outpatient program with medical supervision and electrographic monitoring of patients while they follow an exercise prescription over a period of 4 to 12 weeks after a cardiac event. This phase includes continued education and behavior change as secondary prevention. Stress reduction and adjustment to living with cardiovascular disease are included.
    - Phase III is the maintenance program. Exercise continues in a supervised but unmonitored setting. Lifestyle change is reinforced.
  - Cardiac rehabilitation teams include physicians, nurses, exercise specialists, dietitians, and social workers.

Table 8-4. Deconditioning Effects of Prolonged Bed Rest

Anticipated Change	Result or Comment
Decreased muscle strength and mass	About 10% loss/week
Loss of 600 cc plasma volume	Occurs in first 3 to 7 days of bed rest because of natural diuresis of volume needed to prevent orthostatic hypotension. Results in higher viscosity of blood, increasing risk of DVT.
Venous stasis	Increased risk of DVT
Reduced maximum oxygen consumption	Reduced overall fitness level. Can require weeks to months to return to previous level of fitness.
Higher heart rate and blood pressure for any submaximum work or effort	Heart works harder for any activity. Can require weeks to months to return to previous level of fitness.
Demineralization of bone	Increased risk of osteoporosis

- A medical referral is necessary to enroll in outpatient cardiac rehabilitation.
- Baseline exercise stress testing is required to determine if exertional ischemia or dysrhythmia is present.
- The exercise prescription is followed under medical supervision, with nurse monitoring and input by exercise physiologists on exercise activities and progression of exercise intensity.
- Aerobic exercise, resistance training, and work capacity are included in rehabilitation.
- Health insurance may fully cover Phase II rehabilitation or may require a copayment per visit or program. Phase I is usually a part of inpatient care and Phase III is rarely covered.

Expected Benefits
- The expected benefits of cardiac rehabilitation include reduced CVD morbidity and mortality, increased functional capacity and exercise tolerance, and improvement in patient-reported ability to perform activities of daily living.
- Cardiac rehabilitation has been shown to increase HDL cholesterol levels and modestly reduce triglycerides that are above 200 mg/dL.
- The minimal effect of cardiac rehabilitation on LDL cholesterol suggests a need for concurrent nutritional counseling and drug therapy.
- Oral hypoglycemic agents or insulin may need to be adjusted downward in response to increased sensitivity to insulin, a benefit resulting from routine exercise.
- The cardiovascular physiologic benefits detailed previously also can be found with cardiac rehabilitation.
- One benefit of cardiac rehabilitation is that the RPP with submaximal effort will be less, keeping the person under the threshold where ischemia and symptoms occur. Thus, the person can do more activities before developing cardiac symptoms.
- Cardiac rehabilitation provides the opportunity to assess for an abnormal response to exercise. Table 8–5 lists the abnormal responses.

Table 8-5. Abnormal Response to Exercise

Blood pressure	• A drop in systolic pressure with increasing effort may signal ischemia or failure. • A diastolic increase greater than 10 mm Hg may be prehypertension.
Heart rate	A decrease with increased effort may signal ischemia or failure.
ECG	Ischemia may be evident with • ST segment depression or T wave inversion in two leads from the same set (inferior, anterior, lateral) • New bundle branch block pattern • Arrhythmias
Symptoms	Chest pain, excessive dyspnea or fatigue, calf pain, dizziness
Signs	S3, crackles, cyanosis

Cardiac Rehabilitation Additional Comments

Cardiac rehabilitation includes nutritional counseling, smoking cessation, review of medications, dietary modification, and exercise prescriptions to reduce modifiable risk factors, subsequent coronary events, and rehospitalization.

- Cardiac rehabilitation may be covered by health insurance for a specific number of visits (12 to 36 per single cardiac event), after MI, percutaneous transluminal coronary angioplasty (PTCA), chronic stable angina, or open-heart surgery.
- Self-care and disease management are facets of cardiac rehabilitation programs.
- Cardiac rehabilitation is also appropriate for patients with chronic heart failure and cardiac transplantation.
- Only 10% to 20% of appropriate cardiac candidates participate in outpatient cardiac rehabilitation. More encouragement from physicians and inpatient care providers may improve this rate.
- More than 50% of patients in cardiac rehabilitation are 65 years or older. Preventing and minimizing disability is of prime concern in this age group.

SUMMARY

Efforts to reduce cardiovascular disease risk are multifaceted. This program reviewed information on several important risk factors including smoking, nutrition, and exercise. Primary, secondary, and tertiary risk reduction was discussed. Cardiac rehabilitation provides structured programs to reduce cardiovascular risk for patients with established CVD who are at risk for recurrent cardiac events and death from cardiac causes.

REFERENCES

American Academy of Cardiovascular and Pulmonary Rehabilitation. (2005). *Guidelines for cardiac rehabilitation and secondary prevention* (4th ed.). Champaign, IL: Human Kinetics.

American College of Sports Medicine. (2010). *Guidelines for exercise testing and prescription* (8th ed.). Philadelphia: Lippincott Williams & Wilkins.

American Thoracic Society; American College of Chest Physicians. (2003). ATS/ACCP statement on cardiopulmonary exercise testing. *American Journal of Respiratory and Critical Care Medicine, 167*, 211–277.

Balady, G. J., Williams, M. A., Ades, P. A., Bittner, V., Comoss, P., Foody, J. M., ... American Association of Cardiovascular and Pulmonary Rehabilitation. (2007). Core components of cardiac rehabilitation/secondary prevention programs: 2007 update: A scientific statement from the American Heart Association Exercise, Cardiac Rehabilitation, and Prevention Committee, the Council on Clinical Cardiology; the Councils on Cardiovascular Nursing, Epidemiology and Prevention, and Nutrition, Physical Activity, and Metabolism; and the American Association of Cardiovascular and Pulmonary Rehabilitation. *Circulation, 115*, 2675–2682.

Corvera-Tindel, T., Doering, L. V., Woo, M. A., Khan, S., & Dracup, K. (2004). Effects of a home walking exercise program on functional status and symptoms in heart failure. *American Heart Journal, 147*, 339–346.

Expert Panel on Detection, Evaluation and Treatment of High Blood Cholesterol in Adults. (2001). Executive summary of the third report of the National Cholesterol Education Program (NCEP). Expert Panel on Detection, Evaluation, and Treatment of High Blood Cholesterol in Adults (ATP-III). *JAMA, 285*, 2486–2497.

Flynn, K. E., Piña, I. L., Whellan, D. J., Lin, L., Blumenthal, J. A., Ellis, S. J., ... Weinfurt, K. P. (2009). Effects of exercise training on health status in patients with chronic heart failure: HF-ACTION randomized controlled trial. *JAMA, 301*(14), 1451–1459.

O'Connor, C. M., Whellan, D. J., Lee, K. L., Keteyian, S. J., Cooper, L. S., Ellis, S. J., ... HF-ACTION Investigators. (2009). Efficacy and safety of exercise training in patients with chronic heart failure: HF-ACTION randomized controlled trial. *JAMA, 301*(14), 1439–1450.

Rees, K., Taylor, R. R. S., Singh, S., Coats, A. J. S., Ebrahim, S. (2004). Exercise based rehabilitation for heart failure. *Cochrane Database of Systematic Reviews, Issue 3*. Art. No.: CD003331. DOI: 10.1002/14651858.CD003331.pub2.

Tabet, J. Y., Meurin, P., Beauvais, F., Weber, H., Renaud, N., Thabut, G., ... Ben Driss, A. (2008). Absence of exercise capacity improvement after exercise training program: A strong prognostic factor in patients with chronic heart failure. *Circulation. Heart Failure, 1*, 220–226.

Taylor, R. K., Singh, S., Coats, A. J. S., et al. (2009). Exercise based rehabilitation for heart failure (Review), *The Cochrane Library, Issue 1*. Art. No.: CD003331. DOI: 10.1002/14651858. CD003331.pub2.

Thompson, P. D., Franklin, B. A., Balady, G. J., Blair, S. N., Corrado, D., Estes, N. A. 3rd, ... American College of Sports Medicine. (2007). Exercise and acute cardiovascular events placing the risks into perspective: a scientific statement from the American Heart Association Council on Nutrition, Physical Activity, and Metabolism and the Council on Clinical Cardiology. *Circulation, 115*, 2358–2368.

Williams, M. A., Haskell, W. L., Ades, P. A., Amsterdam, E. A., Bittner, V., Franklin, B. A., ... American Heart Association Council on Nutrition, Physical Activity, and Metabolism. (2007). Resistance exercise in individuals with and without cardiovascular disease: 2007 update: A scientific statement from the American Heart Association Council on Clinical Cardiology and Council on Nutrition, Physical Activity, and Metabolism. *Circulation, 116*, 572–584.

9

Hypertension Management

Hypertension (HTN) is estimated to affect more than 65 million Americans, many of whom do not know they have HTN. Another large proportion of those with HTN are not adequately treated. Better control of HTN could reduce the number of myocardial infarction by 20% to 25%, stroke by 30% to 35%, and heart failure by 50%. This chapter provides a review of the physiology of normal blood pressure and many systems involved with BP regulation. Hypertension is then discussed in detail along with treatments. Because sleep apnea is linked to HTN and stroke, it is included in this chapter. The most important roles for the nurse are in the area of assessment, monitoring, and patient education. Lifestyle change is important in controlling and treating HTN.

NORMAL BLOOD PRESSURE

- Normal blood pressure (BP) for adults over 18 years is less than 120 mm Hg systolic and less than 80 mm Hg diastolic.
- BP is the force exerted by the blood against the walls of the blood vessel and is a function of cardiac output (CO) and systemic vascular resistance (SVR).
  - BP = CO x SVR
- CO is the volume of blood ejected from the heart per minute and is a function of heart rate (HR) and stroke volume (SV).

- SV is the amount of blood ejected from the heart with each contraction; the normal volume at rest is approximately 75 mL.
    - CO = HR x SV
    - Pulse pressure (the difference between SBP and DBP) is an indirect estimate of SV.
- SVR (sometimes referred to as peripheral vascular resistance) is the force within the vascular bed that opposes ejection of blood from the left ventricle.
    - SVR is the major variable determining afterload.
    - Vessel radius is the primary determinant of resistance and the primary sites for SVR are the small arteries and arterioles.

REGULATION OF BLOOD PRESSURE

BP is regulated through the interaction of nervous, cardiovascular, renal, and endocrine functions. Actions of the nervous system and the vascular endothelium are rapid (seconds) and short-term (days), while renal and endocrine actions contribute to long-term (days to weeks) regulation.

Autonomic Nervous System Effects
- Baroreceptors located in the aortic arch and carotid sinus sense change in BP and send either inhibitory or excitatory impulses to the vasomotor control centers in the medulla.
    - When increased BP is sensed, inhibition of sympathetic nervous system (SNS) activity results directly in decreased HR, decreased cardiac contractility, and increased peripheral vasodilation.

Also, increased parasympathetic activity, mediated through the vagus nerve, reduces HR. The net effect of SNS inhibition is to decrease BP.

-
    - When decreased BP is sensed, excitatory impulses are generated. Afferent SNS nerves release the neurotransmitter norepinephrine (NE) into the neuroeffector junction. NE stimulates adrenoreceptors.
    - Adrenoreceptors have been classified into two general groups: α-adrenergic and ß-adrenergic. The net effect of SNS activity is determined by the distribution of sympathetic nerve endings and adrenoreceptors in body tissues.
        - ß_1 adrenoreceptors in the heart increase HR (positive chronotropic effect), contractility (positive inotropic effect), and conductivity (positive dromotropic effect).
        - ß_2 adrenoreceptors in coronary arteries and peripheral arterioles of skeletal muscles produce vasodilation and decrease SVR. ß_2 adrenoreceptors in the lungs produce bronchodilation.
        - Decreased BP in the renal afferent arterioles, decreased sodium chloride concentration in the distal convoluted tubule, and stimulation of ß adrenoreceptors on the juxtaglomerular apparatus (JGA) stimulate renin release. See discussion of the kidney and renin-angiotensin-aldosterone system (RAA) later in this chapter.
        - $\alpha 1$ adrenoreceptors in vascular smooth muscle produce vasoconstriction (increase SVR).

- Cardiopulmonary baroreceptors (also called mechanoreceptors or stretch receptors) are low-pressure receptors located in the heart and pulmonary circulation. Cardiopulmonary baroreceptors sense small changes in cardiac filling pressure and volume. Small increases in cardiac filling pressure and volume inhibit SNS and neurohormonal (RAA) activity, reducing BP and intravascular volume. Small decreases, on the other hand, stimulate SNS and RAA activity, increasing BP and intravascular volume.
- Chemoreceptors located in the carotid and aortic bodies, when stimulated by hypoxia, excite the SNS, producing increased ventilation and venous resistance without significantly altering HR.
- Epinephrine, secreted by the adrenal medulla in response to physical or emotional stress can activate the SNS also.
  - β_1 receptors in the heart increase HR and cardiac contractility (increased CO).
  - β_2 receptors in skeletal and splanchnic arterioles produce vasodilation.
    - Vasodilation of these large beds may decrease SVR.
  - In pharmacological doses (which are higher than physiologic concentrations), epinephrine stimulates receptors in vascular smooth muscle, producing systemic vasoconstriction (but coronary vasodilation) and increasing SVR.

Renal Effects
- The renin-angiotensin-aldosterone (RAA) system regulates BP directly and also through a long-term effect on fluid balance.
  - Renin is released from the JGA of the kidney in response to increased SNS activity, decreased renal perfusion pressure, or decreased sodium concentration in the early distal tubule.
  - Renin acts on angiotensinogen to produce angiotensin I (A-I), an inactive peptide.
  - A-I is converted to angiotensin II (A-II), a potent vasoconstrictor, through the action of angiotensin-converting enzyme (ACE).
    - A-II produces generalized vasoconstriction (increases SVR).
    - A-II potentiates SNS effects (increases SVR and HR).
    - A-II stimulates release of aldosterone from the adrenal cortex.
  - Aldosterone inhibits sodium excretion, causing water retention and increased blood volume.
- Arginine vasopressin (antidiuretic hormone, ADH) is released from the posterior pituitary gland.
  - Increased plasma osmolality is the primary stimulus for ADH release but it may be released also in response to low blood volume and pressure (for example, hemorrhage).
  - ADH enhances water absorption at the distal and collecting tubules of the kidney.

Local Vascular Effects
- Vascular endothelium affects SVR and BP by secreting vasodilator and vasoconstrictor substances.
  - Vasodilating substances include nitric oxide (NO), endothelium-derived relaxing factor, prostacyclin, endothelium-derived hyperpolarizing factor, and bradykinin.
  - Vasoconstricting substances include endothelium-derived contracting factor, endothelin-1, prostanoids, and superoxide anions.

- Certain vascular beds (for example the heart, brain, kidney, and skeletal muscle) alter local vascular resistance to maintain perfusion (autoregulation). The mechanism is unknown but three hypotheses have been proposed.
  - The myogenic hypothesis proposes that increased arterial pressure stimulates contraction of vascular smooth muscle, which increases vascular resistance. Increased resistance in response to increased pressure maintains constant flow.
  - The metabolic hypothesis proposes that metabolic substances liberated from the tissues exert a local vasodilator effect.
  - The tissue pressure hypothesis proposes that increased interstitial pressure passively decreases vessel diameter and flow.

Intravascular Fluid Volume
- Changes in intravascular fluid volume do not directly affect arterial BP but do affect venous pressure and cardiac contractility. The Frank-Starling law of the heart states that stretching of myocardial fibers during diastole increases the force of contraction during systole.
  - Within limits, hypervolemia increases cardiac filling and contractility, thereby increasing CO. If SVR remains constant, increased CO will produce increased BP.
  - Hypovolemia decreases cardiac filling and contractility, decreasing CO. If SVR remains constant, decreased CO will produce decreased BP.

HYPERTENSION

Hypertension in adults over 18 years is defined as sustained SBP of 140 mm Hg or greater, DBP of 90 mm Hg or greater in people who are not taking antihypertensive medication. This definition is based on the average of two or more readings taken at each of two or more visits after an initial BP screening. HTN has been classified by the *Seventh Report of the Joint National Committee on Detection, Evaluation, and Treatment of High Blood Pressure* (JNC 7) as Stage 1 and Stage 2. (See Table 9–1.) You should note that this important guideline is expected to be updated in 2010 when JNC 8 will be published. You will be able to find this information at the National Heart Lung and Blood Institute Web site (www.nhlbi.nih.gov/index.htm). The JNC provides guidelines for defining hypertension, recommending lifestyle changes, and pharmacologic treatment of hypertension.

Primary HTN
- Primary (essential) HTN is elevated BP without a known cause. Primary HTN accounts for 90% to 95% of HTN in adults.
- Most cases of primary HTN result from a complex interaction of genetic, environmental, and demographic factors. Factors associated with primary HTN include
  - Excessive salt and water retention
  - Increased SNS activity; circulating NE levels are usually higher in people with HTN than in those with normal or optimal BP
  - Increased vasoconstrictive response to SNS activity and circulating catecholamines
  - Decreased production of nitric oxide (NO), a potent vasodilator released from the vascular endothelium
  - Inherited cardiovascular risk factors; HTN coexists with hypercholesterolemia and with diabetes; HTN, insulin resistance, dyslipidemia and obesity occur concomitantly and multiply the risk of cardiac and vascular disease

Table 9–1. Classification of Blood Pressure for Adults 18 Years of Age and Older

Category	Systolic (mm Hg)	Diastolic (mm Hg)
Normal	< 120	< 80
Prehypertension	120–139	80–89
Hypertension, Stage 1	140–159	90–99
Hypertension, Stage 2	160+	100+

Adapted from *The Seventh Report of the Joint National Committee on Prevention, Detection, Evaluation, and Treatment of High Blood Pressure* by National Institutes of Health, National Heart, Lung and Blood Institute, 2004, NIH Pub. No. 04-5230, Bethesda, MD: Author.

Secondary HTN

- Secondary HTN is elevated BP with a specific cause that can be identified and corrected.
- Secondary HTN accounts for 5% to 10% of HTN in adults but more than 80% of HTN in children. (Box 9–1 lists common correctable causes of secondary HTN.)
  - Onset of HTN in a person before age 20 or after age 50 suggests secondary HTN.
    - In children, the most common causes of secondary HTN are renal disease and vascular problems.
    - In adults, chronic renal disease, renovascular disease, primary aldosteronism, and the use of oral contraceptives are the most common causes of secondary HTN.

Box 9–1. Selected Causes of Secondary Hypertension

Kidney
Renal parenchymal disease
Chronic nephritis
Polycystic kidneys
Diabetic nephropathy
Acute glomerulonephritis
Renal vascular disease
Renal transplant
Renin-secreting tumors

Endocrine
Adrenal
Primary aldosteronism
Cushing's syndrome
Pheochromocytoma
Hyperparathyroidism
Thyrotoxicosis
Paget's disease of bone

Pregnancy
Preeclampsia
Eclampsia

Drugs and Chemicals
Cyclosporin
Alcohol
Sympathomimetics
Some cold remedies
Cocaine, crack
Some appetite suppressants
Tyramine with monoamine oxidase inhibitors
Nonsteroidal anti-inflammatory drugs
Oral contraceptives
Vascular
Coarctation of the aorta
Anemia
Aortic valvular insufficiency
Neurological
Increased intracranial pressure
Obstructive sleep apnea
Quadriplegia

- – Clinical findings suggestive of secondary HTN include
  - Unexplained hypokalemia, suggesting primary aldosteronism
  - Abdominal or renal bruits, suggesting renovascular disease
  - Labile BP with a history of palpitations, sweating, and tremor, suggesting pheochromocytoma
  - Family history of renal disease, suggesting renovascular disease
  - Decreased BP in the legs in comparison with the arms, suggesting aortic coarctation

Incidence and Demographics

- HTN is common to all human populations (except a few thousand culturally isolated people) and accounts for 6% of deaths in adults worldwide.
- About one in four American adults have HTN. Of those with HTN, 31.6% are unaware of the condition, 27.4% are on medication and have it controlled, 26.2% are on medication but do not have their blood pressure controlled, and 14.8% aren't on medication.
- Ethnicity is related to the prevalence of HTN.
  - The prevalence of HTN is higher in Black and Native American people than in White people.
    - Blacks develop HTN earlier and their average BPs are higher than Whites at all ages.
    - Blacks have a greater rate of stroke (fatal and nonfatal), death from heart disease, and end-stage kidney disease than Whites.
  - In comparison with Whites, the prevalence of HTN in Mexican Americans is slightly lower for men and slightly higher for women.
- The prevalence of HTN increases with age, but systolic and diastolic pressures behave differently over time. These differences account for the high prevalence of isolated systolic HTN (SBP > 140 mm Hg with DBP < 90 mm Hg) in older adults.
  - SBP rises slowly, beginning in the early adult years and continuing into old age.
  - DBP rises steadily in early adulthood, but begins to decline at about age 60.
  - Among Americans 60 years and older, HTN was found in 60% of non-Hispanic Whites, 71% of non-Hispanic Blacks, and 61% of Mexican Americans.
  - Isolated systolic HTN may account for 65% to 75% of HTN in the elderly.
- People with lower educational and income levels tend to have higher BP.

Risk for Cardiac and Vascular Disease

- HTN is a major modifiable risk factor for vascular disease affecting the brain, heart, peripheral vessels, and kidneys.
- Not only the level of BP but also the presence or absence of target-organ damage (TOD) and other risk factors determine the overall risk for cardiac and vascular disease.
  - The presence of TOD or clinical cardiovascular disease (CVD) increases the risk associated with HTN and modifies treatment recommendations.
  - TOD and CVD associated with HTN include
    - Heart diseases: left ventricular hypertrophy, angina, prior myocardial infarction, prior coronary revascularization, and heart failure
    - Stroke or transient ischemic attacks
    - Nephropathy
    - Peripheral arterial disease
    - Hypertensive retinopathy

- The presence of other major risk factors increases the risk associated with HTN and modifies treatment recommendations.
- Major risk factors include
  - Smoking
  - Dyslipidemia
  - Diabetes mellitus
  - Age more than 60 years
  - Gender (men and postmenopausal women)
  - Family history of cardiovascular disease in women before age 65 years and in men before age 55 years

Sequelae and Complications

- Target organ damage
  - Cardiac effects
    - HTN is a major risk factor for coronary heart disease: angina pectoris, myocardial infarction, and sudden death.
    - Sustained HTN increases cardiac work, resulting in concentric left ventricular hypertrophy (LVH) and increased wall thickness.
    - LVH is initially compensatory, but eventually the ventricle dilates and symptoms of heart failure appear.
  - Neurologic effects
    - Retinal effects: Increasing severity of HTN is associated with focal spasm and progressive, general narrowing of the arterioles. Retinal hemorrhage, exudate, and disc edema may be seen on funduscopic examination.
    - Central nervous system effects
      - Cerebral infarction because of atherosclerosis (i.e., stroke)
      - Cerebral hemorrhage because of HTN and development of cerebrovascular microaneurysms
      - Hypertensive encephalopathy is characterized by severe HTN (often exceeding 250/150 mm Hg), headache that is sometimes accompanied by restlessness and confusion, and resolution of symptoms with BP reduction.
        - Nausea, projectile vomiting, and visual blurring may occur.
        - Optic disc edema with retinal hemorrhages and exudates may be observed.
  - Renal effects
    - Decreased glomerular filtration rate and tubular dysfunction because of arteriosclerotic lesions of the afferent and efferent renal arterioles.
    - Proteinuria and microscopic hematuria because of glomerular lesions.
  - Peripheral vascular effects
    - HTN enhances atherosclerosis in the peripheral blood vessels, leading to the development of aortic aneurysm, aortic dissection, and peripheral vascular disease.
- Hypertensive crises are rare situations that require immediate BP reduction to prevent or limit TOD. Examples of TOD associated with hypertensive crisis are hypertensive encephalopathy, intracranial hemorrhage, unstable angina, acute myocardial infarction, dissecting aortic aneurysm, and eclampsia.
  - Hypertensive emergencies are defined as SBP greater than 220 mm Hg and DBP greater than 120 mm Hg.
    - Patients require admission to intensive care for intravenous vasodilator therapy and monitoring.

- Initial goal is to reduce mean arterial BP no more than 25% within several minutes to 2 hours. BP is reduced toward 160/100 mm Hg over next 2 to 6 hours.
        - Past practice of administering sublingual nifedipine to rapidly lower pressure is not recommended because it may cause a stroke because of the sudden drop in cerebral perfusion.
    - Hypertensive urgencies are situations in which it is desirable to reduce BP within a few hours. Examples are more extreme stage 2 HTN (SBP > 180 or DBP > 110 mm Hg), HTN with optic disc edema, progressive target organ complications, and severe peri-operative HTN.

SLEEP APNEA AND HYPERTENSION

- Sleep apnea has a strong relationship with hypertension and with heart failure.
    - Sleep apnea history should be obtained at the onset of hypertension.
    - Those that screen positive should have a sleep polysomnography test performed and continuous positive airway pressure (CPAP) started if indicated.
    - Current guidelines require anyone taking two oral antihypertensive medications but still with uncontrolled hypertension undergo a sleep study.
- Sleep apnea has thee forms.
    - Central sleep apnea in which there is no respiratory drive for seconds
    - Obstructive sleep apnea in which there is respiratory drive but no air movement because of collapse of airway structures
    - Mixed sleep apnea in which both central and obstructive apnea events can be observed
- Obstructive sleep apnea is more commonly seen in obese people but it should be assessed in everyone. Suspect sleep apnea when
    - The person snores,
    - Has daytime sleepiness,
    - Does not feel rested in the morning, and
    - Complains of morning headaches that clear in the first 30 minutes of wakening. This is because of carbon dioxide retention from the apneas. CO_2 retention leads to vasodilation of cerebral vessels but this clears upon awakening with normal breathing.
- Polysomnography (sleep study) entails assessment of respiratory muscle use, airflow, ECG, electro-oculogram (eye movement), electro-myelogram (limb movement), and oxygen saturation.
- Diagnostic criteria for sleep apnea is an apnea-hypopnea index (AHI). The AHI is the total number of apneas (cessation of breathing) and hypopneas (decrease in tidal volume with oxygen desaturation) divided by the hours of sleep.
    - Mild sleep apnea is an AHI of 5 to 15.
    - Moderate sleep apnea is an AHI of 16 to 30.
    - Severe sleep apnea is an AHI above 30.
- Obstructive sleep apnea is commonly treated with CPAP and occasionally with surgery.
- Central sleep apnea can be treated with bilevel positive airway pressure (Bi-PAP).

CLINICAL ASSESSMENT WITH HYPERTENSION

- The purpose of clinical assessment in HTN is to determine risk for cardiac and vascular disease.
  - To accurately measure BP
  - To identify the presence of TOD
  - To identify the presence of other cardiovascular risk factors
  - To identify the presence of cardiac or vascular disease
  - To identify secondary causes of HTN when present
  - To identify coexisting conditions that affect diagnosis, prognosis, or treatment, such as
    - Sleep apnea
    - Pregnancy
    - Substances that may cause HTN
      - Oral contraceptives
      - Sympathomimetics, including cocaine
      - Adrenal steroids
      - Alcohol
      - Excessive salt intake
      - Herbal weight-loss agents containing ephedra
      - Nasal decongestants containing ephedrine
- HTN causes no symptoms until it has become severe and TOD is present.
  - Symptoms related to TOD include fatigue, headache, transient weakness or blindness, loss of visual acuity, chest pain, dyspnea, and claudication.
  - Headache is characteristic of only severe HTN. Nosebleed, blurring of vision because of retinal changes, and TIAs are symptoms of associated vascular disease.
  - Symptoms related to secondary causes of HTN include muscle weakness; episodes of tachycardia, sweating, and tremor; thinning of the skin; and flank pain.
- HTN is easily detected, but cannot be diagnosed from a single BP measurement.
  - BP varies markedly related to time of day, body position, activity, and physical and emotional state.
  - Diagnosis and classification of HTN is based on an average of two or more BPs taken on two or more occasions after an initial screening. (See Table 9–1.)
  - BP should be measured in a standard fashion, using equipment that meets certification criteria.

Physical Examination
- Physical examination of the person with HTN includes
  - Vital signs: variable BP, tachycardia, or bradycardia
  - Heart: size, rhythm, sounds, murmurs
  - Neck: jugular venous pressure, carotid pulses and bruit, thyromegaly
  - Vascular: renal or femoral bruits, ankle brachial systolic pressure index
  - Lungs: respiratory rate, rhythm, and presence of adventitious sounds (crackles or wheezes)
  - Eyes: retinal hemorrhages, exudates, and disc edema
  - Neuro: decreased visual acuity, focal neurological deficits associated with past stroke
  - Abdomen: waist circumference, aortic and renal masses or bruits

Obesity
- Body mass index (BMI) of 27 or higher is closely correlated with HTN. Obesity is defined as BMI of 30 or above.
  - BMI = weight in kilograms divided by height in meters squared
  - BMI = weight in pounds divided by height in inches squared multiplied by 704.5
- Abdominal obesity (waist circumference greater than 40 inches in men and greater than 35 inches in women) is closely correlated with risk for HTN, cardiovascular disease, type 2 diabetes, and dyslipidemia.
- Signs of secondary causes of HTN include abdominal bruit, truncal obesity, excessive hair growth, abdominal striae, and buffalo hump.

Diagnostic Studies
- Diagnostic studies may be done to determine TOD, risk factors, and secondary HTN, or to establish baseline function before initiating therapy.
- Routine tests include urinalysis, complete blood cell count, serum electrolytes, fasting glucose, total and high-density lipoprotein cholesterol, and 12-lead electrocardiogram.
- Additional tests that may be indicated in some patients include creatinine clearance, 24-hour urine for protein and microalbumin, blood calcium, uric acid, fasting triglycerides, glycosylated hemoglobin, thyroid-stimulating hormone, renal or carotid artery Doppler studies, and echocardiography.
- Some clinicians recommend measuring plasma catecholamine and aldosterone level, 24-hour urine for metanephrine, and dexamethasone suppression test to identify secondary causes of hypertension.
- In some patients, renal artery arteriograms may be indicated to look for renal artery stenosis.
- Drug screens may be warranted in hypertensive urgencies or emergencies to determine excessive stimulation because of illegal drugs such as cocaine.

MANAGEMENT OF HYPERTENSION

The goal of treatment for patients with HTN is to prevent TOD and the progression of atherosclerosis by the least intrusive means possible.
- Treatment of HTN is based on individual risk.
- Nonpharmacological management of HTN consists of lifestyle modification. Four lifestyle interventions have been shown in clinical trials to delay or prevent the onset of HTN. These interventions are used in the nonpharmacological management of prehypertension and should be used along with medications for the treatment of stage 1 and stage 2 HTN.
  - Weight reduction
  - Sodium restriction
  - Reduced alcohol intake
  - Physical activity

Lifestyle Interventions
All patients with HTN should be encouraged to adopt lifestyle interventions. Even when lifestyle interventions alone do not control HTN, they may reduce the number and dosage of antihypertensive medications needed. There is some evidence that lifestyle interventions can prevent or delay the onset of HTN.

- Weight reduction. Weight loss has been shown to reduce BP more effectively than any other lifestyle measure.
  - Loss of 10 pounds reduces BP in a large proportion of overweight people with HTN.
  - Weight loss complements pharmacological management of BP.
  - Overweight people should be counseled about calorie restriction and increased activity.
  - Sustaining weight loss is difficult; documented reduction in BP and other cardiovascular risk factors may reward persistence.
- Moderate alcohol use. Excessive alcohol intake is an important risk factor for HTN, can cause resistance to HTN therapy, and increases risk for stroke.
  - Men who drink alcohol should be advised to consume no more than two alcohol-containing beverages a day.
    - One alcohol-containing beverage is defined as 12 oz of beer, 4 oz of wine, 1½ oz of 80-proof liquor, or 1 oz of 100-proof liquor.
  - Women and lighter-weight men who drink alcohol should be advised to consume no more than one alcohol-containing beverage per day.
- Reduced sodium. Clinical trials have shown that reduction of sodium intake lowers BP is some salt-sensitive people with HTN. There is no clinical test to determine which people are salt-sensitive.
  - JNC 7 recommends sodium intake of not more than 6 g of sodium chloride or 2.4 g of sodium per day.
  - About 75% of sodium intake is derived from processed foods. Population-level reduction of sodium in processed food may be more effective than intervention with individuals.
- Diet high in fruits and vegetables. The Dietary Approaches to Stop Hypertension (DASH) Trial found that a diet high in fruits, vegetables, and low-fat dairy products and low in saturated and total fat resulted in a marked decline in both SBP and DBP.
- Physical activity. Regular, moderately intense activity (such as brisk walking) for 30 to 45 minutes on most days of the week has been shown to lower BP.
  - Most people can safely increase their level of activity without extensive medical evaluation.
  - Patients with family history of cardiac disease or other risk factors should be instructed in signs and symptoms of heart attack and stroke and action to take if symptoms occur.
  - Patients with cardiac or other serious disease and those with major risk factors may need a more through evaluation or referral to a medically supervised exercise program.
  - Increased activity increases weight loss and improves lipid profile.
- Control of other risk factors. Although smoking cessation and improving lipid profile do not improve a patient's BP, they reduce overall risk of morbidity and mortality from atherosclerotic disease.
- Avoid illegal drugs or over-the-counter drugs/herbals with ephedrine or ephedra.
- Reduce caffeine in the diet.

Pharmacological Management

- The decision to initiate pharmacological therapy is based on the degree of BP averaged from at least two readings taken at two or more visits after initial screening. Once this is established, medications should be prescribed.
- Reducing BP with drugs has been shown to protect against stroke, coronary events, heart failure, progression of renal disease, more severe BP elevation, and all-cause mortality.
- The beneficial effect of drug therapy has been seen across age, gender, race, BP level, and socioeconomic status.

- Seven classes of drugs are used in managing HTN. (Drugs are discussed in Chapter 15.)
  - Diuretics—primarily the thiazide types
  - Adrenergic inhibitors
    - α-adrenergic blockers
    - Centrally acting inhibitors
    - Central α-adrenergic agonists
    - ß-adrenergic blockers
    - Combined α- and ß-adrenergic blockers
  - Vasodilators
    - Arterial: hydralazine
    - Venous: nitrates
  - Calcium channel blocking agents
  - ACE inhibitors
  - Angiotensin II receptor blockers
  - Renin inhibitor
- According to JNC 7 guidelines, if there are no indications for another class of drug, a diuretic or ß-adrenergic blocker is recommended for initial treatment of uncomplicated HTN. In clinical trials, diuretics and ß blockers have been shown to reduce morbidity and mortality in patients with HTN.
- Other classes of drugs are recommended for initial treatment when specific indications exist.
  - For patients with HTN and insulin-dependent diabetes mellitus (DM), ACE inhibitors or angiotensin-receptor blockers (ARBs) are recommended for initial therapy. These two categories of drugs are now being given to persons with either form of DM with normal blood pressures to protect the kidney from developing proteinuria.
  - For patients with HTN and heart failure, ACE inhibitors, ß blockers and diuretics are recommended.
  - In older adult patients with isolated systolic hypertension, diuretics and long-acting dihydropyridine calcium antagonists (e.g., amlodipine) are recommended.
  - For patients with myocardial infarction and HTN, ß blockers and ACE inhibitors (with systolic dysfunction) are recommended.
- For most patients with HTN, an initial trial of lifestyle modification followed by initiation of low-dose drug therapy is appropriate. If necessary, dose of the initial drug can be increased and other agents with different mechanism of action can be added.
- In patients with stage 2 HTN, initial drug therapy is started with two drugs, one usually a thiazide diuretic.
  - Patients with an average SBP of 200 mm Hg or higher require immediate therapy, as do those with average DBP of 120 mm Hg or higher. If symptomatic or if TOD is present, these patients may require hospitalization and the use of parenteral antihypertensive agents.
- Management of HTN is modified by individual patient characteristics, including membership in specific groups.
  - HTN in women
    - Women taking oral contraceptives experience a small but detectable increase in SBP and DBP.
    - Clinical HTN is two to three times more prevalent in women taking oral contraceptives than among those not taking these drugs.
    - HTN that occurs in nonpregnant women and HTN that occurs before the 20th week of gestation or persists more than 6 weeks after delivery are considered chronic.

- Gestational HTN occurs in the third trimester and is not associated with signs of eclampsia.
    - Preeclampsia is elevated BP associated with proteinuria and edema.
    - Eclampsia is a HTN emergency that occurs during pregnancy.
    - Neither ACE inhibitors nor angiotensin II blockers should be used to treat hypertension in pregnant women. A central α-agonist (e.g., methyldopa) is the drug of choice during pregnancy.
- HTN in older adults
    - Isolated systolic hypertension (SBP > 140 mm Hg with DBP < 90 mm Hg) is common in older adults.
    - Target BP is the same as for younger adults (< 140/90 mm Hg), although an interim goal of 160/90 mm Hg may be necessary.
    - Among older adults, SBP is a better predictor of events (CHD, CVD, heart failure, stroke, end-stage renal disease, and all-cause mortality) than DBP.
    - Treatment includes lifestyle modification and drugs. Diuretics are the preferred first-line drug therapy unless there is specific indication for another drug.
        - Treatment reduces stroke, clinical cardiovascular disease (CCD), CVD, heart failure, and mortality.
    - Falsely high BP readings may occur because of excessive vascular stiffness. This may be seen with high BP without TOD and lack of response to treatment.
    - High risk of orthostatic HTN exists among older adults. Always measure BP and pulse while standing, as well as while sitting or supine.
- HTN and coexisting disease
    - Reduce BP gradually in people with cerebrovascular disease to avoid orthostatic hypotension.
    - HTN is major risk factor for carotid atherosclerosis, peripheral arterial disease, and aneurysm. Data are not available to determine if treatment of HTN reduces the risk of these processes. Data show reduced risk of death from aortic dissection.
    - In people with diabetes mellitus and HTN, the goal is to reduce BP below 130/85 mm Hg. ACE and ARB therapy is recommended in normotensive people with DM to reduce the risk of renal complications.
        - Lifestyle modification, especially weight loss and exercise
        - ACE inhibitors, α blockers, calcium channel antagonists, or low-dose diuretics are preferred agents.
    - In people with renal disease and HTN, control of HTN (< 130/85 mm Hg) slows the progression of renal failure.
        - Lifestyle modification, especially sodium restriction.
        - ACE inhibitor is the preferred drug class.
    - Lower target BP may be desired in patients with existing coronary heart disease or heart failure.
        - After MI, ß blocker is the preferred drug class.
        - For patients with heart failure, ACE inhibitors and combined α–ß blockers are preferred.
- After BP has been controlled on drug therapy for 1 year, drug dosage reduction should be attempted.

Nurses' Role

- Nurses' role in managing HTN depends on the individual nurse's preparation, work experience, and clinical setting.
- Nursing diagnoses are derived from the comprehensive assessment. Common diagnoses among patients with HTN include
  - Deficient knowledge about disease process and management
  - Ineffective therapeutic regimen management
  - Noncompliance (specify)
  - Deficient fluid volume related to diuretic therapy
- General therapeutic goals for people with HTN include
  - Achieve and maintain individually determined target BP
    - In people with average risk, SBP less than 140 mm Hg and DBP less than 90 mm Hg
    - If tolerated, further lowering of BP may prevent stroke, preserve renal function, and prevent or slow the progression of heart failure.
    - Lower target BP (130/85) has been established for people with diabetes, renal disease, or heart disease.
  - Understand and implement lifestyle interventions.
  - Comply with therapeutic regimen.
- Frequently used nursing interventions when caring for patients with HTN include
  - Exercise promotion
  - Nutritional counseling
  - Teaching: diet, disease process, health behaviors, medication, prescribed activity, treatment regimen
  - Weight reduction assistance
  - Patient contracting
  - Smoking cessation assistance
- Dependent upon individual patient assessment and practice setting, the following indicators of nursing outcomes may be appropriate.
  - Compliance behavior
  - Circulation status
  - Knowledge: Diet, disease process, health behaviors, medication, prescribed activity, treatment regimen
  - Neurological status
  - Nutritional status
  - Tissue perfusion: Abdominal organs, cardiac, cerebral, peripheral, pulmonary
  - Vital signs status
- Collaborative strategies to enhance adherence to HTN therapy
  - Educate patients
    - Assess understanding of diagnosis and treatment.
    - Discuss concerns and clarify misunderstandings; assess for unpleasant secondary drug effects.
    - Inform patient of actual and desired BP level.
    - Provide specific written information.
    - Emphasize that HTN is symptomless and the importance of continued therapy.

- Individualize treatment
    - Include patient in decision-making.
    - Simplify and minimize cost of treatment.
    - Incorporate treatment into daily life.
    - Encourage self-monitoring of BP.
        - BP of people with HTN tends to be lower when measured at home.
        - Average readings of 135/85 mm Hg or greater are considered elevated.
    - When weight loss is desired, discourage quick weight-loss regimens, fasting, and unscientific methods.
- Provide reinforcement
    - Trend BP over time.
    - Give positive feedback for behavioral and BP improvement.
    - Solicit questions and concerns.
    - Use appointment reminders and contact patients to confirm.
    - Schedule more frequent appointments with nonadherent patients. Consider nurse-initiated telephone follow-up.
    - Consider clinician–patient contracting.
    - Involve family member, if appropriate.

SUMMARY

This chapter provided an overview of hypertension including a discussion of physiology and regulation of blood pressure. Assessment and treatment guidelines were presented. It is important that the nurse assess and continuously monitor for HTN. Too many people are not treated adequately, resulting in unnecessary high incidence of cerebrovascular accident (CVA), MI, and heart failure. Another important role of the nurse is to assist the patient in the process of making lifestyle changes. Patient advocacy can save lives.

REFERENCES

Alli, O., Jacobs, L., & Amanullah, A. M. (2008). Hypertensive crisis. How to tell if it's an emergency or an urgency. *Reviews in Cardiovascular Medicine, 9*(2), 111–124.

Calhoun, D. A., Jones, D., Textor, S., Goff, D. C., Murphy, T. P., Toto, R. D., ... Carey, R. M. (2008). Resistant hypertension: Diagnosis, evaluation, and treatment. A scientific statement from the American Heart Association Professional Education Committee of the Council for High Blood Pressure Research. *Hypertension, 51*(6), 1403–19.

Izzo, J. L., Sica, D. A., & Black, H. R. (2008). *Hypertension primer: The essential of high blood pressure.* Philadelphia: Lippincott William & Wilkins.

National Institutes of Health, National Heart, Lung and Blood Institute. (2004). *The seventh report of the Joint National Committee on Prevention, Detection, Evaluation, and Treatment of High Blood Pressure.* NIH Publication 04-5230. Bethesda, MD: Author.

Perez, M. I., & Musini, V. M. (2008). Pharmacological interventions for hypertensive emergencies: A Cochrane systematic review. *Journal of Human Hypertension, 22*(9), 596–607. Epub 2008 Apr 17.

Rosendorff, C., Black, H. R., Cannon, C. P., Gersh, B. J., Gore, J., Izzo, J. L. Jr., ... American Heart Association Council on Epidemiology and Prevention. (2007). Treatment of hypertension in the prevention and management of ischemic heart disease: A scientific statement from the American Heart Association Council for High Blood Pressure Research and the Councils on Clinical Cardiology and Epidemiology and Prevention. *Circulation, 115,* 2761–2788.

Thomas, R. J., Weiss, M. D., Mietus, J. E., Peng, C. K., Goldberger, A. L., & Gottlieb, D. J. (2009). Prevalent hypertension and stroke in the Sleep Heart Health Study: Association with an ECG-derived spectrographic marker of cardiopulmonary coupling. *Sleep, 32*(7), 897–904.

10

Dyslipidemia Management

Management of dyslipidemia is essential to the prevention and treatment of atherosclerosis. High levels of low-density lipoprotein cholesterol (LDL-C), low levels of high-density lipoprotein cholesterol (HDL-C), and high levels of triglycerides increase the risk of developing this condition. This chapter will review normal lipid profiles, lipid pathways, and lipid subclasses. In addition, treatment guidelines and drug and lifestyle therapies will be presented. The Adult Treatment Panel III (ATP III) report contains the National Cholesterol Education Program's (NCEP) evidence-based clinical guidelines for lipid testing and management. This chapter presents screening guidelines for coronary heart disease (CHD) risk and the metabolic syndrome, the ATP III guidelines for primary and secondary prevention of atherosclerosis, and the implications of dyslipidemia management for nursing practice. A new set of guidelines is due for publication in 2010 so check the National Heart Lung and Blood Institute Web site (http://www.nhlbi.nih.gov/index.htm) for the ATP IV report in the future.

UNDERSTANDING LIPOPROTEIN STRUCTURE, FUNCTION, AND METABOLISM

- Structure of lipids includes
  - Core composted of cholesterol ester and triglyceride (TG)
  - Coat containing apoproteins A, B, C, E, J, and Apo(a); unesterified cholesterol; and phospholipids

- Cholesterol is an important component of cell walls and needed throughout the body for cell stability and regeneration of all forms of tissues.
- Cholesterol is defined based on size of molecules, density, protein content, and major apoproteins. Table 10–1 describes the various forms of lipoproteins.
  - Chylomicrons rapidly enter the plasma from the gut after meals. This is the largest but least dense molecule. It is triglyceride rich.
  - Very low density lipoproteins (VLDL) serve the role of providing a source of triglyceride when fat is not readily available from the diet. The liver can secrete VLDL that is not quite as large but is slightly more dense than chylomicrons. Through several metabolic processes the VLDL is converted to Intermediate density lipoprotein (IDL) and eventually to low density lipoproteins (LDL). As these processes occur, the triglyceride content of the lipid molecule decreases and cholesterol increases. The overall size decreases but the molecule becomes more dense.
  - LDL molecules are usually 4% to 8% triglyceride content but this can increase when there is a higher level of serum triglycerides. LDL particles serve as the major carrier of cholesterol to the body tissues for cell membrane use. LDL-C level has the greatest strength of all the lipid particles for predicting CHD.
  - High-density lipoprotein (HDL) level is inversely related to development of CHD, theorized to result from reverse cholesterol transport (transport of cholesterol from the tissue to the liver). High HDL is protective for the development of CHD.
  - Not all LDL and HDL is the same in terms of structure and function. New information on the subclasses of the various lipoproteins and which ones are more specific to CHD risk will be discussed later in this chapter.

Table 10–1. Plasma Lipoprotein Composition

	Origin	Density (g/mL)	Size (nm)	% Protein	Apoprotein Major (Minor)
Chylomicrons	Intestines	< 0.95	100–1000	1–2	B48 (A-I, Cs)
VLDL	Liver	< 1.006	40–50	10	B100 (AI, Cs)
IDL	VLDL	1.006–1.019	25–30	18	B100, E
LDL	IDL	1.019–1.063	20–25	25	B100
HDL	Tissue	1.063–1.210	6–10	40–55	A-I (A-II, A-IV)
Lipoprotein (a)	Liver	1.051–1.082	25	30–50	B100, (a)

Adapted from "Lipoprotein disorders and cardiovascular disease," by J. Genest, P. Libby, & A. M. Gotto, 2005, in D. P. Zipes, P. Libby, R. O. Bonow, & E. Braunwald (Eds.), *Braunwald's heart disease: A textbook of cardiovascular medicine* (pp. 1013–1033), Philadelphia: Elsevier Saunders.

- Lipids are metabolized by means of two pathways: exogenous and endogenous. Both are active processes, one for the lipids that our body produces (genetically programmed) and the other for the lipids that we ingest (lifestyle). Either one or the interaction of both can be responsible for the overall lipid status of the person.
  - Exogenous pathway
    - Chylomicrons formed from dietary TG and cholesterol
    - Lipoprotein lipase from adipose and muscle removes TG, leaving chylomicron remnants (cholesterol)
    - Remnants reach the liver where cholesterol is released and
      - Stored as esters in hepatocytes
      - Released in bile ash cholesterol or bile acids
      - Used to form membranes or endogenous lipoproteins
  - Endogenous pathway
    - VLDL formed in liver from TG and cholesterol from caloric intake
    - VLDL released in plasma
    - Lipoprotein lipase cleaves TG
    - Remnant is IDL, which is taken up in liver and results in free cholesterol or remains in circulation where TG removed, leaving LDL
    - LDL transports endogenous cholesterol ester to liver
    - Apolipoprotein B is found in LDL and VLDL
    - HDL involved in transport of cholesterol from periphery to liver
  - A third pathway is nonspecific, the result of macrophage participation in lipoprotein degradation with deposits in select sites including arterial walls and tendons.
    - Clinically this can be seen as eruptive xanthomas (growths often on the elbow) or xanthelasmas (deposits on the upper eyelid).
    - Aggressive treatment may be needed to arrest or remove these deposits.

HYPERLIPIDEMIA

Hyperlipidemia is often described as having heredity or secondary cause.
- Hereditary causes are primarily the result of
  - Familial hypercholesterolemia
  - Familial hyperchylomicronemia
  - Dysbetaliproteinemia
  - Familial combined hyperlipidemia
- Fredrickson's Classification of Genetic Hyperlipidemias is presented in Table 10–2.
- Secondary causes of hyperlipidemias include
  - Metabolic: diabetes, glycogen storage deficits, lipodystrophy
  - Renal: chronic renal failure, glomerulonephritis
  - Hepatic: obstructive liver disease, cirrhosis
  - Hormonal: estrogen, progesterone, growth hormone, hypothyroidism, corticosteroids
  - Lifestyle: obesity, physical inactivity, high-fat diet, increased alcohol intake
  - Medications: corticosteroids, exogenous estrogens, testosterone, thiazide diuretics, selective beta blockers, cyclosporine, antiretrovirals

Table 10–2. Fredrickson's Classification of Genetic Forms of Hyperlipidemia

Type I	Exogenous hyperlipidemia: total cholesterol normal, triglyerides and chylomicrons increased
Type IIa	LDL and total cholesterol increased
Type IIb	LDL, VLDL, total cholesterol, triglyerides increased
Type III	Dysbetalipoproteinemia: IDL, total cholesterol, and triglyerides increased
Type IV	Endogenous hyperlipidemia: glucose intolerance
Type V	Mixed hyperlipidemia

- Serum lipoprotein laboratory testing has traditionally only measured total cholesterol, HDL-C, and triglycerides. LDL is estimated based on the Friedewald Formula.
  - There is a fairly consistent ratio between VLDL and triglycerides. This is expressed as VLDL – C = triglycerides ÷ 5.
  - Most cholesterol is carried on three lipoproteins: HDL, LDL, and VLDL, so total cholesterol = HDL + LDL + VLDL.
  - If we measure triglyceride level, we can calculate an estimate of the VLDL.
  - If we measure total cholesterol, HDL, and TG, we can calculate an estimate for the LDL.
  - When TG is elevated (usually > 250 mg/dl), it is unwise to use this formula to estimate the LDL because there is too much error in the estimation.
  - At times it is important to know the non-LDL level and that is calculated as non–LDL-C = HDL + (triglycerides ÷ 5).
  - The 2004 Update in the ATP III guidelines recommended that LDL-C be directly measured and not calculated; however, this has not been universally adopted. More direct measurement of LDL and subparticles is expected to be done over the next few years.
- Hypertriglyceridemia is often associated with type 2 diabetes mellitus (DM) and pancreatitis. If the patient has DM, improved blood sugar control will lower TG levels and should be done in conjunction with TG-lowering medications

SCREENING FOR ATHEROSCLEROSIS RISK

In all adults (20 years and older), a fasting lipoprotein profile (total cholesterol, LDL-C, HDL-C, and TG) should be obtained once every 5 years. New guidelines recommend screening children between the ages of 2 and 10 years. A 12-hour fast prior to the blood draw improves the accuracy of TG. Because LDL is most often calculated based on triglyeride levels, the LDL may not be accurate if the person is not fasting. Total cholesterol and HDL measurement is not as sensitive to fasting state as triglycerides. Other atherosclerosis risk factors should also be assessed. (Assessment and management of cardiac and vascular risk is discussed in Chapters 7 and 8 of this manual.)

- Modifiable risk factors
  - Cigarette smoking
  - Uncontrolled diabetes mellitus (Hemoglobin A1C > 6%)
  - Uncontrolled hypertension
  - Obesity

  - – Sedentary lifestyle
  - – Atherosclerotic dyslipidemia
    - • Low HDL cholesterol (< 40 mg/dL)
    - • High LDL cholesterol (> 160 gm/dL)
    - • High triglycerides (> 150 mg/dL)
- • Nonmodifiable risk factors
  - – Family history of early myocardial infarction (MI) or sudden death (first-degree male relative before 55 years or first-degree female relative before 65 years)
  - – Increased age: men older than 45 years and women older than 55 years
  - – Early onset of menopause because of total abdominal hysterectomy
- • People with multiple risk factors should be screened more frequently than every 5 years, regardless of gender or race.
  - – Rapid-result machines can give an entire lipid panel from a drop of blood within 5 minutes.
- • Risk reduction is an important component of prevention and treatment of atherosclerosis and CHD.
- • The presence of risk factors determines the acceptable level of blood lipids and the level at which pharmacological reduction should be initiated.

ATP III GUIDELINES

The purpose of the guidelines is to provide direction to healthcare providers in the prevention and treatment of dyslipidemia in people with and without CHD.

ATP III Classification
- • For the general adult population, ATP III classification of LDL, total, and HDL cholesterol (mg/dL) is the following:
  - – LDL cholesterol
    - • Under 100 is optimal.
    - • 100 to 129 is near but above optimal.
    - • 130 to 159 is borderline high.
    - • 160 to 189 is high.
    - • 190 or above is very high.
  - – Total cholesterol
    - • Under 200 is desirable.
    - • 200 to 239 is borderline high.
    - • 240 or above is high.
  - – HDL cholesterol
    - • Under 40 is low.
    - • 60 or above is high (desirable).
- • Major risk factors (exclusive of LDL cholesterol) that modify LDL treatment goals
  - – Cigarette smoking
  - – Hypertension
  - – Low HDL cholesterol
  - – Family history of premature CHD
  - – Age (men 45 years and older; women 55 years and older)

- LDL treatment goals related to risk
  - For people with clinical CHD or CHD risk equivalents, the LDL goal is under 100 mg/dL.
  - For people with more than two major risk factors, the LDL goal is under 130 mg/dL.
  - For people with no or one major risk factor, the LDL goal is under 160 mg/dL.

CHD Risk Equivalents

- CHD risk equivalents include
  - Other forms of clinical atherosclerotic disease (i.e., peripheral arterial disease, abdominal aortic aneurysm, symptomatic carotid artery disease)
  - Diabetes
  - Multiple risk factors that confer a 10-year risk for CHD of 20% or more.
    - For people with two or more risk factors, data from the Framingham Heart Study are used to estimate the 10-year risk of CHD.
    - Points are assigned by gender for age, total cholesterol, HDL cholesterol, smoking, and blood pressure.
      - Point total predicts 10-year risk for CHD.
      - 10-year risk for CHD of 20% or more is a CHD equivalent and reason for more intensive lowering of LDL cholesterol
    - The Framingham scoring method is included in the ATP III guidelines, which can be downloaded from the Web site of the National Heart Lung and Blood Institute (www.nhlbi.nih.gov).

Therapeutic Lifestyle Changes

- The ATP III report recommends a multifaceted approach to CHD risk reduction designated "therapeutic lifestyle changes (TLC)."
  - Reduced intake of saturated fats (less than 7% of total calories) and cholesterol (less than 200 mg per day)
  - Use of plant stanols and sterols (2 g per day) and increased soluble fiber (20 to 30 g per day)
    - Plant stanols and sterols are naturally occurring food substances that are combined with small amounts of canola oil and added to foods.
    - Currently, regular and "light" spreads fortified with plant stanols and sterols are available commercially.
  - Soluble fiber is found in oats, legumes, grains, vegetables, and fruits. Dietary intake is preferred over supplements.
  - Weight reduction
  - Increased physical exercise

IMPLICATIONS FOR NURSING PRACTICE

- Nurses screen, monitor, and teach individuals and groups about the management of dyslipidemia and atherosclerotic risk.
  - Screening occurs in community and acute care settings.
    - Patients admitted to the hospital with a cardiovascular event should be screened within 24 hours of admission.
  - Individual risk assessment and modification is essential.
  - Routine monitoring of the lipid profile allows the person to observe improvement and reinforces behavior change.
    - Providing laboratory results, together with target goals, in writing enables the patient to monitor his or her progress over time.
- Nurses and dietitians are responsible for teaching people about therapeutic lifestyle changes.
- Nurses monitor the therapeutic and side effects of pharmacotherapy and promote patient adherence.

TREATMENT OF DYSLIPIDEMIA

Primary Prevention
- Primary prevention consists of screening and therapeutic lifestyle changes (TLC).
- TLC dietary recommendations include
  - Total fat (saturated, polyunsaturated, and monounsaturated) should not exceed 25% to 30% of total calories.
    - Saturated fat should constitute less than 7% of total calories.
    - Polyunsaturated fats may be up to 10% of total calories.
    - Monounsaturated fats may be up to 20% of total calories.
  - Carbohydrates (primarily whole grains, fruits, and vegetables) may be up to 50% to 60% of total calories.
  - Fiber should be 20 to 30 grams per day.
  - Protein should constitute approximately 15% of total calories.
  - Cholesterol should be less than 200 mg per day.
  - Total calories consumed should be balanced with energy expended to achieve and maintain desirable body weight.
  - When TG is elevated, advise the patient to decrease sugar and alcohol intake.
- If the target lipid levels are not achieved after 6 weeks with the TLC diet, plant stanols and sterols are added.
- If target lipid levels are not achieved after 12 weeks, pharmacotherapy is initiated. LDL-lowering drugs reduce the risk for major coronary events and coronary death.
- At each visit, TLCs are reviewed and reinforced, even after drug treatment is begun.
- Pharmacologic therapy should be started if patient is unresponsive to TLC; if the patient is at high risk, medications are started along with TLC.
- The primary target is to treat LDL-C to goal.
- The secondary targets are to raise HDL-C and lower TG if not at goal.
  - Exercise can raise HDL-C.
  - Reducing intake of simple carbohydrates and alcohol can lower TG.

Secondary Prevention
- Cholesterol treatment goals for people with clinical CHD or CHD equivalents are more stringent.
  - LDL cholesterol should be less than 100 mg/dL or, in the very high risk group, less than 70 mg/dL.
- Lipid profile should be obtained within 24 hours of hospital admission for an acute coronary event and therapy should be initiated before discharge.
  - Current guidelines recommend starting HMG-CoA reductase inhibitors (statins) on all patients after CHD is diagnosed.
  - ATP III guidelines recommend starting a fibric acid derivative or nicotinic acid, if appropriate for secondary target therapy.
- Lipid profile should be reevaluated 6 and 12 weeks after initiating drug treatment.
- Therapeutic lifestyle changes and reduction of other risk factor reduction should be encouraged also.

Drug Therapy
- Drugs used to treat dyslipidemia are described in detail in Chapter 15.
- HMG-CoA reductase inhibitors, also known as statins, decrease mortality, reduce the risk of major coronary events by 30%, and stimulate plaque regression in coronary heart disease.
  - Statins are most effective when taken at bedtime.
  - Statins decrease LDL (18% to 55%), increase HDL (5% to 15%), and decrease triglycerides (7% to 30%).
  - Statins can be combined with nicotinic or fibric acids if necessary.
  - Statins are contraindicated in people with active or chronic liver disease.
  - Liver enzymes are assessed after 6 weeks and every 6 months during treatment. Discontinue the statin if liver function tests (LFTs) are more than three times the upper limit of normal (ULN).
  - Statins also can reduce the inflammatory marker high-sensitivity C-reactive protein (hs-CRP) and are thought to reduce inflammation at the site of an atherosclerotic lesion, resulting in a more stable lesion that is less likely to rupture and cause an MI.
  - Patients must be taught to report symptoms of muscle aches or weakness.
    - Myalgia with normal creatine kinase (CK) may occur in up to 5% of those on a statin.
    - Myopathy is muscle aches with CK more than 10 times ULN, which occurs in less than 0.1%.
    - Rhabdomyolysis—breakdown of the muscle cells with CK above 10,000 IU/L—is rare (< 0.01%).
    - The highest risk for rhabdomyolysis is in elderly, women, small frame, dehydrated, hypothermia, acidosis, chronic disease, infection, alcohol abuse, extreme exercise, and cytochrome P450 interactions.
- Bile acid sequestrants
  - Decrease LDL (15% to 30%) and increase HDL (3% to 5%) without affecting triglycerides.
  - May be added to statin therapy in people who do not reach target levels on statins alone.
  - Side effects include gastrointestinal (GI) distress and constipation.
  - May interfere with absorption of other drugs.

- Nicotinic acid
  - Decrease LDL (5% to 25%) and triglyceride (20% to 50%) and increase HDL (15% to 35%).
  - Side effects include flushing, hyperglycemia, hyperuricemia (gout), upper GI distress, and hepatotoxicity.
- Fibric acids (gemfibrozil, fenofibrate, clofibrate)
  - Decrease LDL (5% to 20%) and triglyceride (20% to 50%) and increase HDL (10% to 20%).
  - Side effects include dyspepsia, gallstone, and myopathy. Unexplained non-CHD deaths were seen in clinical trials.
  - Contraindicated in severe renal or hepatic disease.
- Cholesterol absorption inhibitors (ezetimibe)
  - Work on the brushy border of the small intestine, inhibiting the absorption of cholesterol and other sterols.
  - This drug can achieve 18% LDL-C–lowering alone and can be used if a statin is not tolerated.
  - It can also be added to a statin to achieve lower LDL-C if on maximal statin dose.
- Omega-3 polyunsaturated fatty acids (PUFA) are found in the diet in oily fish or can be provided as supplements.
  - Increase HDL-C and can be used with statins and other pharmacotherapies.
  - Similar PUFAs are found in nuts (e.g., walnuts, almonds).

METABOLIC SYNDROME

Metabolic syndrome is present in approximately 22% of the adult (20 years and older) population. People with the metabolic syndrome have an increased risk of developing atherosclerosis and a higher incidence of cardiac events than those without this syndrome. Metabolic syndrome is a growing problem in children and adolescents.

- The metabolic syndrome consists of lipid and nonlipid factors. The presence of any three of the five factors makes the diagnosis of metabolic syndrome. The factors are
  - Triglyceride 150 mg/dL or higher
  - HDL cholesterol below 40 mg/dL in men and below 50 mg/dL in women
  - Abdominal obesity (waist circumference over 40 inches in men and over 35 inches in women)
  - Elevated BP (130/85 mm Hg or higher)
  - Glucose intolerance (fasting blood glucose above 110 mg/dL).
- Treatment of metabolic syndrome is a secondary target in managing dyslipidemia. That is, after LDL cholesterol is reduced, further risk reduction can be achieved by treating the metabolic syndrome.
- Likewise, weight reduction and hyperglycemia and hypertension treatment should be aggressive to reduce the risk of CHD.

Table 10-3. Treatment Recommendations Based on Direct Measurement of Lipid Subclasses

Elevated LDL	Statin
Elevated Lp(a)	Niacin
Elevated IDL	Statin + niacin, fibrate
Pattern B, A/B	Omega-3 fatty acids, niacin, fibrate, statin
Low HDL2	Omega-3 fatty acids, niacin, fibrate
VLDL, Triglycerides	Omega-3 fatty acids, niacin, fibrate, some statins

NEW APPROACHES TO LIPID ASSESSMENT

- While several different methods exist, subparticles in lipoproteins are generally determined through electrophoresis, which separates the serum cholesterol based on the size of particles.
- LDL is most often calculated and not directly measured. When calculated it predicts 40% of the variance in CHD. However, when LDL is measured directly the prediction increases to 90%.
  - LDL, HDL, VLDL, triglycerides, non-HDL (LDL + VLDL) have same range as traditional tests.
  - Subclass measurement of HDL (2a, 2b, 3a, 3b, and 3c) and LDL (I, IIa, IIb, IIIa, IIIb, IVa, IVb) are measured along with lipoprotein (a), IDL, and VLDL.
    - Smaller LDL particles are more atherogenic than larger LDL particles.
    - HDL-2 is larger and most protective while HDL-3 is smaller, denser, and least protective.
  - Pattern A, which is desirable, can be determined.
  - Pattern B, which has the highest risk for atherosclerosis and metabolic syndrome, is identified.
- Therapies can be more appropriately prescribed based on subclasses. Table 10–3 provides the overview of treatment based on knowledge of subclasses.

SUMMARY

This chapter provided an overview of lipids, lipid metabolism, and risk in cardiovascular disease. Current treatment goals and therapies are part of the ATP III guidelines. The fourth edition will be published in the near future so be sure to stay updated on this information. More data on the use of subclasses of lipid components will continue to drive risk reduction efforts.

REFERENCES

Berra, K. (2008). Lipid lowering therapy today: Treating the high-risk cardiovascular patient. *Journal of Cardiovascular Nursing, 23*(5), 414–421.

Expert Panel on Detection, Evaluation, and Treatment of High Blood Cholesterol in Adults. (2001). Executive summary of the third report of the National Cholesterol Education Program (NCEP) Expert Panel on Detection, Evaluation, and Treatment of High Blood Cholesterol in Adults (Adult Treatment Panel III). *JAMA, 285*, 2486–2497.

Genest, J., Libby, P., & Gotto, A. M. (2005). Lipoprotein disorders and cardiovascular disease. In D. P. Zipes, P. Libby, R. O. Bonow, & E. Braunwald (Eds.), *Braunwald's heart disease: A textbook of cardiovascular medicine* (pp. 1013–1033). Philadelphia: Elsevier-Saunders.

Gissi-HF Investigators, Tavazzi, L., Maggioni, A. P., Marchioli, R., Barlera, S., Franzosi, M. G., ... Tognoni, G. (2008). Effect of n-3 polyunsaturated fatty acids in patients with chronic heart failure (the GISSI-HF trial): A randomised, double-blind, placebo-controlled trial. *Lancet, 372*(9645), 1223–1230.

Grundy, S. M., Cleeman, J. I., Merz, C. N., Brewer, H. B. Jr., Clark, L. T., Hunninghake, D. B., ... American Heart Association. (2004). Implications of recent clinical trials for the National Cholesterol Education Program Adult Treatment Panel III Guidelines. *Circulation, 110*, 227–239.

Hughes, S. (2007). Dyslipidemia. In D. Moser & B. Reigel (Eds.), *Cardiac nursing: A companion to Braunwald's heart disease* (pp. 418–430). St. Louis, MO: Elsevier-Saunders.

Jarvis, C. M., Hayman, L. L., Braun, L. T., Schwertz, D. W., Ferrans, C. E., Piano, M. R. (2007). Cardiovascular risk factors and metabolic syndrome in alcohol and nicotine dependent men and women. *Journal of Cardiovascular Nursing 22*(3), 429–435.

Ridker, P. M., Danielson, E., Fonseca, F. A., Genest, J., Gotto, A. M. Jr, Kastelein, J. J., ... JUPITER Study Group. (2008). Rosuvastatin to prevent vascular events in men and women with elevated C-reactive protein. *New England Journal of Medicine, 359*, 2195–2207.

Pagana, K. D. (2007). What's the latest on lipoproteins? *American Nurse Today, 2*(11), 41–42.

11

Pathophysiologic Processes

Pathophysiology is the study of disrupted function and the mechanisms of disease. Pathophysiologic processes interfere with the provision of basic cellular survival needs (oxygen, nutrients, waste removal, electrolyte and acid–base balance) and cause cellular injury and death, which disrupt tissue, organ, and system function. This chapter reviews the pathophysiology of major cardiac and vascular conditions.

PATHOPHYSIOLOGIC STIMULI

Stimuli
- Hypoxia, lack of sufficient oxygen to maintain aerobic metabolism, is the most common cause of cellular injury.
- Ischemia, lack of sufficient blood supply to tissues, is the most common cause of cellular hypoxia. Ischemia injures tissues faster than hypoxia does because insufficient nutrients are supplied to tissues (restricting anaerobic metabolism) and lactic acid builds up.
- Physical agents: mechanical trauma, pressure or temperature gradients, and irradiation
- Chemical agents: drugs and poisons (alcohol)
- Microorganisms and their toxins
- Genetic defects
- Nutritional imbalances: protein, vitamin, or mineral deficiency
- Cellular and chemical components of immune and inflammatory responses

Response

Cellular response to pathophysiologic stimuli occurs along a continuum from adaptation through injury to death. Cellular structure and function is disturbed or destroyed.

CELLULAR STRUCTURE AND FUNCTION

Cytoplasm, the internal compartment of the cell, contains organelles and cytosol.

Organelles
- Organelles (little organs) are membrane-bound compartments within the cell that have specialized functions.
  - Mitochondria generate cellular energy through aerobic metabolism.
  - Endoplasmic reticulum (ER) provides a large surface within the cell on which chemical reactions can occur.
  - Ribosomes synthesize protein.
  - Golgi apparatus (GA) processes and packages chemicals for transport to more distant cells. The GA also produces polysaccharides, modifies some activating enzymes, and produces lysosomes.
  - Lysosomes contain digestive enzymes and peroxisomes contain oxidative enzymes. Peroxisomes play a major role in lipid metabolism.
  - Nucleus contains large quantities of deoxyribonucleic acid (DNA), which forms the genes that regulate and differentiate cell function.
- Cytosol is the fluid medium in which the organelles are suspended.

Plasma and Intracellular Membranes
- Plasma membrane surrounds the entire cell and separates intracellular and extracellular fluid compartments. Characteristics of the plasma membrane include the following:
  - Consists of a double layer of lipid molecules (the lipid bilayer).
  - Proteins, which are anchored on or in the lipid bilayer, transport, and exchange material between the cell and its environment.
  - Damage to or altered function of the plasma membrane is a common, early response to pathophysiologic stimuli.
- Cell junctions are specialized regions on the plasma membrane that link individual cells into tissues and allow small molecules to pass from cell to cell. Three kinds of junctions have been identified.
  - Desmosomes hold cells together and maintain structural stability.
    - Cardiac intercalated discs maintain the functional integration of myocardial cells.
  - Tight junctions prevent the leakage of small molecules between adjacent cells.
  - Gap junctions coordinate the activity of adjacent cells.
    - Synchronize contraction of myocardial cells.
    - Facilitate the rapid spread of action potentials in neural tissues.
  - Opening or loosening of cell junctions allows potassium to leak out of and water to move into injured cells.
- Intracellular membranes surround the organelles and allow specific functions to occur within each.

- Substances can move across the plasma and intracellular membranes by passive or active processes.
  - Passive movement does not require cell energy.
    - Diffusion is the movement of a substance from a region of higher concentration to a region of lower concentration down a concentration gradient.
    - Osmosis is the net movement of water across a semipermeable membrane, which separates compartments with different solute concentrations. Water moves into the compartment with the higher solute concentration.
    - Filtration is the net movement of water because of a pressure gradient. Water moves from an area of higher pressure to one of lower pressure.
    - Facilitated diffusion uses a carrier protein to move a substance across a semipermeable membrane. Glucose uses insulin (carrier protein) to move into cells.
  - Active movement is energy-dependent. When pathophysiologic processes interfere with energy production (adenosine triphosphate, ATP), active movement slows or ceases.
    - The sodium-potassium pump (Na+–K+–ATPase) maintains fluid and electrolyte balance between extracellular and intracellular fluid (cytosol).
      - Failure of the sodium-potassium pump produces cellular swelling—intracellular sodium concentration increases and draws water into the cell (osmosis).
    - An active calcium transport system (Ca++–ATPase) maintains differential calcium concentrations in the cytosol and organelles.
      - Failure of the calcium transport system interferes with muscle contraction, cell signaling, and plasma membrane function.
      - Calcium ions are important in the regulation of cardiac muscle contraction.
        - Calcium is released from the sarcoplasmic reticulum and transverse tubules.
        - Calcium is required for actin and myosin filaments to contract.
    - An active hydrogen transport system (H+–ATPase) is one mechanism used to maintain acid–base balance.

Electrical Properties of Cells

- An electrical gradient (membrane potential) exists across the plasma membrane of all living cells.
  - The electrical charge within resting cells is more negative than the charge outside cells because of the abundance of intracellular ions with a negative charge.
  - Cardiac, skeletal muscle, and nerve cells are excitable cells. Excitable cells are capable of generating and propelling an action potential along the plasma membrane.
    - Resting membrane potential in excitable cells is minus 70 to minus 90 mV. Excitable cells are polarized when at their resting potential.
    - In resting cardiac cells, there is a slow inward flow of positively charged ions. When the membrane potential reaches threshold (minus 60 to minus 70 mV), specialized channels open in the plasma membrane and positively charged ions rush into the cell.
      - Reduction of cell membrane potential to a less negative value is depolarization.
      - Restoration of the cell to its resting membrane potential is repolarization.

Cardiac Action Potential (AP)

- Myocardial cell action potential (see Figure 11–1)
  - Phase 0—depolarization—is characterized by the rapid upstroke.
    - Membrane channels open and sodium ions rush into the cell.
    - Membrane potential changes from approximately –90 millivolts (mV) at rest to +20 mV.
  - Phase 1 represents a brief period of repolarization.
    - Inward sodium movement slows and slow inward calcium movement begins.
    - Membrane potential changes from approximately +20 mV to +5 mV.
  - Phase 2 is the plateau phase during which cardiac contraction occurs.
    - Slow inward calcium current.
    - Slow downward drift of membrane potential from approximately +5 to –5 mV.
  - Phase 3 is repolarization.
    - Potassium moves out of cell.
    - Membrane potential changes from approximately –5 to –80 mV.
  - Phase 4 is the resting membrane potential.
    - Corresponds to diastole.
    - Approximately –80 to –90 mV.
- Specialized conduction cells: sinoatrial (SA) and atrioventricular (AV) nodes
  - Slow spontaneous rise in resting membrane potential because of a slow inward sodium leak (Phase 4).
    - Catecholamines increase heart rate (HR) by increasing rate of rise to threshold.
    - Acetylcholine (vagal neurotransmitter) reduces rate of rise and slows HR
  - When membrane reaches threshold (approximately –55 mV), rapid depolarization (Phase 0) occurs.
  - No plateau phase; immediate repolarization (Phase 3).
- Pathophysiologic processes that interfere with plasma membrane permeability or deplete cellular energy affect the electrical properties of cells.
  - Cardiac dysrhythmia results from interference with the generation or propagation of cardiac APs.
- Antidysrhythmic drugs are grouped according to their effects on the cardiac AP. (See Chapter 15.)

Figure 11–1. Action Potential of a Cardiac Muscle Cell

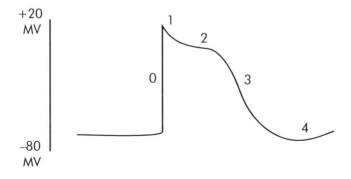

Cellular Energy Metabolism

- Adenosine triphosphate (ATP), the major carrier of cellular energy, is required for many cellular processes: muscle contraction, active transport, and biochemical synthesis, for example.
- ATP is generated from chemical processes during the metabolism of food (carbohydrates, fats, and proteins).
  - Aerobic metabolism and energy generation occur in the mitochondria.
    - Fats, proteins, and carbohydrates are broken down and combined with molecular oxygen to form carbon dioxide and water.
    - Krebs cycle (also called the citric acid or the tricarboxylic acid cycle) is the final common pathway for metabolism of pyruvate (from glucose), amino acids (from proteins), and fatty acids (from fat).
    - Oxidative phosphorylation is the process in which inorganic phosphate couples with adenosine diphosphate (ADP) to form ATP.
    - The net gain of energy from aerobic metabolism of one mole of glucose is 38 moles of ATP.
  - Anaerobic metabolism occurs in the cytoplasm.
    - Glucose is converted to pyruvate and ADP is converted to ATP in the process, called glycolysis.
    - The net gain of energy from anaerobic metabolism of one mole of glucose is two moles of ATP and two moles of pyruvate.
      - If oxygen is present, pyruvate moves into the Krebs cycle.
      - In the absence of oxygen, pyruvate is converted to lactic acid, builds up, and stops the metabolic process.
    - Anaerobic metabolism generates much less energy (one mole of glucose yields two moles of ATP) than aerobic metabolism (1 mole of glucose yields 38 moles of ATP).
    - Despite inefficient energy production, anaerobic metabolism prevents cell injury for a few minutes under hypoxic conditions.

Cellular Reproduction and Regeneration

- Most cells have the ability to reproduce through mitosis.
- Labile cells (for example, vascular endothelial cells and platelets) regenerate frequently and have a short life span.
- Stable cells (for example, osteophytes) retain the ability to regenerate but do so only under special circumstances.
- Permanent cells do not regenerate or regenerate very slowly (for example, nerve and muscle cells).

Cellular Communication

- Receptors on the plasma membrane bind with messenger molecules to produce a specific response.
  - Primary messengers include hormones, neurotransmitters, and local mediators.
  - When messengers and receptor bind, four types of cellular response may occur.
    - Change in membrane permeability and the electrical properties of cells
    - Alter contraction of muscle cells
    - Alter secretion
    - Alter cellular metabolism

- Other receptors, when activated, regulate intracellular responses through the release of secondary messengers.
  - G-protein–linked receptors increase the intracellular concentration of cyclic adenosine monophosphate (AMP).
    - β_1 receptors in the plasma membrane of myocardial cells bind with norepinephrine and activate cyclic AMP to increase the force of contraction.
  - Inositol-phospholipid (IP3) linked receptors increase intracellular calcium and activate protein kinase C, which activates other intracellular proteins.
    - Muscarinic receptors of myocardial cells may act by way of the IP3 system.
    - Muscarinic receptors are part of the parasympathetic autonomic system.
- Autonomic nervous system regulates cardiovascular function.
  - Sympathetic nervous system (SNS)
    - Preganglionic SNS neurons release the neurotransmitter acetylcholine (ACh).
    - Postganglionic SNS neurons release norepinephrine (NE) at the effector site.
    - Receptors are present on the target cells: α_1, α_2, β_1, and β_2.
      - Myocardial cells have β_1 receptors that, when stimulated, increase HR, contractile force, and conduction velocity.
      - Arterioles, including coronary arteries, have α and β_2 receptors.
        - When stimulated, α receptors produce vasoconstriction.
        - When stimulated, β_2 receptors produce vasodilation.
    - The number or density of receptors activated determines the intensity of response.
      - β_1 receptors in cardiac tissue can be up- or down-regulated as a response to frequent bombardment or infrequent stimulation.
        - Down-regulation occurs when receptor sites are overstimulated for a prolonged period of time and the receptors tire. As a protective mechanism, the receptors move intracellular result in a functional decrease in receptors available for stimulation.
        - Up-regulation occurs when the receptors that have moved intracellular return to their normal position on the cell surface, resulting in a functional increase in receptor sites available for stimulation and you can get over-expression of the receptor activity.
      - Distribution of receptors in vascular beds is variable; for example, skin, mucosa, and cerebral arterioles have primarily α receptors.
  - Parasympathetic nervous system
    - Parasympathetic postganglionic neurons release the neurotransmitter ACh, which acts on muscarinic receptors.
      - Myocardial cells have muscarinic receptors that, when stimulated, decrease HR, contractile force, and conduction velocity.

CELLULAR INJURY AND DEATH

Apoptosis

Apoptosis (programmed cell death) is designed to eliminate unwanted cells through an internally programmed series of events. It can be a normal process during embryologic development or can be initiated by toxins. When unchecked it can lead to problems.

- Stimuli of apoptosis include injurious agents, withdrawal of growth factors or hormones, and the action of specific death substances (e.g., tissue necrosis factor).

- Intracellular proteins can inhibit or promote the cell's death.
- Execution enzymes (caspase) initiate a cascade of cellular degradation that results in the formation of apoptotic bodies that contain organelles and cytosol.
- Phagocytes devour the apoptotic bodies. The dead cells leave without a trace—little or no inflammation occurs.

Necrosis
Necrosis refers to cell or tissue death characterized by cellular swelling and the breakdown of proteins and organelles. General mechanisms include
- Energy depletion and decreased ATP generation
- Formation of toxic oxygen-derived free radicals (OFR)
- Disruption of calcium homeostasis and increased calcium concentration in the cytosol
- Defects in plasma membrane permeability
- Irreversible damage to mitochondria

As cells undergo necrosis, scar tissue develops in the area; scar tissue is not able to respond to electrical stimulation and does not have intrinsic contractile ability.

VASCULAR STRUCTURE AND FUNCTION

Wall Structure
- Basic constituents of the vascular wall are endothelium, smooth muscle, and the extracellular matrix, which is made up of elastic elements and collagen.
- Endothelial cells (vascular endothelium) have multiple functions.
    - Maintain vessel permeability
    - Release anticoagulant substances: prostacyclin, thrombomodulin
    - Release a balance of antithrombotic (plasminogen activator) and prothrombotic (von Willebrand factor, tissue factor, plasminogen activator inhibitor) substances
    - Modulate vascular tone and blood flow
    - Regulate immune and inflammatory reactions by controlling leukocyte interaction with the vessel wall
    - Modify lipoprotein deposit and metabolism within the vessel wall
    - Regulate growth of smooth muscle cells in the vessel wall
- Smooth muscle cells determine lumen size and vascular resistance, i.e., vasoconstriction and dilation. Smooth muscle cells may also
    - Synthesize collagen and elastin
    - Elaborate growth factors and cytokines
    - Migrate to the intima and proliferate

Arteries
- Arteries have three concentric layers.
    - Intima: closest to the lumen, made up of vascular endothelial cells
    - Media: middle layer of smooth muscle encased in the internal and external elastic lamina
    - Adventitia: outer layer made up of connective tissue and encasing nerve fibers and the vasa vasorum
- Vasa vasorum (vessels of the vessel) perforates the adventitia and external elastic lamina to nourish the media. The intima obtains oxygen and nutrients directly from circulating blood.

Small Vessels

- Arterioles, the smallest branches of the arterial tree, are the principal source of vascular resistance and convert blood flow from pulsatile to steady current.
- Capillaries have thin walls primarily made up of endothelium supported by a thin basement membrane.
- Postcapillary venules

Veins

- Veins are large caliber, thin-walled vessels.
  - Large capacity—approximately two-thirds of circulating blood is in the veins.
  - Relatively little support; easily compressed.
  - Valves prevent reverse flow, particularly in the extremities.

Lymphatics

- Lymphatics are thin-walled, endothelium-lined channels that drain interstitial fluid to the blood.
- Lymph is drained through a series of lymphatic ducts that eventually drain into the right or left subclavian vein. Lymph enters the venous circulation shortly before reaching the right atrium of the heart.

CARDIAC STRUCTURE AND FUNCTION

- The heart is a four-chamber, four-valve organ designed to pump venous blood to the lungs for oxygenation and arterial blood to body to supply oxygen and other substances to body tissues. (See Figures 11–2 and 11–3.)
  - The muscle weighs approximately 350 grams and is the size of the person's fist.
  - The heart generally is positioned obliquely in the mediastinum between the right and left lung.
- The heart has three layers:
  - The epicardium or outer layer, part of the pericardium
  - The thick, muscular myocardium anchored with a fibrous skeleton
  - The endocardium or inner lining of the chamber
- The heart is surrounded by the pericardium.
  - Between the two layers of this sac (visceral and parietal layers), there is about 10 cc to 30 cc of pericardial fluid, which helps to prevent friction during cardiac movement.
  - The pericardium attaches to structures in the mediastinum. Functions of the pericardium are
    - Prevent displacement of the heart during acceleration, deceleration, gravitation pull, or movement.
    - Provide a physical barrier to protect against infection and inflammation.
    - Contains the pain receptors and baroreceptors important in the control of blood pressure

Chambers of the heart
- Chambers of the heart (see Figure 11–2) include
  - Right atrium (RA) receives blood from superior and inferior vena cava. It is a smooth, thin-walled (2 mm), low-pressure chamber collecting venous blood returning to the heart.

Figure 11–2. The Heart Chambers and Valves

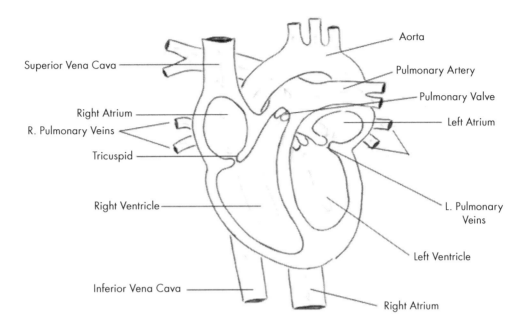

- Right ventricle (RV) is slightly thicker (3 mm to 5 mm), triangularly shaped, and constitutes most of the lower, anterior surface of the heart. The inflow portion receives blood from the right atrium and the outflow portion pushes blood into the pulmonary artery with contraction. The inner surface is trabeculated; that is, it has a strand of tissue projecting into the chamber because of papillary muscle formations.
- Left atrium (LA) receives blood from two right pulmonary veins and two left pulmonary veins. It is a thin-walled chamber like the right atrium.
- Left ventricle (LV) is also triangular in shape; it overlies the right ventricle but composes more of the posterior portion of the heart. It is much thicker (13 mm to 15 mm) with higher pressures (6 to 7 times the RV pressure) and trabeculated.
- The muscular septum divides the right and left sides of the heart.
  - The atrial septum separates the RA and LA.
  - The ventricular septum separates the RV and LV.

Heart Valves
- The valves of the heart provide for unidirectional flow of blood through the heart and vessels.
- There are four valves in the heart. (See Figure 11–2.) The mitral and tricuspid are referred to as atrioventricular valves and the aortic and pulmonic are semilunar valves.
  - The tricuspid valve separates the RA and RV.
    - There are three leaflets with thin, fibrous chordae tendineae attached.
    - The chordae tendineae connect the leaflets to the papillary muscles in the RV wall.
    - The tricuspid valve opens and closes with the tensing and relaxing of the papillary muscles.

– The pulmonic valve separates the RV and pulmonary artery and is called a semilunar valve.
  • It is constructed of three cusps.
  • It opens when pressure from the ventricle exceeds the pressure in the artery during ventricular contraction.
  • The pulmonic valve closes when pressure in the RV drops to the same pressure in the artery during relaxation of the ventricle.
– The mitral valve separates the LA and LV.
  • It has two leaflets with chordae tendineae.
  • It functions in the same way as the tricuspid valve.
– The aortic valve separates the LV and aorta.
  • It has the same semilunar valve structure as the pulmonic valve.
  • It functions the same way as the pulmonic valve.

Conduction System and the Cardiac Cycle

• The cardiac cycle describes the electrical and mechanical events occurring during each heartbeat.
• Electrical events are because of specialized tissue that conducts the electrical signal responsible for depolarization of muscle tissue that results in contraction of the myocardium.
  – The sinoatrial (SA) node is the pacemaker of the heart. It sends out the impulse in a rhythmic function across the RA and LA, resulting in atrial contraction. It is located in the upper anterior portion of the RA just under the superior vena cava.
  – The atrioventricular (AV) node is located in the lower portion of the RA septal wall and receives the impulse from the atrium. Here the impulse is slowed slightly to allow for atrial contraction.
  – The bundle of His stretches across the lower RA septal wall to the ventricular septum. It brings the impulse to the lower portion of the heart.
  – The bundle branches to the right and left bundles and carries the impulse to RV and LV.
  – Purkinje fibers are spread across the endocardial layer of the RV and LV. When the impulse reaches this area, the Purkinje fibers depolarize the ventricles, resulting in contraction of the RV and LV and the ejection of blood into the arteries.
• The SA node has the property of automaticity, which allows for regular firing of the specialized tissue to initiate the action potential. Other sites in the conduction system have the same property but will initiate the pacing impulse at a slower rate.
• Electrical events precede mechanical events in the cardiac cycle.
  – Each beat of the heart is one cardiac cycle.
  – Mechanical events include:
    • Systole or contraction with the ejection of blood
    • Diastole or relaxation with passive filling of the chambers
    • Stroke volume (SV) is the amount of blood ejected from the ventricle with a heart beat.

Hemodynamics

- Hemodynamics includes understanding the pressure and volume relationships in the heart.
  - Cardiac output (CO) is the volume of blood ejected from the heart in 1 minute and is determined by heart rate (HR) and SV (CO = HR x SV). Normal resting CO is 5 to 8 liters per minute based on body size. With extreme exercise in a healthy person it can increase to 20 to 30 liters per minute.
  - SV is determined by three factors.
    - Preload is the stretch of the ventricular fibers due the volume of blood in the RV or LV.
      - According to the Frank-Starling law, the greater the stretch, the stronger the contraction and thus the greater the SV.
      - However, there is a maximum point past which the contraction is weaker and SV falls.
      - For example, when a person is greatly dehydrated, the blood volume is decreased, SV is less, and HR must increase or else CO falls. But when rehydrated, SV, HR, and CO return to normal.
    - Afterload is the amount of resistance that the heart must overcome to eject the blood. This is a reflection of the degree of peripheral vascular resistance or hypertension that occurs. The more resistance, the harder it is to eject blood.
    - Contractility consists of all of the other factors that compose the cardiac muscle's ability to contract normally.
- Pathologic conditions will decrease CO by limiting SV because of muscle damage, ischemia, or valve problem.
- Many medications are aimed at decreasing preload (diuretics), decreasing afterload (antihypertensives), or increasing contractility (inotropes).
- Right and left side circulation is synchronized so that right and left atrial systole occurs almost simultaneously and right and left ventricular systole occur nearly simultaneously. Figure 11–3 illustrates the flow of blood through the heart.

Figure 11–3. Circulation of Blood Through the Heart

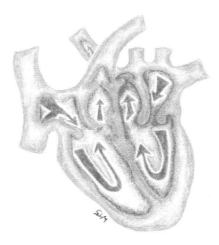

Coronary Blood Flow

- The coronary arteries lie on the epicardial surface of the myocardium. They are the first blood vessels off the aorta just above the aortic valve. The arteries burrow in the myocardium and the endocardial surface of the heart is the last to receive blood flow. (See Figure 11–4.)
- Coronary arteries supply the blood flow to the myocardium.
  - The right coronary artery (RCA) lies in the grove between the RA and RV and wraps around the right lateral wall to the posterior of the heart. It then runs down the ventricular septum to supply blood to the inferior wall of the LV. It also supplies the RA and much of the RV along with the SA and AV nodes.
  - The left main coronary artery divides shortly after origin into the left anterior descending (LAD) and the left circumflex (CX) arteries.
    - The LAD runs in the anterior septal groove and supplies the septum, anterior LV, and anterior RV. It also supplies the left and proximal right bundle branches of the conduction system.
    - The CX artery supplies the LA and the lateral wall of the LV and the high posterior wall of the LV.
    - In some people, the CX supplies the inferior wall of the LV instead of the RCA. This is referred to as left dominance.

Figure 11–4. Coronary Arteries

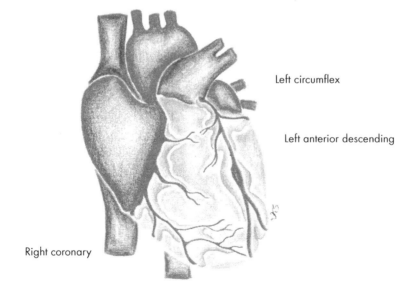

Left circumflex

Left anterior descending

Right coronary

CARDIAC MUSCLE CELLS

Cardiac muscle cells (myocytes) have five major components:
- Cell membrane (sarcolemma) and T tubules for conduction
- Sarcoplasmic reticulum, a calcium reservoir for excitation-contraction coupling
- Contractile elements
- Mitochondria
- Nucleus

Sarcomere
Sarcomere, the contractile unit of cardiac muscle, is an orderly arrangement of actin and myosin together with the regulatory proteins, troponin and tropomyosin.

Intercalated Discs
- Intercalated discs that permit both mechanical and ionic coupling promote functional integration of myocytes.
    - Gap junctions, plasma membrane channels, directly link the cytoplasmic components of neighboring cardiac cells.

CEREBRAL CIRCULATION

- The cerebral circulation begins with the carotid and vertebral vessels that arise from brachiocephalic trunk, a branch off the aorta. There is a right and left version of this circulation. (See Figure 11–5.)
- The common carotid artery branches into the internal and external carotid arteries.
    - The external carotid supplies the face.
    - The internal carotid supplies the anterior portion of the brain and gives rise to the anterior and middle cerebral arteries.
- The vertebral artery gives rise to the basilar artery and the posterior cerebral artery.
- The Circle of Willis is a special connection of arteries in the brain. The right and left circulations are connected as well as the anterior and middle cerebral branches of the internal carotids and the posterior cerebral arteries from the vertebral circulation.

Figure 11–5. Cerebral Circulation

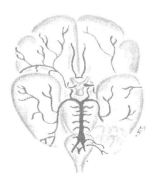
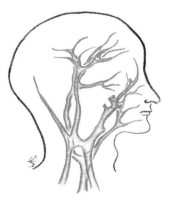

VASCULAR CELL RESPONSE TO INJURY

Injurious Stimuli
- Cytokines and inflammatory products
- Hemodynamic stress and lipids
- Microorganisms
- Components of the complement cascade
- Hypoxia

Endothelial Cell Response
- Endothelial cells are activated by vascular injury and may
  - Elaborate adhesion molecules and other inflammatory mediators,
  - Elaborate growth factors that contribute to vascular stenosis,
  - Elaborate vasoactive substances that produce vasoconstriction or vasodilation, and
  - Elaborate pro- or anticoagulant substances.
- Endothelial functions and response to injury are areas of active research.

Smooth Muscle Cell Response
- Vascular injury stimulates smooth muscle cell growth by disrupting the balance between inhibition and stimulation.
- Intimal wall thickening is an exaggerated healing response that can cause stenosis or occlusion of small vessels.

HYPOXIA AND ISCHEMIA

- Hypoxia, lack of sufficient oxygen at the tissue level, is the most common cause of cellular injury.
  - Molecular oxygen must be present for aerobic metabolism to occur.
  - As cellular oxygen tension decreases, mitochondrial energy production is reduced.
  - At a critical level, the cell shifts to anaerobic metabolism.
- Ischemia—lack of sufficient blood supply—accelerates tissue damage from hypoxia because of lack of fuel for anaerobic metabolism and the accumulation of metabolic waste products. Under resting conditions, tissues extract different amounts of oxygen from the blood. For example, myocardial cells extract 70% to 75% of the available oxygen, whereas peripheral muscle cells extract 30%. When stressed, peripheral cells increase oxygen extraction but myocardial cells cannot.

Causes of Hypoxia and Ischemia
- Decreased oxygen-carrying capacity (decreased amount or altered function of red blood cells and hemoglobin)
- Decreased oxygen saturation (due to pulmonary disease, fever, or acidosis)
- Impaired oxygen delivery (hypoperfusion or ischemia)
  - Stenosis or narrowing of blood vessels because of plaque formation
  - Thrombosis or embolism occluding vessels
  - Weakening and rupture of vessels
  - Decreased force of cardiac contraction

Effects of Hypoxia and Ischemia
- Energy depletion and decreased ATP synthesis because of shift to anaerobic metabolism
- Anaerobic metabolism leads to accumulation of lactic acid and cellular acidosis
- Reduced activity of Na+–K+ pump produces cellular swelling
- Reduced protein synthesis and lipid deposition
- End result is cellular necrosis

Functional Impact
- Coronary occlusion
  - Myocardial cells cease to contract within 60 seconds
  - Continued energy depletion leads to plasma and intracellular membrane damage
  - Irreversible injury to heart muscle occurs after 30 to 40 minutes
- Cerebral ischemia
  - Irreversible injury to brain cells by hypoxia occurs after 4 to 6 minutes.
  - Survival of brain cells depends, in part, on duration of ischemia, presence of collateral circulation, and the magnitude and rapidity of flow reduction.

Clinical Manifestations
- Cardiac dysfunction: dysrhythmia, decreased contractility
- Cerebral dysfunction: decreased level of consciousness, aphasia, motor deficits
- Pain: intermittent claudication, angina

Reperfusion Injury
- Reperfusion injury is cell damage that occurs after blood flow is returned to ischemic tissue. Reperfusion injury may be clinically significant in myocardial infarction (MI), after thrombolytic or angioplasty procedures, and stroke.
  - Reperfusion results in production of OFRs (oxygen-derived free radicals).
    - OFRs are highly toxic to vascular endothelium and to mitochondria.
    - OFRs damage the myocardial or brain cell and also the microvasculature.
  - Cytokines and adhesion molecules produced by ischemic cells initiate inflammation and further cell injury.
  - Reperfusion dysrhythmia may be because of increased calcium load or to OFRs.

INFLAMMATION

Inflammation is a defensive response of the body to cellular injury.

Causes of Inflammation
- Microorganisms
- Physical trauma with the release of blood into tissues
- Direct irritation because of physical, mechanical, or chemical injury
- Immune reaction, including autoimmune

Phases of Inflammation

- Purpose of inflammation is to rid the body of the causative agent and reduce injury.
- Acute inflammation begins immediately after cell injury and lasts a few minutes to several days.
  - Vascular phase
    - Neural reflex produces vasoconstriction of arterioles near site of injury.
    - Vasodilation (hyperemia) and increased blood flow follow vasoconstriction.
    - Plasma proteins leak into tissues and generate an osmotic pull that causes edema (swelling).
    - Movement of fluid into tissues (extravasation) increases red blood cell concentration and slows capillary circulation.
    - Endothelial cells lining capillaries and venules retract, producing spaces between cells (vascular permeability).
  - Cellular phase
    - Slowed capillary circulation and fluid extravasation cause white cells to line up along the vascular endothelium.
    - Adhesion molecules under the influence of inflammatory mediators cause the white cells to adhere to the vascular endothelium.
    - Lymphokines are released at the site of injury and attract white cells (chemotaxis).
    - White cells (first neutrophils, later macrophages) ingest invading organisms, dead cells, and cellular debris (phagocytosis).

Inflammatory Mediators

- A large number of substances—some not yet discovered, others not well characterized—mediate inflammation.
  - Vasoactive proteins
    - Histamine and serotonin, released from mast cells and platelets, cause arteriolar dilation and increase permeability of venules.
    - Prostaglandins potentiate the vascular action of histamine and serotonin and are involved in pain and fever response.
    - Platelet activating factor (PAF) increases vascular permeability, activates platelets, and increases leukocyte aggregation and adhesion.
  - Cytokines, produced by many cell types, modulate the function of other cells. Interleukin-1 (IL-1) and tumor necrosis factor (TNF) are major inflammatory cytokines.
    - IL-1 and TNF induce the synthesis of adhesion molecules and growth factors. They increase the thrombogenicity of the endothelial surface.
    - IL-1 and TNF induce systemic responses including fever, loss of appetite, sleepiness, and the release of corticosteroids.
    - TNF is a primary mediator of the hemodynamic effects of septic shock.
  - Nitric oxide (NO), a potent vasodilator, is released from vascular endothelium.
  - Intermediary substances in the complement cascade increase vascular permeability and vasodilation, white cell adhesion, and chemotaxis, and enhance phagocytosis. Terminal elements of the complement cascade break down plasma and intracellular membranes and cause cell lysis.

- The clotting system forms a fibrinous mesh at the site of inflammation, which traps microorganisms and prevents the spread of infection. Fibrin forms a clot that stops bleeding and provides a framework for healing and repair.
- Kinins (especially bradykinin) promote vasodilation and vascular permeability, and contribute to the pain response.

Resolution
- Acute inflammation resolves through cell regeneration and scarring or becomes chronic.
- Chronic inflammation may follow acute inflammation or may occur as a distinct process.
  - Dense infiltration of lymphocytes and macrophages
  - Macrophages may wall off an infected site, producing a granuloma

Functional Impact
- Vasculitis is a general term for inflammation of blood vessels.
  - Arteritis or angiitis are terms for inflammation of an artery.
  - Phlebitis is inflammation of a vein.
- Myocarditis, pericarditis, and endocarditis are inflammatory processes affecting cardiac function.
- Atherosclerosis is viewed currently as a chronic inflammatory process.

ATHEROSCLEROSIS

Definition
- Atherosclerosis is the process of lipid deposition within the intimal layer of large and medium-sized arteries.
- Arteriosclerosis involves deterioration of the intima and media of smaller arteries and arterioles. (See Figure 11–6.)

Figure 11-6. Coronary Lesion

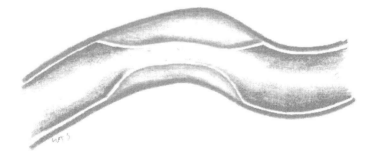

Lesion Progression
- Fatty streak is an early, detectable lesion that can occur within first decade of life.
  - Mainly intracellular lipid accumulation
  - No obstruction to blood flow; clinically silent
- Atheromatous plaque develops from
  - Extracellular lipid accumulation within the intima
  - Fibrous cap made up of smooth muscle cells encapsulates the lipid deposits
  - Shoulder of the cap is a common site of rupture
    - Macrophages are active at the shoulder
  - May be clinically silent or symptomatic
- Fibroatheroma
  - Lipid core and fibrotic layers
  - May be mainly calcified or mainly fibrotic
  - May be clinically silent or symptomatic
- Complicated lesions culminate in
  - Calcification that leads to arterial stiffness and reduces accommodation to pulsatile flow.
  - Areas of rupture and ulceration that may dislodge debris and cause embolization.
  - Hemorrhage into the plaque that may produce hematoma, which impinges on the vessel lumen.
  - Superimposed thrombosis at the site of injury may occlude the vessel lumen.
  - Complicated lesions may be clinically silent or symptomatic.

Inflammatory Response Hypothesis
- Damage to vascular endothelium by established and emerging cardiovascular risk factors (e.g., hyperlipidemia, hypertension, increased homocysteine).
- Chronic inflammatory response of the arterial wall
  - Increased endothelial permeability that allows low-density lipoprotein cholesterol (LDL) to move into the intimal layer. (See Figure 11–7.)
  - LDL is oxidized and attracts macrophages.
  - Macrophages take up LDL and become foam cells.
  - Enzymes are released that weaken the fibrotic cap.
- Progressive development of plaque is associated with continuation of the inflammatory response.

Location of Lesions
Atheromatous plaque can occur in any artery; however, certain sites are affected more commonly.
- Lower abdominal aorta is most common
- Other sites in descending order of frequency
  - Coronary arteries
  - Popliteal arteries
  - Descending thoracic aorta
  - Internal carotid arteries
  - Vessels of the Circle of Willis

Figure 11–7. Lesion Development

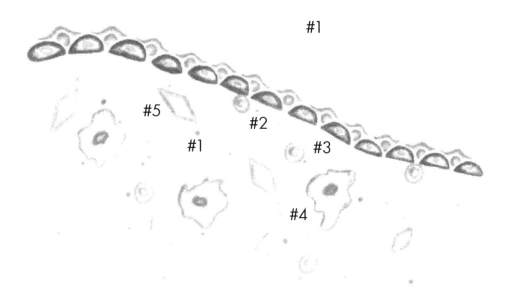

1. Lipid infiltration into intimal layer of vessel
2. Inflammatory cytokines gather
3. Lipid oxidation
4. Macrophage engulfs oxidized LDL
5. Smooth muscle cells migrate from medial layer to intima
6. Apoptosis

Functional Impact
- Atheromatous plaque protrudes into vessel lumen and decreases blood flow.
- Plaque encroaches on the medial layer and weakens the vessel wall, leading to aneurysm, vessel rupture, or thrombosis.
- Complicated lesions become friable and embolize, occlude vessel lumen, or thrombus develops at the site.

THROMBOSIS AND EMBOLISM

- Thrombosis is the formation of blood clot within the vasculature.
- An embolus is a piece of thrombus that breaks off and travels within the bloodstream.
  - Other substances (e.g., fat, air) may enter the bloodstream, travel as a bolus, and occlude smaller vessels.
- Thrombosis depends on three general components.
  - Endothelial injury
  - Platelet adhesion
  - Activation of the coagulation cascade

Causes of Thrombosis and Embolism
- Triad of Virchow: three factors that increase the risk of thrombosis
  - Injury to the vessel wall
  - Decreased blood flow
  - Hypercoagulability
- Elevated plasma homocysteine is toxic to the vascular endothelium, promotes thrombosis, increases collagen production, and decreases availability of nitric oxide (NO).
  - Nutritional deficiency of B vitamins is associated with high homocysteine level.

Effects of Thrombosis and Embolism
- Thrombus narrows vessel lumen and reduces blood flow, producing distal hypoperfusion and ischemia.
- Embolism travels through the bloodstream and occludes more distal vessels.
  - Venous embolism travels to the pulmonary vasculature, where it becomes trapped.
  - Arterial embolism reduces or blocks arterial blood supply distal to its origin.
- Thrombus within a vessel produces a local inflammatory reaction.

Functional Impact
- Myocardial infarction (MI)
- Ischemic and thrombotic stroke
- Deep vein thrombosis (DVT)
- Acute arterial insufficiency
- Pulmonary embolism

ALTERED VASCULAR FUNCTION

Arterial
- Coronary heart disease (CHD)
  - Atherosclerosis of the coronary arteries is the primary mechanism. (See Figure 11–6.)
  - Plaque or atheroma partially occludes the vessel lumen.
    - Asymptomatic until occluding 75% or more of blood supply
      - Initially, myocardial cells avoid ischemia through autoregulation of coronary blood flow.
      - Collateral circulation develops among smaller arteries and may adequately nourish myocardium under nonstress conditions.
  - Pathophysiology of myocardial ischemia
    - Myocardial ischemia results when myocardial oxygen demand exceeds supply.
    - Factors that increase oxygen demand:
      - Increased heart rate
      - Increased systolic wall tension
      - Increased contractility
    - Myocardial cells shift to anaerobic metabolism and the resulting accumulation of lactic acid impairs cardiac contractility.
    - Ischemia is reversible if the oxygen imbalance is corrected.

- Pathophysiology of MI
  - Infarction results from prolonged ischemia. Cell death characterizes MI.
  - Infarction is irreversible and the necrotic cells are replaced by scar tissue.
  - Replacement of myocardial cells with scar tissue impairs cardiac function.
    - Reduced contractility and abnormal wall motion
    - Increased ventricular compliance (stiffening), which impedes diastolic filling
    - Reduced stroke volume and ejection fraction
    - Increased left ventricular end diastolic pressure
  - Acute MI has a central area of necrosis that is surrounded by an area of injury; an area of ischemia surrounds the area of injury.
    - Signs of infarction, injury, and ischemia may be observed on the electrocardiogram.
    - When myocardial cells die, they liberate intracellular proteins (troponin and myosin) and enzymes (lactic dehydrogenase and creatine kinase) that can be used diagnostically.
- Cerebrovascular insufficiency
  - Transient ischemic attacks (TIA) result in temporary neurologic dysfunction.
    - Duration 15 minutes to 24 hours
    - Caused by thrombosis that narrows an atherosclerotic cerebral vessel
    - Major risk factor for subsequent ischemic stroke
  - Stroke results from the occlusion of cerebral arteries by thrombosis or embolism or from hemorrhage. Figure 11–5 provides a view of the cerebral circulation.
  - Ischemic stroke is caused by thrombosis or embolism. Ischemia is the etiology of 84% of strokes.
    - The central ischemic core is surrounded by a larger area called the ischemic penumbra.
    - Oxygen to the core is depleted within 10 seconds of occlusion and irreversible neuron damage occurs within 2 to 4 minutes.
    - The ischemic penumbra remains potentially viable for longer periods.
  - Pathophysiology of ischemic stroke
    - Mitochondria in ischemic cells are unable to generate sufficient ATP; there is a shift to anaerobic metabolism with accumulation of lactic acid and OFR.
      - Within the ischemic core, cellular acidosis leads to cell death.
    - Within the ischemic penumbra, cellular ionic gradients are disrupted, leading to cellular swelling, a shift in electrolyte balance, and the accumulation of glutamate, the major excitatory neurotransmitter.
      - Excitotoxicity (accumulation of glutamate in ischemic tissue) causes cell damage by over-stimulation and persistent opening of calcium channels, producing toxic intracellular calcium concentration.
    - Increased intracellular calcium concentration activates prostaglandins, cytokines, leukotrienes, and NO.
    - Cell products destroy plasma and intracellular membranes and cause breakdown of the blood—brain barrier, increased vascular permeability and edema, and cell death.

- Thrombotic stroke
  - Thrombus forms on atherosclerotic plaque and occludes the blood vessel; occurs most commonly at curves and bifurcations.
    - Vessels affected commonly include the internal carotid artery, vertebral and basilar arteries, the middle cerebral artery (MCA), the posterior cerebral artery (PCA), and the anterior cerebral artery (ACA).
  - Site of occlusion determines the clinical manifestations.
    - Collateral circulation may compensate for obstruction proximal to the Circle of Willis; obstruction distal to the Circle of Willis results in infarction.
    - Thrombotic stroke may progress to cerebral infarction.
    - Location and amount of intracerebral damage determines recovery.
- Embolic stroke
  - Heart is the main source of emboli; less common sources include fat, air, or tumor emboli.
  - Embolus lodges most frequently in the MCA.
  - A large embolus may break into smaller ones that occlude smaller, more distal branches.
- Hemorrhagic stroke
  - Intracerebral hemorrhage is caused most frequently by hypertension (HTN).
    - Elevated blood pressure weakens the vessel and leads to rupture.
    - Charcot-Bouchard aneurysms that form at the bifurcation of small intracerebral arteries in people with HTN are a frequent source of bleeding.
    - In large bleeds, the blood forms a mass that compresses and disrupts surrounding brain tissue.
    - Blood in the parenchyma of the brain causes extensive neuronal destruction.
      - Blood is reabsorbed eventually.
      - Remaining area is filled with connective (scar) tissue.
- Subarachnoid hemorrhage: bleeding into the subarachnoid space
  - Most result from congenital malformation of cerebrovascular beds
  - May accompany cerebral tumor, trauma, atherosclerosis, or infection
- Cerebral aneurysm: a congenital weakness in the middle layer of the vessel results in a saccular out-pouching at the weakened area.
  - Fusiform cerebral aneurysms result from weakening of the middle layer of the vessel because of atherosclerosis.
- Arteriovenous malformations (AVM) are developmental defects of cerebral vasculature.
  - Veins connect with the artery without an intermediate capillary bed.
  - Higher pressure in the arterial circulation is transmitted to the weaker venous system and causes rupture.
- Occlusive disease of extremities produces ischemia in distal tissues.
  - Iliac bifurcation of the aorta and the femoral popliteal narrowing are the most common sites.
  - Gradual occlusion results in development of collateral circulation that prevents symptoms for a variable period of time.
    - Collateral circulation is native, undeveloped blood vessels that enlarge and develop in response to inflammatory mediators of ischemia.

- Aortic and large artery aneurysm
  - Fusiform aneurysm is a circumferential arterial dilation usually related to atherosclerosis and weakening of the middle layer of the arterial wall.
    - Abdominal aortic aneurysms arise below the renal arteries and may extend to include the iliac arteries.
    - Thoracic aneurysms are located in the ascending aorta, aortic arch, or descending segment of the thoracic aorta.
  - Aortic dissection occurs when tearing and degeneration of the medial layer allow blood to separate the aorta's intimal layer from the adventitial layer.
    - Hematoma forms in the area of separation.
    - Aortic dissection is associated with HTN and with Marfan syndrome.
  - Saccular aneurysms are outpouching on one side of aorta.
    - Saccular aneurysms are associated with syphilis and congenital malformations.
    - Risk of rupture
- Raynaud's phenomenon
  - Episodic constriction of the small arteries or arterioles of the extremities, causing intermittent pallor and cyanosis of the skin of the fingers, toes, ears, or nose.
    - Pallor is caused by spasm of the arterioles and possibly the venules that produces decreased or absent capillary flow.
    - Cyanosis results from capillary dilation and slow blood flow.
    - Vasoconstriction may be followed by hyperemia because of a reactive vasodilation.
- Vasculitis is inflammation of the vessel wall. Two most common mechanisms are immune-mediated inflammation and direct invasion of the vessel wall by infectious pathogens.
  - Large vessels; may involve medium-sized arteries also
    - Infective aortitis: invasion of the aortic wall by bloodborne pathogens
    - Takayasu's disease: inflammation of the aorta and its upper branches
      - Ischemic symptoms involving the upper extremities and central nervous system may occur.
      - Etiology is unknown.
    - Giant-cell arteritis occurs mainly in the cerebral arteries (especially the temporal artery) but may affect the aorta.
      - The affected artery is infiltrated with granulomatous inflammations that contain giant cells. (Giant cells are fused epithelial cells.)
      - Granulomas become foci for necrosis in the vessel wall.
      - The affected artery becomes swollen, nodular, and tender.
  - Medium vessels
    - Polyarteritis nodosa
      - Inflammation may lead to weakening of vessel wall and aneurysm formation.
      - Etiology unknown
    - Kawasaki's disease
      - Usually occurs in children before age 12 years
      - Coronary arteries often affected
    - Thromboangiitis obliterans (Buerger's disease)
      - Segmental thrombosing inflammation of medium-sized and small arteries
      - Principally affects the tibial and radial arteries; may extend to veins and nerves of the extremities
      - Strong association with cigarette smoking
      - Clinical manifestations: cold sensitivity, instep claudication, chronic ulcers, and pain at rest

- Small vessels: arterioles, venules, and capillaries
  - Wegener; granulomatosis
  - Churg-Strauss syndrome
  - Microscopic polyarteritis
  - Hypersensitivity drug reactions

Venous

- Venous thrombosis: thrombotic occlusion of vein or venule
  - Thrombus develops as a result of endothelial dysfunction, which causes imbalance of the procoagulant and anticoagulant substances, and slowed blood flow.
  - Venous thrombosis obstructs venous blood flow from distal tissues.
    - Collateral circulation may partially compensate.
    - Venous pressure distal to the occlusion rises and produces edema.
    - Cellulitis, a diffuse infection of the skin and soft tissues, may occur.
  - Thrombus may completely and permanently occlude the vessel or it may resolve.
- Venous insufficiency and stasis occur when something, usually incompetent venous valves, interferes with blood flow against gravity.
  - Elevated venous pressure produces edema, hyperpigmentation, dermatitis, induration, stasis cellulitis, and venostasis ulcers.
  - Venous insufficiency may develop after venous thrombosis.
- Varicose veins are dilated, elongated, and tortuous superficial veins of the lower extremities.
  - Incompetent valves and increased venous pressure produce varicose veins.
  - Varicose veins can lead to chronic venous insufficiency.

ALTERED CARDIAC FUNCTION

Dysrhythmia

- Cardiac dysrhythmia disrupts the orderly sequence of cardiac contraction.
- Mechanism of cardiac dysrhythmia
  - Enhanced automaticity: increased rate of depolarization of cardiac muscle cells.
  - Depressed automaticity: decreased rate of depolarization of cardiac muscle cells.
  - Reentry occurs when an impulse is able to excite previously depolarized cardiac tissue through anatomic or functional circuits.

Valvular Heart Disease (VHD)

Reduced opening (stenosis) or inadequate closing (insufficiency) of the valves interferes with the normal forward flow of blood.

- Stenosis: valve orifice narrows and valve leaflets fuse, thereby obstructing blood flow.
  - Pressure rises in the chamber behind the stenotic valve.
  - Myocardial fibers hypertrophy to generate more force to push blood through the stenotic valve.
- Insufficiency: valve cannot close completely because of scarring and retraction of the valve leaflets.
  - Blood flows backward (regurgitation) through the insufficient valve.
  - The chamber that receives the regurgitant flow must pump an increased blood volume (normal filling volume plus regurgitant volume).
  - Myocardial fibers hypertrophy and the chamber dilates.

- Mixed lesions: both stenosis and insufficiency occur in the same valve.
  - Usually signifies advanced disease
- Rheumatic fever is the most common cause of VHD worldwide.

Heart Failure
- Heart failure (HF) is a clinical syndrome that results from the heart's inability to pump enough blood to meet the body's metabolic demand. It can be the result of ischemia, hypertension, viral infection, toxins, or idiopathic.
- Two forms exist:
  - Systolic dysfunction can be caused by damaged cardiac muscle, which contracts weakly so the chambers do not empty properly. This is noted by a reduced SV and left ventricular ejection fraction.
  - Diastolic dysfunction can be caused by hypertension. The LV does not relax sufficiently to provide enough filling. Overall SV is reduced, but there is a preserved ejection fraction because the percent of blood ejected with each beat is still a normal proportion. So, diastolic heart failure is also called heart failure with preserved ejection fraction.
  - In either form of heart failure, CO declines while venous return to the ventricles remains the same or increases.
- Systemic responses to decreased CO include:
  - Increased sympathetic activity
    - Increased HR and contractile force
    - Systemic vasoconstriction
  - Renin release from the kidney
    - Renin converts angiotensinogen to angiotensin I (A-I).
    - Angiotensin converting enzyme (ACE) converts A-I to angiotensin II (A-II), a potent vasoconstrictor.
    - A-II stimulates release of aldosterone from the adrenal cortex.
      - Aldosterone promotes sodium and water reabsorption in the kidney tubule, producing increased blood volume.
    - Increased circulating level of A-II acts in conjunction with signals from the atrial baroreceptors to release antidiuretic hormone (ADH) from the posterior pituitary.
      - ADH promotes water reabsorption through the distal tubule of the kidney.
  - Myocardial oxygen balance
    - Oxygen demand is increased because of increased HR, force of contraction, and muscle wall stress.
    - Oxygen supply is reduced because of decreased CO.
  - Atrial and ventricular tissues release atrial natriuretic peptide (ANP) and brain natriuretic peptide (BNP), respectively.
    - ANP and BNP promote diuresis through a direct effect on the kidney.
    - ANP also suppresses aldosterone, renin, and ADH release.
    - The effect of ANP and BNP is small and probably overwhelmed by factors that promote sodium and water retention and vasoconstriction.

- Cardiac responses to increased blood volume are initially compensatory but beyond a critical point contribute to inadequate systemic perfusion.
  - The Frank-Starling law states that within normal limits, the more the heart is filled during diastole, the greater the force of contraction during systole.
    - This mechanism enhances CO up to a critical point, beyond which further stretch on myocardial fibers increases cardiac energy requirements beyond what can be supplied.
    - Beyond this critical point, increased volume and pressure are transmitted in a retrograde fashion to the pulmonary circulation and may result in pulmonary congestion and edema.
  - Dilation of cardiac chambers (acute response)
    - Ventricles dilate in acute HF
    - Dilation increases myocardial oxygen demand and decreases the effectiveness of cardiac contraction.
  - Myocardial hypertrophy (chronic response)
    - Hypertrophy results from increased cardiac workload, commonly HTN.
    - Hypertrophy increases myocardial oxygen demand. When oxygen supply to the hypertrophied muscle is inadequate, ischemia and cardiac dysfunction result.
- Cardiomyopathy: primary abnormality of the myocardium
  - Dilated cardiomyopathy (DCM): progressive cardiac hypertrophy, dilation, and contractile dysfunction *Thinning*
    - Etiology: viral, alcohol or other toxicity, pregnancy-associated, genetic influences
    - Clinical features
      - May occur at any age, commonly affects those 20 to 60 years old
      - Slowly progressive HF
      - Mortality without transplant: 50% within 2 years, 75% within 5 years
      - Embolism and dysrhythmia are common complications
  - Hypertrophic cardiomyopathy (HCM): myocardial hypertrophy, abnormal diastolic filling, and intermittent left ventricular outflow obstruction
    - Etiology: strong genetic basis *← Thickening*
    - Clinical features
      - Reduced CO and increased ventricular pressure cause a secondary increase in pulmonary venous pressure.
      - Focal myocardial ischemia occurs because muscle hypertrophy exceeds intramural arterial blood supply.
      - Atrial fibrillation with mural thrombosis and possible embolization
      - Ventricular dysrhythmia and sudden death
  - Restrictive cardiomyopathy (RCM): decreased ventricular compliance resulting in impaired filling
    - May be idiopathic or associated with radiation fibrosis, amyloidosis, sarcoidosis, or metastatic tumor
    - Clinical features similar to HCM *Ridged o/t scarring*

Inflammatory Heart Disease

- Infective endocarditis occurs when microorganisms invade the lining of the heart.
  - Causative agents include bacteria, fungi, rickettsiae, viruses, and parasites.
  - May be acute or subacute
    - Acute bacterial endocarditis (ABE) occurs most commonly in intravenous drug users. Most common causative organism is *Staphylococcus aureus*.
    - Subacute bacterial endocarditis (SBE) is caused by organisms of low virulence. The most common causative organism is *Streptococcus viridans*. It usually affects a damaged heart (e.g., congenital or acquired valvular disease).
  - Bloodborne organisms attach to the endocardial lining of the heart and become enmeshed in fibrin and platelets (vegetations). Vegetations lodge on valve cusps and may embolize throughout the vasculature.
  - Clinical features:
    - Fever most consistent sign; may be accompanied by chills, lassitude, and weakness.
    - Complications
      - Cardiac: valvular insufficiency or stenosis and HF; with artificial valves, partial disruption with paravalvular leak may occur.
      - Embolic: cerebral infarct or abscess, MI, spleen or kidney abscess
      - Renal: embolic infarction, glomerulonephritis because of trapping of antigen-antibody complexes, leading to renal failure
- Myocarditis: inflammatory processes that injure myocardial cells.
  - Viral infection: Coxsackie virus most common; cytomegalovirus (CMV) and human immunodeficiency virus (HIV) less common
  - Occurs in approximately two-thirds of patients with Lyme disease
  - Allergic and immune process
  - Clinical features:
    - Variable presentation: may be asymptomatic or present with sudden HF and dysrhythmias
    - Usually self-limited but may progress to DCM
- Pericarditis may be secondary to physical trauma (after heart surgery), infection (viral or bacterial), or immune-mediated inflammation (e.g., post-MI, drug hypersensitivity).
  - Fluid (blood, effusion, or pus) accumulates in the pericardial sac and interferes with cardiac filling.
  - With slow accumulation, pericardial sac may accommodate up to 500 mL without symptoms. If rapid accumulation, collections of as little as 60 mL to 90 mL may impair cardiac filling and produce potentially fatal cardiac tamponade.

SUMMARY

This chapter provided an overview of the anatomy of the heart and circulation. A brief overview of cellular function provided the basis for understanding the major cardiovascular pathologies. The next chapter describes many of the common cardiac diagnoses along with common treatments.

REFERENCES

Barrett, K. E., Barman, S. M., Boitano, S., & Brooks, H. (2009). *Ganong's review of medical physiology* (23rd ed.). New York: McGraw Hill.

Crawford, M. H. (2009). *Cardiology: Current diagnosis and treatment.* New York: McGraw Hill.

Hansson, G. K. (2005). Inflammation, atherosclerosis, and coronary artery disease. *New England Journal of Medicine, 352,* 1685–1695.

Hill, J. A., & Olson, E. N. (2008). Cardiac plasticity. *New England Journal of Medicine, 358,* 1370–1380.

Gary, R., & Davis, L. (2008). Diastolic heart failure. *Heart and Lung, 37,* 405–416.

Labus, D. (2008). *Cardiovascular care made incredibly easy.* Philadelphia: Springhouse.

McCance, K. L., & Heuther, S. E. (2005). *Pathophysiology: The biologic basis for disease in adults and children* (5th ed.). St. Louis, MO: Mosby.

McPhee, S. J., & Hammer, G. D. (2009). *Pathophysiology of disease: An introduction to clinical medicine* (6th ed.). New York: McGraw-Hill.

Moser, D., & Reigel, B. (2008). *Cardiac nursing: A companion to Braunwald.* St. Louis, MO: Elsevier-Saunders.

Pepine, C. J., & Nichols, W. W. (2007). The pathophysiology of chronic ischemic heart disease. *Clinical Cardiology, 30* (Suppl. I), 14–19.

Porth, C. M., & Matfin, G. (2009). *Pathophysiology: Concepts of altered health states* (8th ed.). Philadelphia: Lippincott Williams & Wilkins.

Woods, S. L., Sivarajan-Froelicher, F. S., Motzer, S. A., & Bridges, E. J. (2010). *Cardiac nursing* (6th ed). Philadelphia: Lippincott Williams Wilken.

Zipes, D. P., Libby, P., Bonow, R. O., & Braunwald, E. (2009). *Braunwald's heart disease: A textbook of cardiovascular medicine* (8th ed.). Philadelphia: Elsevier-Saunders.

12

Cardiac and Vascular Assessment

Information included in this chapter relates to the patient with cardiac or vascular disease. The chapter focuses on key symptoms of cardiac and vascular disease and examination of body systems directly related to these symptoms. Excellent health assessment textbooks are available to readers requiring a more comprehensive or more basic review. In addition, this chapter provides a review of common cardiovascular diagnostic tests.

BASIC PRINCIPLES

Assessment is the process of data collection and interpretation. Sources of data include the history, physical examination, laboratory testing, and diagnostic imaging.

- Historical (subjective) information and physical (objective) findings direct appropriate laboratory and diagnostic testing.
- Assessment data are used to formulate clinical diagnoses (both nursing and medical), establish patient goals, plan care, and evaluate outcomes.
- Patient condition (stage of illness) and the purpose of the encounter determine areas that are included in an assessment.
- Elements of the history and physical examination are the same whether performed by a physician, nurse, or other clinician.

Data Quality

Quality of the data obtained through assessment is related to the rapport established between the clinician and patient.

- Create a comfortable environment.
  - Ensure privacy.
  - Comfortable temperature, sufficient lighting, minimal noise.
- Focus on the patient as a unique individual.
  - Refuse interruptions.
  - Review available records before the encounter; avoid repeating elements obtained by other clinicians.
  - Be aware of cultural needs; avoid stereotypes.
  - Attend to both verbal and nonverbal cues.
  - Establish equal-status seating (i.e., both comfortably seated at the same eye level).
- If documenting in an electronic medical record be sure to
  - Position the computer so that you can provide face-to-face contact.
  - Focus your attention on the patient so that you spend the least amount of time facing the computer.
  - Be familiar with the computer screens so that you do not need to read them for each patient question during history-taking.

SUBJECTIVE INFORMATION (HISTORY)

Subjective information is usually obtained through the patient interview. The patient is the expert on his or her experience and is the primary source of information. Often the situation includes several symptoms and you must take complex data to drill down to the primary symptom and determine which ones are associated or incidental events. Secondary sources of data include family interview and record review. Secondary data sources may be needed during periods of acute illness, when the complaint is syncope, or whenever the patient is unable to provide information.

Symptom Analysis

For each symptom presented by the patient, the clinician attempts to determine the following characteristics. Pain is used as an example.

- Quality: describes the character of the symptom
  - Dull, sharp, squeezing, or aching pain
- Quantity: describes the severity, intensity, or amount of the symptom in measurable terms
  - Pain rated on an 11-point scale
  - 0: pain free; 10: worst possible pain
  - Documented as fraction or ratio (e.g., 6/10)
- Location: describes the specific bodily location where the symptom is experienced; includes any area of radiating pain
  - Substernal chest pain radiating to the left arm, jaw, throat, or back
  - Have patient point to area(s) of pain

- Timing: describes the evolution of the symptom over time; includes onset, frequency, and duration
  - Timing for each episode; for example, "sudden onset of chest pain rapidly reaching maximal intensity (6/10) and resolving over approximately 10 minutes."
    - Discrete, intermittent episodes versus sustained pain that waxes and wanes
  - Course of disease; for example, "Initially experienced occasional episodes of chest pain 4 years ago, over the past 6 months has experienced chest pain more frequently (two or three times per week)."
- Precipitating factors: describes events that initiate the symptom, such as activity or emotional upset
- Aggravating factors: describes what makes the symptom worse, such as position change or jarring
  - Pain associated with acute pericarditis may be exacerbated by lying down or by movement; sitting up and leaning forward may alleviate it.
  - Angina is usually worse with activity.
- Alleviating factors: describes what relieves the symptom, such as medications or heat; may include past treatments, such as angioplasty or surgery
- Associated symptoms: symptoms rarely occur in isolation; recognition of patterns of symptoms leads to clinical diagnoses

Key Signs and Symptoms of Cardiac Disease

A full description is elicited for each symptom that is present.

- Chest pain
  - Visceral pain is deep, diffuse, and poorly localized.
    - Cardiac: angina, myocardial infarction, and acute pericarditis
    - Esophageal: spasm, gastroesophageal reflux
    - Pulmonary embolism and infarction
    - Vascular: dissecting aortic aneurysm
  - Chest wall pain is reproduced or intensified by palpation.
    - Skin and subcutaneous structures: herpes zoster
    - Musculoskeletal: costochondritis, strain of pectoral muscle
- Cough may be associated with cardiac or pulmonary disease.
  - Note whether it is productive and the color of the phlegm.
  - Note if it worsens at night or with activity. Cardiac disease or asthma can cause either.
  - Cough when in the recumbent position can be the equivalent of dyspnea and a sign of heart failure.
- Shortness of breath or breathlessness is an abnormal awareness of breathing.
  - Dyspnea on exertion: he clinician attempts to quantify the degree of exertion that reliably induces dyspnea. For example, dyspnea occurs with climbing 10 steps at moderate pace.
  - Orthopnea is breathlessness that occurs in a supine position and prompts the patient to elevate the head and thorax.
    - Orthopnea is suggestive of left ventricular failure.
    - The clinician may quantify the orthopnea by the number of pillows used (e.g., two-pillow orthopnea) or if the person must sleep sitting up in a chair.

- Paroxysmal nocturnal dyspnea (PND) is breathlessness that occurs after a period of recumbence and usually with sleep. The patient reports being awakened with a suffocating sensation necessitating assuming an upright position. Sometimes patients report that they need to go to an open window or exit the building for relief. PND is associated with heart failure.
- Palpitations describe abnormal awareness of the heartbeat; may be related to rapid rate or irregular rhythm.
- Cyanosis is a bluish discoloration of the skin caused by the presence of 5 or more grams of reduced (unoxygenated) hemoglobin in 100 mL of blood.
  - Central cyanosis is present in high blood-flow areas, such as the tongue and soft palate. Central cyanosis is usually associated with inadequate oxygenation.
  - Peripheral cyanosis occurs in low or slow blood-flow areas, such as the fingers, toes, and lips. Peripheral cyanosis may be present in normal people because vasoconstriction from the cold as well as in patients with low cardiac output.
- Nocturia is increased urine formation during sleep and recumbency as a result of better renal perfusion. In general, awakening once per night to void is within normal limits; awakening two or more times per night is abnormal.
- Fatigue is a sense of weariness or mental exhaustion.
  - Fatigue is a nonspecific but worrisome symptom. It may be present in cardiac patients with heart failure, myocardial ischemia, and sleep apnea.
  - It is the seventh most common complaint in primary care practices and may be unrelated to cardiac or vascular disease.
  - If cardiac-related, it is an indication that the person is not able to keep up with the previous activity level and this may be because insufficient cardiac output (CO) increase for the effort needed.
  - Fatigue may also be because of sleep apnea.
    - If so, it also may be manifest by
      - Daytime sleepiness
      - Nighttime snoring
      - Early morning headaches that are relieved within 30 minutes of awakening
      - Often obesity or a thick neck is associated with obstructive form of sleep apnea
    - Sleep apnea is associated with uncontrolled hypertension and heart failure. Recognition and treatment will improve the cardiac conditions.
- Syncope is sudden loss of consciousness associated with muscle weakness (fainting).
  - True syncope has three stages.
    1. The prodromal stage usually begins in the erect position and the patient feels weak and unsteady; dimming of the vision, nausea, vomiting, and pallor are common.
    2. The syncopal stage consists of muscle weakness and impaired consciousness. The patient usually falls to the ground, but it is a gradual fall and usually does not result in serious injury.
    3. Recovery stage occurs while the patient is in the horizontal position. Gradually color comes back and the patient awakens with an immediate awareness of the surroundings, but muscle weakness persists.

- – Syncope must be differentiated from "near syncope" in which the patient does not experience loss of consciousness.
  - – Patients may experience light-headedness and muscle weakness before losing consciousness from myocardial ischemia, transient ischemic attacks, cerebrovascular accidents, or cardiac dysrhythmia.
- Abdominal fullness or bloating may occur with fluid retention or ascites. The person may not be able to eat as much at one sitting (early satiety). Some develop postprandial angina if there is atherosclerosis in the mesenteric arteries causing ischemia to the gut.

Key Signs and Symptoms of Vascular Disease

There is considerable overlap among symptoms of cardiac and vascular disease. This is explained, in part, by the overlap of pathophysiological processes. While the following symptoms may be seen in patients with cardiac disease, they are more commonly observed among those with vascular disease.

- Pallor is an absence of normal coloration, which may be localized or generalized. When localized it reflects vascular disease. There are many causes of generalized pallor, including anemia.
- Swelling of feet or ankles results from an abnormal accumulation of fluid in the interstitial tissue. It may reflect systemic illnesses, such as heart failure or cirrhosis, or vascular diseases, such as acute or chronic thrombophlebitis and chronic venous insufficiency.
  - – A weight gain of 10 lb, which is indicative of approximately 5 L of fluid, precedes visible edema in most patients. This is why patients with heart failure are instructed to monitor their weight daily at home.
  - – Bilateral edema is associated with systemic process.
  - – Unilateral edema is associated with localized process such as lymphedema.
- Amaurosis fugax is monocular blindness of less than 10-minute duration. Patients may describe a sensation that a blind is falling over their field of vision. This is a symptom of reduced cerebral circulation.
- Intermittent claudication is pain or weakness in the muscle of one or both legs that occurs after walking a fixed distance.
  - – If the patient stops walking, the pain or weakness resolves, only to recur after walking a similar distance.
  - – If the patient continues walking, intense muscle cramping occurs.
  - – There are no symptoms at rest.
- Raynaud's phenomenon is a syndrome of peripheral vasospasm with intermittent cutaneous pallor or cyanosis. Precipitating factor is usually exposure to cold. It is often associated with autoimmune disorders such as scleroderma.
- Gangrene is death of tissue because severe hypoxia that may occur because blockage of major arteries or severe peripheral vasospasm.
  - – Gas gangrene is because the toxin released during an infection by a species of Clostridium.
- Acute epigastric abdominal pain can have many causes, including dissecting aneurysm and mesenteric ischemia.
- Pain and numbness in the feet (neuropathy) that is generally constant may indicate peripheral neuropathy, which can occur with vascular disease as well as diabetes mellitus.

Review of Systems (ROS)

Systematically review symptoms associated with all body systems. Major health assessment textbooks include lists of major symptoms associated with each body system.

- Cardiac ROS: heart trouble, high blood pressure, rheumatic fever, heart murmurs, chest pain or discomfort, palpitations, dyspnea, orthopnea, paroxysmal nocturnal dyspnea, edema, past electrocardiogram or other heart test results.
- Vascular ROS: Intermittent claudication, leg cramps, varicose veins, past clots in veins.

Functional Assessment

Nurses collect data about functional patterns also. For each pattern, the nurse elicits information about usual pattern and recent changes. Assessment aids in the identification of strengths and resources, as well as problems and symptoms.

- Health perception—Health management: patient perceptions and concerns about current health and activities used to manage and maintain health
- Nutrition—Metabolism: information about food consumption, preparation, and preferences
- Elimination: patterns of urination and defecation; may include urinary incontinence, constipation, etc.
- Activity—exercise: current level of activity, as well as recent changes because of symptoms or treatment
- Cognitive—perceptual: the special senses—hearing, seeing—as well as memory, thinking, and judgment. Affect (e.g., depression) and information about preferred learning style may be included in this pattern.
- Sleep/rest: symptoms of sleep apnea such as snoring and early morning headache
- Self-perception—Self-concept: thoughts and feelings associated with self-evaluation and general satisfaction with body image and personality
- Roles and relationships: family structures, work role, and changes related to illness
- Sexuality: function and satisfaction; many drugs as well as cardiac and vascular illnesses and emotional response have a negative effect on sexual function; patients may be reluctant to discuss concerns unless the nurse asks these questions.
- Coping—stress: usual ways of coping; may include affect (e.g., depression)
- Values—beliefs: religious and spiritual beliefs and practices

Cardiac and Vascular Risk Factors

The presence of atherosclerosis risk factors is included in the history. Information on the risk factors is found in Chapters 7 through 10.

Medications

- Include all medications currently taken—prescribed, over-the-counter, herbs, and supplements.
- Note allergies and sensitivities.
  - Allergy to iodine (shellfish or previous contrast medium) should be specifically elicited.

PHYSICAL EXAMINATION

Basic Principles
- Organization of the examination
  - Systematic head-to-toe sequence assures completeness.
  - Side-to-side comparison helps to evaluate normality. In some situations (e.g., muscle strength, range of motion), patient-to-examiner comparison helps evaluate normality.
  - The usual sequence of examination techniques is inspection, palpation, percussion, and auscultation.
    - Abdominal exam sequence is inspection, auscultation, palpation, and percussion.
    - Not all techniques are used for all systems; for example, skin examination uses inspection and palpation only.
- Comfort of the patient and clinician
  - Clinician usually stands on the patient's right side.
  - Privacy and draping to assure comfort and dignity.

Special Equipment
- Stethoscope is essential for auscultation.
  - Double or single tubing no more than 30 to 40 cm long and 4 mm in diameter. (Longer and wider tubing may distort sounds.)
  - Ear pieces fit snugly but comfortably in the ear canals. Ear piece opening is directed toward the ear canal.
  - Use the diaphragm to detect high-pitched sounds (e.g., breath sounds, bowel sounds, some cardiac sounds). Use the bell to detect low-pitched sounds (e.g., bruits, some cardiac sounds).
- Sphygmomanometer must fit properly to give accurate readings.
  - The inflatable bladder should have a width of about 40% and a length of about 80% of the upper arm circumference.
  - Cuffs are generally available in adult, obese, and child sizes. Measure the size of the arm circumference and select the cuff that is designed for that arm size.
  - Cuffs that are too short or too narrow may give falsely high readings, while cuffs that are too large will give a falsely low reading.
  - A Doppler device can be used to obtain the sound associated with a systolic pressure when obtaining lower extremity pressures or when there is difficulty auscultating the sound.
- An ophthalmoscope is a light source with lens and mirrors, which is used to examine internal eye structures. Examination of the undilated pupil may be difficult. In general, nurses do not use drugs to dilate the pupil for funduscopic examination.
- Pulse oximeter is a photoelectric device that noninvasively measures arterial oxygen saturation.

General Survey

- Includes height, weight, body mass index (BMI), and vital signs: temperature, pulse, respiration, and blood pressure (T, P, R, and BP).
  - Ideal body weight (IBW) ranges can be read from standardized tables.
    - General rule for women: IBW = 100 lb for first 5 feet of height plus 5 lb per inch above 5 feet
    - General rule for men: IBW = 105 lb for first 5 feet of height and 6 lb per inch above 5 feet
  - BMI describes relationship between height and weight.
    - BMI = weight (in kg) divided by height (in meters squared).
    - BMI = weight (in lb) divided by height (in inches squared) multiplied by 704.5.
    - BMI values of 20 to 24.9 are optimal; 25 to 29 are overweight; 30 to 34 are obese; and 35 or above is morbidly obese.
  - Accurate blood pressure (BP) and pulse is fundamental to the physical examination of the cardiac and vascular patient. The following steps will help to assure accuracy.
    - Patients should be seated in a chair with their backs supported. Arms should be bared and supported at heart level.
    - Patients should refrain from smoking and caffeine ingestion for 30 minutes prior to measurement.
    - Measurement should begin after at least 5 minutes of rest.
    - The bladder within the cuff should encircle at least 80% of the arm. Cuff width should be at least 40% of arm circumference.
    - Mercury sphygmomanometer measurements were the gold standard but are not used clinically for environmental safety reasons. A recently calibrated aneroid manometer or a validated electronic device can be used.
    - Both systolic (first appearance of sound) and diastolic (disappearance of sound) pressure should be recorded.
      - Auscultatory gap, a period of silence that occurs during Korotkoff sounds, is of no clinical importance—except that if you miss its existence you may report an erroneously low (or normal) systolic pressure.
      - Auscultatory gaps have been reported in patients with hypertension, aortic valve disease, bradycardia, and heart failure.
      - To be sure you have inflated the cuff above systolic pressure, keep your finger on the pulse while you are inflating the cuff the first time. When you reach systolic pressure the pulse disappears.
    - BP should be measured in both arms initially. The arm with the higher reading should be used for subsequent measurements.
    - Two or more readings separated by 2 minutes should be averaged. If the readings differ by more than 5 mm Hg, additional readings should be obtained and averaged.
    - Patient should be informed of the reading and advised of the need for periodic reassessment.
    - There is growing support for use of the lower arm for BP measurement if the cuff size is appropriate and all other measurement standards are followed.

- Arterial pulses are palpated in the radial, brachial, femoral, carotid, posterior tibialis, and dorsalis pedis arteries.
  - Assess and compare characteristics of arterial pulses on the right and left side of the body.
  - A 3- or 4-point scale may be used to describe the pulse.
    - If using a 3-point scale, the results would be recorded as: 0 (absent), 1+ (weak or thready), 2+ (normal), and 3+ (full and bounding).
    - If using a 4-point scale, the results would be recorded as: 0 (absent), 1+ (thready), 2+ (weak), 3+ (normal), and 4+ (full and bounding).
    - To ensure that the reader knows which scale you used, write the finding as the numerator over the scale used as the denominator (e.g., 3+/4).
    - Note that with each scale, the highest number is abnormally strong and the second to the highest number is normal.
  - Abnormal arterial pulses
    - Water hammer (Corrigan) pulse is a rapidly rising and falling pulse associated with aortic insufficiency. It transmits a tapping sensation to the palpating fingers.
    - Pulsus parvus is a low-amplitude pulse associated with stenosis of any of the heart valves and any form of low-output heart failure.
    - Pulsus tardus is a slow-rising pulse associated with aortic stenosis.
    - Unequal right and left carotid and radial pulses may be seen in aortic dissection. Other causes of unequal pulses (right to left) include supravalvular aortic stenosis, thoracic outlet syndrome, and local occlusive disease of the peripheral artery.
    - Pulsus alternans is the alternation of stronger and weaker beats in a regular rhythm associated with severe heart failure.
      - Regular rhythm differentiates pulsus alternans from atrial or ventricular bigeminal rhythms.
    - Pulse deficit is the difference between apical and radial artery pulse rate associated with atrial fibrillation and nonperfusing ectopic impulses.
- Allen Test is a special examination technique used to determine patency of the palmar arch in the hand. Adequacy of the ulnar artery and palmar arch is assessed before puncturing the radial artery for blood samples.
  - The patient is asked to make a tight fist with one hand.
  - The examiner occludes both the radial and ulnar arteries.
  - The patient is asked to release the fist while the examiner maintains arterial occlusion; the palm is pale.
  - The examiner releases pressure over the ulnar artery. If the artery and arch are patent, the palm flushes within 3 to 5 seconds.
- Pulse pressure, the difference between systolic and diastolic pressure in mm Hg, is an indirect indicator of stroke volume. Pulse pressure is normally approximately one third of systolic pressure.
  - May be increased during exercise and in people with valvular heart disease (aortic insufficiency).
  - May be decreased in people with heart failure or intravascular volume deficits.
  - If less than 25% of systolic pressure, indicates increased afterload, especially in the setting of heart failure.

— Mean arterial pressure (MAP) is the diastolic BP plus one-third of the pulse pressure. MAP represents average pressure within the vessels throughout the cardiac cycle. MAP = (SBP + 2DBP) ÷ 3
— Postural (orthostatic) hypotension occurs when blood pressure drops upon standing and compensatory mechanisms are insufficient to prevent symptoms.
  • Postural change in BP and pulse should be assessed in patients who are elderly, have diabetes mellitus, take antihypertensive medications including diuretics, and anyone complaining of dizziness or syncope.
  • Attention to the following points will assure accuracy and allow meaningful interpretation of results.
    — Have patient rest in a recumbent position for at least 10 minutes before the initial measurement of BP and pulse.
    — Check supine pressure and pulse before upright measurement. Always check both BP and pulse in each position. Do not remove the cuff between measurements.
    — Have the patient assume an upright position. (In some cases, BP may be measured in a seated position, although standing is preferred.)
      ▪ Measure BP and pulse immediately and after 2 minutes.
      ▪ If orthostasis is strongly suspected and not immediately apparent, take the BP and pulse every 2 minutes five times while the patient remains standing.
    — Be alert for signs or symptoms of patient distress, including dizziness, weakness, blurred vision, and syncope.
  • Normal postural response on standing
    — Transient increase in pulse (5 to 10 beats per minute)
    — Decrease in systolic BP (< 10 mm Hg)
    — Increase in diastolic BP (approximately 5 mm Hg)
  • The pattern of postural change consisting of increased pulse, decreased systolic BP (15 mm Hg or more), decreased diastolic BP, and increased heart rate suggests intravascular volume depletion.
  • Orthostatic hypotension must be differentiated from autonomic insufficiency. Constant pulse rate when the patient's position changes from supine to standing suggest autonomic insufficiency.
— Paradoxical pulse (also called BP paradox) is an exaggeration of the normal decrease in systolic BP during inspiration.
  • Steps to assess paradoxical pulse:
    — Have patient comfortable and breathing normally.
    — Inflate and gradually deflate the cuff until the first Korotkoff sound is heard during expiration.
    — Continue slowly deflating the cuff until sounds are heard during both inspiration and expiration.
  • Normal pressure differential from expiration to inspiration is less than 10 mm Hg.
  • Paradoxical pressures should be measured on all patients in the cardiac care unit and in those with pericarditis or a temporary pacing wire. It can also be abnormal with the exaggerated respiratory effort seen during an asthma attack.

- Ankle-brachial index (ABI) is the ratio of systolic BP measured in the lower leg (ankle) to that measured in the arm (brachial).
  - Normal ABI is 0.95 or higher.
  - ABI below 0.80 is definitely abnormal.
  - Abnormal ABI is seen with arterial insufficiency.
  - The lower the ABI, the poorer the perfusion of the limb.
  - The systolic pressure in the leg is taken with the cuff over the calf and using the dorsalis or pedal pulse Doppler systolic measurement.

Skin, Hair, and Nails

Inspection and palpation of the skin, hair, and nails may reveal abnormalities associated with specific cardiac and vascular conditions.

- Capillary refill: pressure-induced blanching of the nail is used to assess peripheral blood flow. After blanching, the nail bed should resume its normal color within 2 seconds of pressure release. Capillary refill is slowed in low-flow states.
- Quincke pulsation: Visible pulsation seen at the pink-white junction with pressure-induced blanching of the fingernail. Associated with aortic insufficiency may be accompanied by involuntary head bobbing.
- Splinter hemorrhages under the nails, purpura and ecchymoses, Janeway lesions, and petechiae are skin signs that may be seen with infective endocarditis.
  - Janeway lesions are painless, circular or oval, nontender macules that appear and fade over a week or two.
- Clubbing is enlargement of the connective tissue in the terminal phalanges of the fingers and toes.
  - Clubbing is often associated with cyanosis.
  - Hypoxia does not explain its occurrence in many conditions.
- With arterial insufficiency, skin of the lower legs may appear pale, shiny, and relatively hairless. Pulses may be diminished or absent. Postural change in skin color may be observed.
  - With the patient recumbent, raise both legs to about 60 degrees until maximal pallor develops (approximately one minute).
  - Have the patient sit up with legs dependent. Normally, color returns within 10 seconds and veins fill within 15 seconds. When arterial flow is insufficient:
    - Pallor may persist for more than 10 seconds, or
    - Dusky redness (rubor) may develop.
- Hemosiderin (brown) staining may be seen over the lower legs in the presence of chronic venous insufficiency.

Head, Eyes, Ears, Nose, and Throat

- Examination of the eyes and ears
  - Inspection
    - Corneal arcus: a thin, grayish-white circle around the iris, may be a sign of hyperlipidemia and precocious atherosclerosis in white people under age 50. After age 50, loses significance.
    - Xanthelasma: slightly raised, yellowish plaques of cholesterol in the skin that appear along the eyelids. May be associated with hyperlipidemia but may be a normal variant.
    - A deep, diagonal crease running across the ear lobe may be associated with coronary heart disease. This does not apply to Native Americans.

- Examination of the retinal circulation is the only opportunity for direct visualization of blood vessels.
  - Normal retinal arteries and veins appear to arise from the optic disc.
    - Arteries are lighter in color than veins and have a more prominent light reflex.
    - Vein-to-artery ratio is 3:2.
    - Retinal background is a uniform reddish-orange color.
    - The macula is located directly temporal to the optic disc and appears darker than the surrounding retina.
  - Diabetic retinopathy
    - Nonproliferative diabetic retinopathy (NPDR) occurs early and produces microaneurysms, dot-and-blot hemorrhages, hard exudates, and macular edema.
    - Proliferative diabetic retinopathy (PDR) is responsible for most of the visual loss from diabetes. In response to retinal ischemia, new vessels form (neovascularization) in the area of the optic disc. These new vessels are fragile and if untreated may bleed into the vitreous. Retinal detachment may occur.
  - Hypertensive retinopathy
    - Changes because atherosclerosis
      - Arteriolar sclerosis causes thickening of the vessel wall; the central light reflex thickens. As sclerosis progresses, the light reflex occupies most of the vessel, producing "copper wire" vessels.
      - There may be zones where the vein, passing beneath the thickened arterial wall, is invisible producing A-V (arteriovenous) nicking. A-V nicking can lead to retinal venous occlusions and decreased central visual acuity.
    - Changes because elevated BP
      - Moderate acute rise in BP results in arteriolar constriction. Severe acute elevation (diastolic pressure > 120 mm Hg) causes necrosis of the vessel wall, producing exudates, flame-shaped hemorrhages, and whitish swelling and edema of large areas of the retina.
      - In most severe BP elevation, optic disc swelling is seen.
  - Response of pupils to light and assessment of extraocular movements are included in the examination of cranial nerves.
- Examination of vascular structures in the neck
  - Carotid arteries
    - Inspection, palpation, and auscultation
      - Carotid pulsation may be visible and palpable in the neck just medial to the border of the sternomastoid muscle.
        - Abnormally vigorous pulsation may be seen and felt in aortic insufficiency and in high-output states.
        - Carotid pulsation can be used to time intracardiac events, but there is a short time lag.
      - Palpate each carotid pulse in the lower third of the neck.
        - Palpate low in the neck and singly to avoid carotid sinus stimulation and reflex slowing of the heart rate.

      – Auscultate each carotid artery for bruits, a swooshing sound (like a murmur) made by turbulent blood flow because carotid artery stenosis.

               * Avoid excessive pressure with the stethoscope because external pressure may create turbulent flow.

               * Bruits are usually low-pitched sounds best heard with the bell.

               * Referred cardiac murmurs are more intense lower in the neck.

   – Jugular veins reflect intravascular volume and cardiac function. They are best viewed with tangential lighting to cast shadows with pulsations.

      • Internal jugular venous pressure (JVP) reflects right atrial (central venous) pressure and volume.

         – Position patient comfortably with head slightly elevated and the sternomastoid muscle relaxed.

               * Start with the head of the bed or table elevated to at least 30º and adjust the angle to maximize visibility of jugular pulsation in the lower neck.

               * The internal jugular vein lies deep under the sternomastoid muscle. The vein itself is not visible. A diffuse, wavelike pulsation is seen in the soft tissue of the neck. (Figure 12–1 illustrates the arterial and venous pulse of a cardiac cycle.)

         – Measure the height of the highest pulsation seen with reference to the sternal angle.

               * Normal venous pressure is 3 cm or less above the sternal angle. This is the equivalent of 10 cm.

               * Increased JVP is seen in right-sided heart failure, constrictive pericarditis, tricuspid stenosis, and superior vena caval obstruction.

               * Decreased JVP is an indication of intravascular volume depletion (dehydration or over-diuresis).

Figure 12–1. Illustration of the Timing of the ECG, Arterial Waveform, Venous Waveform, and the Heart Sounds

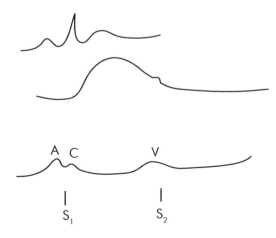

- The amplitude and timing of the jugular venous pulsation reflect the phases of the cardiac cycle.
  - The a wave precedes S1 and reflects atrial filling during diastole. Conditions that produce overloading of the right atrium (e.g., tricuspid stenosis, pulmonary hypertension, right heart failure) create giant a waves.
    - Cannon a waves occur when the right atrium contracts against closed atrioventricular valves. Presence of cannon a waves can help differentiate ventricular tachycardia from supraventricular tachycardia.
  - The x descent follows S1 and reflects early systole.
  - The v wave coincides with S2 and the y descent marks early diastole.
  - Giant v waves are seen with regurgitation of blood from the ventricle into the atrium and veins. This is found with mitral and tricuspid insufficiency.
- Abdominojugular test (also known as hepatojugular reflux)
  - Apply pressure with the palm of the hand over the abdomen for 30 to 60 seconds.
  - Observe jugular venous pulsation.
    - Increase in the height of the jugular pulsation above the sternal angle associated with abdominal pressure is a positive test.
    - There is a normal increase in the height of jugular pulsation during inspiration. This increase is augmented and sustained during expiration for a positive test.
  - A positive test is associated with right-sided heart failure.

Chest and Thorax

The breast exam, in both males and females, is part of the examination of the chest and thorax. Readers are directed to one of the health assessment texts for information about the breast examination. Here we will focus only on cardiac and pulmonary examination of the chest.

- Cardiac exam
  - Chest wall regions (see Figure 12–2)
    - Aortic valve area: second intercostal space (ICS) at the right sternal border
    - Pulmonic valve area: second ICS at the left sternal border (LSB)
    - Second pulmonic area: third ICS at the LSB
    - Tricuspid valve area: fourth ICS along the lower LSB
    - Mitral valve area (apical area): fifth ICS at the left midclavicular line (MCL)
  - Inspection and palpation
    - Apical pulsation (also known as point of maximal impulse [PMI]) is the lowest and left-most visible (or palpable) pulsation on the precordium.
      - Reflects contraction of the left ventricle and is the best guide to heart size.
      - Normal apical pulsation is localized to the fourth or fifth ICS at or medial to the left MCL. The normal impulse is not larger than a nickel.
    - Right ventricular pulsation may be visible or palpable in the lower sternal areas. This is most often because right ventricular enlargement or hypertrophy.
    - Visible or palpable pulsation in the epigastrium usually originates from the aorta, liver, or right ventricle.
  - Percussion was used in the past to assess heart size; rarely used today.

Figure 12–2. Auscultation Sites on the Chest

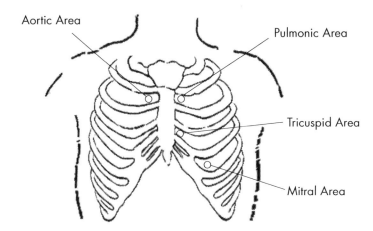

- Auscultation of the precordium should be compulsively systematic.
  - Begin at the mitral area (apex) or at the aortic area (base) and gradually move the stethoscope over the entire precordium, listening attentively in each area.
  - Examine all areas with the diaphragm of the stethoscope first, then the bell.
  - Listen with the patient first in the recumbent and then in the sitting position.
    - Having the seated patient lean forward brings the heart closer to the chest wall and may bring out soft sounds (e.g., pericardial friction rub or diastolic murmur of aortic insufficiency).
    - Turning the recumbent patient to the left side brings the heart closer to the chest wall and may bring out left-sided events (for example S3 or mitral clicks and murmurs).
  - Audible sounds should be identified as occurring during systole or diastole.
    - At normal heart rates, systole is shorter than diastole.
    - S1 marks the beginning of systole. It occurs as the mitral and tricuspid valves close and are the louder sound when listening in the mitral and tricuspid areas of the chest.
    - S2 marks the beginning of diastole. It occurs as the aortic and pulmonic valves close and are the louder sound when listening in the aortic and pulmonic areas of the chest.
    - S1—systole—S2—diastole—S1
- Heart rate (HR) and rhythm are determined during cardiac auscultation.
  - Normal HR is 60 to 100 beats per minute (BPM).
    - Tachycardia is above 100 BPM.
    - Bradycardia is below 60 BPM.
  - Normal heart rhythm is regular.
    - Minor variation in rate associated with respiratory phase may be normal (sinus dysrhythmia) because HR increases during inspiration and decreases during expiration.
    - Atrial or ventricular extrasystoles may cause sporadic irregularity.
    - Atrial fibrillation may cause total irregularity (irregularly irregular).

- Left-side events and valve closure precede the right by a fraction of a second that is usually not detected. If the pause is long enough, it may be audible and produce splitting of S1 or S2. A split S2 may be physiological (normal) or pathological (abnormal), while a split S1 is always abnormal.
    - Physiological splitting of S2 is heard during inspiration, but not during expiration. Reversal of this normal pattern is associated with heart disease. It is more apparent in children and adults under age 30.
    - Pathological splitting of S1 is associated with right bundle branch block (RBBB) and ventricular extrasystoles.
    - Pathological splitting of S2 is associated with atrial septal defects, right and left bundle branch block, and pulmonary hypertension.
        - S1 is lower pitched and of longer duration than S2.
        - S1 precedes the carotid pulsation and S2 follows this pulse.
        - S1 is loudest at the apex and is best heard with the diaphragm of the stethoscope. S2 is loudest at the base and is also best heard with the diaphragm.
- Extrasystolic sounds (see Table 12–1 for a pictorial description of extra heart sounds)
    - Transients
        - Aortic or pulmonic ejection sounds may be heard with aortic or pulmonary valve stenosis. The sounds are best heard with the diaphragm at the base of the heart.
        - Systolic click, associated with mitral valve prolapse, is heard during mid to late systole.
    - Systolic murmurs
        - Innocent systolic murmur is commonly heard in children and adolescents.
        - Benign systolic murmurs are soft, short, and low-pitched. They have no hemodynamic significance.
        - Loud systolic murmurs may be because ventricular septal defect, pulmonary or aortic stenosis, or mitral or tricuspid insufficiency.
- Extradiastolic sounds
    - Transients—the third (S3) and fourth (S4) heart sounds
        - S3 and S4 are low-pitched sounds best heard with the bell of the stethoscope.
        - S3 is normal when heard in children and young adults (younger than 40 years).
        - In people older than 40 years, S3 is abnormal. It is often heard in left-sided heart failure.

Table 12–1. A Representation of Timing of Extra Heart Sounds

	Systole	Diastole	Systole	Diastole	
Normal heart sounds	S_1	S_2	S_1	S_2	S_1
Split S_2	S_1	A_2P_2	S_1	A_2P_2	S_1
Ventricular gallop S_3	S_1	S_2 S_3	S_1	S_2 S_3	S_1
Atrial gallop S_4	S_1	S_2	S_4 S_1	S_2	S_4 S_1

- S4 is expected when ventricular filling is augmented by atrial contraction or the ventricle is stiff and not able to accept the extra volume of blood during atrial contraction.
  - Ventricular filling may be augmented in hypertension, myocardial infarction, thyrotoxicosis, and anemia.
  - S4 depends on atrial contraction and is never heard during atrial fibrillation.
- • Diastolic murmurs
  - Always abnormal
  - Aortic or pulmonary valve insufficiency
  - Mitral or tricuspid valve stenosis
- Pericardial rub, associated with pericarditis, is characteristically scratchy, creaking, or grating.
  - • Triphasic associated with atrial systole, ventricular systole, and diastole.
  - • Best heard with the diaphragm of the stethoscope along the LSB as the patient leans forward.
  - • Differentiate pericardial rub from pleural rub by asking patient to hold his or her breath. Pericardial rub persists; pleural rub is abolished by breath-holding.
- Heart murmurs indicate turbulent flow and are frequently produced by abnormal heart valves. Table 12–2 lists the valve disorders and their associated murmurs. The following characteristics of murmurs should be assessed.
- Phase of the cardiac cycle—systole or diastole
  - • Diastolic murmurs are associated with disease.
  - • Systolic murmurs may be normal in some cases.
- Loudness or intensity is graded on 6-point scale. Systolic murmurs of grade III or more are usually hemodynamically and clinically significant.
  - Grade I: Heard only with concentration; distinct but faint.
  - Grade II: Faint but heard immediately.
  - Grade III: Comparable loudness to heart sounds.
  - Grade IV: Loud; may be associated with palpable thrill (buzzing sensation).
  - Grade V: Very loud; may be heard with only one edge of the stethoscope in contact with the chest wall. Thrill is present.
  - Grade VI: Very loud; may be heard with stethoscope off the chest. Thrill present.
  - • Location and radiation help determine the cause and significance of the murmur. Note the area where the murmur is loudest and any area of radiation.
    - For example, grade III or VI systolic murmur, loudest at the apex, and radiating to the left axilla.

Table 12–2. Auscultation Findings with Common Left-Sided Valve Disorders

	Listening Site	Timing	Radiation
Mitral regurgitation	5th ICS MCL	Systole	Axiliary area
Mitral stenosis	5th ICS MCL	Diastole	Axiliary area
Aortic insufficiency	2nd ICS LSB	Diastole	Neck
Aortic stenosis	2nd ICS LSB	Systole	Neck

- Lung exam
  - Inspection: observe the rate, depth, and effort of breathing.
    - Normal respiratory rate is 14 to 20 breaths per minute.
    - Expiration is normally slightly longer than inspiration, but prolonged expiration signifies airway disease.
    - Some abnormal respiratory patterns include the following:
      - Tachypnea: respiratory rate above 20
      - Hyperpnea: abnormally deep, large-volume breaths
      - Bradypnea: respiratory rate below 14
      - Cheyne-Stokes breathing: periods of deep breathing alternate with periods of apnea. There is a waxing and waning to the cycle. May be seen in left heart failure and during sleep in those with central sleep apnea.
      - Biot breathing: unpredictable irregularity of respiratory rate and depth; usually associated with brain damage.
      - Hyperventilation is the elimination of excessive CO_2. It is diagnosed by analysis of CO_2 content in the blood and not by observation of breathing pattern.
  - Palpation: Palpate any areas of chest pain and tenderness. Check for vocal fremitus (vocal vibrations transmitted through the chest wall to the ball of the hand). Compare side to side.
    - Fremitus is reduced when there is an obstructed bronchus, pleural effusion, pneumothorax, or a very thick chest wall.
    - Fremitus is increased when lung tissue is consolidated (e.g., pneumonia).
  - Percussion: Direct or indirect percussion helps determine whether lung structures are air-filled, fluid-filled, or solid. Compare side to side. Normal, air-filled lung produces a resonant percussion note.
    - Dull percussion note is heard when fluid or solid tissue replaces air-filled lung.
    - Hyperresonance is heard with over-inflated lungs (e.g., emphysema).
  - Auscultation: Normal lung sounds are normal when heard in normal places and abnormal when heard in abnormal places. Compare side to side.
    - Vesicular sounds are soft, relatively low-pitched sounds heard over the lung periphery. Inspiratory phase sounds longer than expiratory phase.
    - Bronchovesicular sounds are louder than vesicular sounds, normally heard in the region between the scapulae. Inspiratory and expiratory phases sound equal in duration.
      - Bronchovesicular sounds heard in the periphery may represent pneumonia or tumor.
    - Bronchial breath sounds are loud, relatively high-pitched, and heard over the manubrium, if at all. Expiratory phase sounds longer than inspiratory phase. There may be a slight pause between the inspiratory and expiratory phases.
      - Bronchial sounds that are heard in other locations might represent pneumonia or tumor.

- Adventitious (i.e., added) sounds are superimposed on normal lung sounds and are abnormal.
  - Crackles (also known as "rales") are discontinuous sounds that are intermittent and brief. They may be heard during inspiration, expiration, or both.
    - Note respiratory phase and lung region where heard.
    - Crackles may clear with cough; have patient cough to see if they change.
    - Crackles are abnormal and may be because pneumonia, fibrosis, atelectasis, heart failure, or bronchitis.
  - Wheezes are relatively high-pitched, continuous sounds. Wheezes suggest narrowed airways (e.g., asthma, COPD, bronchitis.)
  - Rhonchi are relatively low-pitched, continuous sounds. Rhonchi suggest the presence of secretions in the large airways.

Abdomen
- Waist circumference is associated with increased risk for cardiovascular disease and diabetes.
  - Waist circumference above 40 inches in men and above 35 inches in women indicates abdominal fat distribution and increased risk.
- Listen for bruits over the aorta, iliac, and femoral arteries and in each upper abdominal quadrant.
  - Bruits with both systolic and diastolic components are associated with arterial stenosis.
  - A systolic-phase bruit may be a normal finding.

Peripheral Circulation: Extremities
- Compare arm to arm and leg to leg.
  - Observe and compare size, temperature, symmetry, pigmentation, scars, and ulcers.
- Edema: an abnormal accumulation of fluid in the interstitial space
  - Weight gain of 10 pounds, indicative of 5 L of fluid, precedes visible edema.
  - Daily weights provide the best serial measure of edema.
  - Edema fluid accumulates in areas of dependency.
    - For ambulatory or seated patients, edema accumulates in feet and lower legs.
    - For bedridden patients, edema accumulates in the sacral or lumbar regions
  - Anasarca: generalized edema
  - Grading of edema—not all edema is pitting.
    - Edema causes swelling that may obscure the veins and bony prominences.
    - To check for pitting edema, press firmly for at least 5 seconds
      - Over the dorsum of each foot
      - Behind each medial malleolus
      - Over the shins
    - Severity of edema can be graded on a 5-point scale from 0 (none) to 4 (very severe).
    - Leg circumference can be measured, compared side-to-side, and monitored over time to assess changes in the amount of edema.
  - Long-standing edema may induce pigmentation (brownish), inflammation (redness), induration, and fibrosis of the skin and subcutaneous tissues. Edema reduces skin mobility and resiliency.

- Varicose veins are dilated, tortuous superficial veins with incompetent valves.
- Thrombophlebitis is inflammation of the vein with associated thrombus.
  - Homans sign is positive in only about 35% of patients with deep venous thrombosis (DVT) of the lower legs.
    - With the patient's knee flexed, the examiner abruptly dorsiflexes the ankle.
    - Sign is positive if pain is experienced in the calf or popliteal region. May be positive also in people with lumbar-sacral disc pathology.
- Venous insufficiency is a syndrome that involves destruction of the venous valves and obliteration of thrombosed veins.
  - Pain, if present, is described as a dull ache or heaviness.
  - Brownish discoloration of skin may occur.
  - Edema that increases with dependency and decreases with elevation may be present.
  - Chronic venous insufficiency (CVI) may cause ulceration of the lower leg around the ankle.
    - Skin surrounding the ulcer may be pigmented (brownish) or inflamed (reddened) and edematous.
    - CVI ulcers can be very painful.
    - Ulcer may have irregular shape and uneven borders
    - Venous ulcers are commonly located on the anterior or medial aspect of the lower leg.
- Arterial insufficiency is a syndrome of hypoperfusion.
  - Pain is present in the affected extremity.
    - Intermittent claudication is relieved with rest.
    - When pain is continuous, it is less severe with the affected extremity in the dependent position.
  - Skin of the lower extremity is dry, thin, and shiny with little hair present.
  - Toenails are thick and brittle.
  - Foot and extremity are cool and pale.
    - Elevation pallor and dependent rubor (redness)
  - Pulses are weak or absent.
    - Iliac or femoral bruits may be present.
  - Chronic arterial insufficiency may cause ulceration of the toes, feet, or ankles.
    - Skin surrounding the ulcer may be atrophic. The ulcer has smooth edges and a "punched out" appearance.
    - Pain may be severe unless masked by neuropathy.
    - Gangrene may be associated.

Neurological Exam

Neurological examination answers two important questions. Are right- and left-sided findings symmetrical? And, if findings are abnormal, does the causative lesion lie in the central or peripheral nervous system?

- Mental status and speech
  - Altered mental status is associated with hypertensive encephalopathy, stroke, and multi-infarct and vascular dementia.
  - Stroke is the most common cause of acquired speech defect in adults.
    - Dysarthria: defect in the muscular control of the speech apparatus
    - Aphasia: disorder in producing or understanding language

- Levels of consciousness
  - Alert: When spoken to in a normal tone of voice, patient opens eyes and responds fully and appropriately to stimulus.
  - Lethargic: When spoken to in a loud voice, patient may open eyes but falls back to sleep immediately.
  - Obtunded: When physically shaken, patient opens eyes, but responds slowly and is somewhat confused.
  - Stupor: Arouses only with application of a painful stimulus. Verbal response is slow or absent.
  - Coma: Eyes remain closed; no evidence of response to stimuli.
- Cranial nerves
  - CN II and III: optic and oculomotor
    - Observe pupil size and symmetry and test response to light (direct and consensual).
    - Test visual acuity.
  - CN III, IV, and VI: oculomotor, trochlear, and abducens
    - Test extraocular movements in the six cardinal directions of gaze.
    - Identify nystagmus (rapid eye movements).
    - Look for ptosis and lid lag.
  - CN V: trigeminal
    - While palpating temporal and masseter muscles, have patient clench and unclench his or her teeth. Notice the strength of muscle contraction.
    - Test for sensation of the forehead, cheek, and chin area.
    - Test corneal reflex.
  - CN VII: facial
    - Observe the facial musculature at rest and during conversation for asymmetry.
    - Ask the patient to do the following maneuvers; notice any weakness or asymmetry.
      - Smile and show teeth.
      - Close eyes tightly and don't let the examiner open them.
      - Puff out both cheeks.
      - Stick out tongue.
  - CN VIII: acoustic
    - Assess hearing—whisper test or finger rub.
    - If hearing loss is present, test for lateralization and compare air and bone conduction.
  - CN IX and X: glossopharyngeal and vagus
    - Observe voice quality.
    - Observe swallowing.
    - Observe movement of the soft palate and the pharynx.
    - Test the gag reflex.
  - CN XI: spinal accessory
    - Ask the patient to shrug both shoulders up against your hands. Observe the strength and contraction of the trapezius muscles.
  - CN XII: hypoglossal
    - Inspect the tongue for fasciculation.
    - Ask patient to protrude tongue and move it from side to side; look for asymmetry.

- Motor strength and function
  - Observe for involuntary movements.
  - Observe muscle size and contours—look for symmetry and atrophy.
  - Check muscle strength and spontaneous movement.
    - Paresis: impaired strength or weakness
    - Plegia: paralysis or absence of strength
- Sensation
  - Peripheral neuropathy—numbness in foot, leg, or hand
- Reflexes
  - Deep tendon reflexes are graded on a 5-point scale: 0 (no response), 1+ (diminished response), 2+ (normal or average response), 3+ (brisker than average response), and 4+ (very brisk hyperactive response with clonus).

DIAGNOSTIC TESTS

Sensitivity and Specificity
An ideal diagnostic test would be 100% sensitive and 100% specific. No diagnostic test is ideal.
- Sensitivity of a test is the ability of the test to detect patients with the disease in question (i.e., how often false negatives occur). For example, troponin I is 98% to 99% sensitive for MI; elevated troponin level is rarely seen in other conditions. (Clinical controversy suggests troponin may be elevated in patients after cardiac surgery or with end-stage renal disease.)
- Specificity of a test is how well test abnormality is restricted to those people who have the disease in question (i.e., how often false positives occur). An electrocardiogram (ECG) is 100% specific for MI. ECG changes associated with MI are only seen in patients who actually have MI. Sensitivity and specificity are inversely correlated, thus increasing sensitivity decreases specificity and vice versa.
- Combinations of tests are used to enhance sensitivity and specificity.
  - The combination of elevated troponin I and characteristic ECG changes makes the diagnosis of MI.

LABORATORY TESTS USING BLOOD

Obtaining Venous Sample
To enhance the reliability of venous samples:
- Avoid hemolysis, which will cause a false hyperkalemia.
  - Dry skin with gauze after antiseptic preparation.
  - Minimize duration of tourniquet.
  - Use double-ended needle and vacuum tube, if possible.
  - Use appropriate size needle; small needle when drawing multiple samples increases risk of hemolysis.
  - Remove needle from syringe, if used, before putting blood into tube.
- Do not draw blood from an arm where a solution is infusing intravenously.
- Color of the tube stopper reflects additives. Be sure to use the correct tube for each test.

Reference Values Are Laboratory-Specific

Interpret test results in light of the range provided.

- Variables that affect test results:
    - Age and gender: There may be different ranges established for men and women or for age groups.
    - Time of day: Most hormones show diurnal variation, so time of day affects results.
    - Drug interference
    - Time since food consumption: Some tests must be obtained with the patient in the fasting state.
- Reference range is established by testing a large number of healthy people and ranking results.
    - Values above a cutoff point (often 95%) are considered abnormal.
    - Because all tests in the reference group were done on healthy people, 5 out of 100 healthy people will have an abnormal result and be considered unhealthy statistically.

Cardiac Markers

Enzymes are proteins that catalyze chemical reactions in cells. Some enzymes are present in nearly all cells; others are specific to cells of certain organs.

- Cardiac enzymes
    - Creatine kinase (CK) is an enzyme present in brain, myocardial, and skeletal muscle cells. It is released from cells after irreversible injury; the presence of CK in the blood indicates cardiac, cerebral, or skeletal muscle injury.
        - CK isoenzymes are specific to each type of tissue.
            - CK-MB (CK-2) is from myocardial cells.
            - CK-BB is from brain cells.
            - CK-MM is from myocardial and skeletal muscle cells.
        - Enzyme release and clearance follows a predictable pattern after injury, which can be used diagnostically.
            - Reference range for total CK is 30 IU/L to 180 IU/L.
            - Reference range for CK-MB is 0 IU/L to 5 IU/L or 0% to 5% of total CK.
            - Total CK and CK-MB levels rise within 4 to 6 hours after a myocardial infarction (MI), peak within 12 to 24 hours, and (if there is no further injury) return to normal within 3 to 4 days.
            - Peak levels after MI are more than six times the normal value. Smaller elevations may be seen after reperfusion by angioplasty or thrombolysis and after electrical cardioversion.
            - Total CK and CK-MB are highly sensitive (93% to 100%) tests for MI. Total CK is a less specific (57% to 88%) test than CK-MB (specificity of 93% to 100%).
                - Intramuscular injection and skeletal muscle injury elevate total CK.
        - CK and CK-MB are repeated every 6 to 8 hours to establish the pattern.

- Cardiac proteins
  - Myoglobin, a protein found in myocardial and skeletal muscle, is released into blood after cell injury. Blood levels elevate in 1 to 3 hours after MI, peak in 8 to 12 hours, and return to normal in 12 to 30 hours.
    - Myoglobin is more sensitive than but not as specific as CK-MB for MI.
    - Because of early elevation, myoglobin is used in conjunction with cardiac enzyme elevation or ECG changes to make decisions for thrombolysis or early angioplasty.
    - Reference range: levels are undetectable in uninjured persons.
  - Troponin is found in both myocardial and skeletal muscle.
  - Three isotopes have been identified. Troponin I and T are found in myocardium; levels elevate in 4 to 6 hours after MI and remain elevated for 5 to 7 days.
    - Troponin I is 98% to 99% sensitive for MI.
    - Reference range: levels are undetectable in uninjured persons.

Coagulation Tests

- Platelets are elements of the blood that clump and stick to rough surfaces when clotting is necessary.
  - Reference range: 150,000/mm^3 to 400,000/mm^3
  - Bleeding time (how long it takes blood to clot in the body) is a simple test of platelet function.
    - Reference range: 3 to 7 minutes.
    - Aspirin therapy reduces platelet adhesion and prolongs bleeding time.
    - Aspirin effect on platelets is not reversible and lasts approximately 10 days.
    - Bleeding test may not be a reliable indicator of platelet function; use varies by practice region.
- Prothrombin time (PT) and international normalized ratio (INR) are used to initiate and maintain anticoagulation therapy with warfarin (Coumadin®).
  - PT is used to initiate therapy; after a stable dose is achieved (approximately 1 week), the INR is used for monitoring.
  - Reference range: PT 10 to 13 seconds or 70% to 100%.
  - Therapeutic range for PT is 2 to 2.5 times the control.
  - In most cases, the therapeutic INR range extends from 2 to 3.5. Ranges have been established for specific conditions.
    - For DVT prophylaxis, INR range of 1.5 to 2.0
    - For DVT treatment, INR range of 2.0 to 3.0
    - For prevention of embolism in atrial fibrillation, INR range of 2.0 to 3.0
    - For pulmonary embolism treatment, INR range of 3.0 to 4.0
    - For mechanical valve prophylaxis, INR range of 2.5 to 3.5
  - Most antibiotics taken with warfarin enhance the effect on PT and INR.
    - Aspirin and other antiplatelet medicines may be used with warfarin.
    - Caution patients about increased bleeding tendency with these combinations.
  - Instruct patients to avoid variable intake of vitamin K and to observe for and report signs of bleeding.
- Partial thromboplastin time (PTT) and activated PTT (aPTT) are used when patients receive unfractionated heparin.
  - Reference range: PTT 60 to 70 seconds; aPTT 20 to 35 seconds.
  - The therapeutic range for both the PTT and aPTT is 1.5 to 2.5 times baseline.
  - Laboratory monitoring is not required for patients receiving low molecular heparin.

Plasma Lipoproteins

- Elevated total and low-density lipoprotein (LDL) cholesterol increase atherosclerosis risk.
- Elevated high-density lipoprotein (HDL) cholesterol is protective (i.e., associated with lower atherosclerosis risk.)
- Classification of plasma cholesterol levels in the general adult population:
  - Total cholesterol
    - Desirable: below 200 mg/dL
    - Borderline high: 200 to 239 mg/dL
    - High: 240 mg/dL or above
  - LDL cholesterol
    - Optimal: below 100 mg/dL
    - Near optimal: 100 to 129 mg/dL
    - Borderline high: 130 to 159 mg/dL
    - High: 160 to 189 mg/dL
    - Very high 190 mg/dL or above
  - HDL cholesterol
    - Low: below 40 mg/dL
    - High: 60 mg/dL or above
- When patients are hospitalized with acute coronary syndromes or coronary procedures, a lipid profile should be measured on admission or within the first 24 hours.
  - LDL-lowering therapy should be initiated before or on discharge.
  - Therapy may need adjustment after 12 weeks.
- Random total cholesterol may be used for screening; fasting specimen (12 hours) is needed for diagnosis and treatment monitoring.
- There is a movement toward obtaining measured rather than calculated LDL-C and to obtain the subclasses of LDL and HDL for more specific risk identification (see Chapter 10).

Drug Levels

- Drug levels are quantitative tests used to monitor the effectiveness of drug therapy.
- Therapeutic drug monitoring is used when a drug has a low therapeutic to toxic dose range, such as digoxin and lithium.
- Serum concentrations must be interpreted within the clinical context.
  - Symptoms of digoxin toxicity can occur despite a therapeutic drug level if the patient has hypokalemia.
  - Digoxin may control heart rate effectively at less than therapeutic levels.
- To ensure accurate interpretation of results, note the drug name and dosage, time of last dose, route of administration, time blood was drawn, patient's age and clinical characteristics (e.g., creatinine clearance indicates renal function).

Additional Blood Tests of Interest

- B-type natriuretic protein (BNP) is a substance secreted when the atrial or ventricular tissue is overstretched. It is a mild compensatory measure to waste more sodium, which is followed by water. Elevated levels of BNP indicate fluid overload as seen with an acute exacerbation of heart failure.
- Electrolyte disorders can be associated with diuretic use or fluid overload. Monitor potassium and sodium levels and correlate with the underlying pathology. Potassium-sparing diuretics can result in hyperkalemia, especially in the presence of angiotensin converting enzyme inhibitors (ACE-I).

- Anemia of chronic disease can occur with heart or renal disorders and should be evaluated.
- Renal function should be monitored because some medicines may need to be dose-adjusted for elevated creatinine, associated decreased clearance, or decreased glomerular filtration rate (GFR).
  - The most common reason for a rise in creatinine in a person with heart disease is over-diuresis.
  - Similar drug categories also may worsen renal disease.
- Liver function tests need to be monitored in association with many of the cardiac medications that are prescribed (e.g., statins, fibrates, amiodarone).

NONINVASIVE DIAGNOSTIC TESTING

Chest X-Ray
- Two views of the chest, posterior to anterior (PA) and left lateral (LL).
- Provides information about the heart, lungs, and thoracic vascular and bony structures.
  - Size and contour of cardiac chambers
  - Presence of acute and chronic pulmonary disease
  - Dilation and calcification of thoracic vessels
- Correlation with clinical context and comparison with previous chest films provides the most useful information.
- X-ray is used for screening purposes and followed by other extensive diagnostic tests.
- X-ray gives a two-dimensional view.
- The heart should be no larger than one-third the width of the thorax. See Figure 12–3 for x-rays of a normal heart and an enlarged heart with failure.

Figure 12–3. Normal Chest X-Ray and Patient With Heart Failure

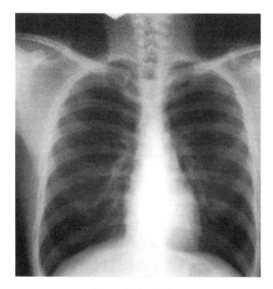 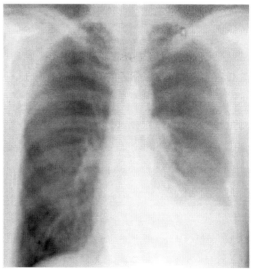

Normal Chest X-Ray   Patient With Heart Failure

Computed Tomography (CT) Scan

- A narrow x-ray beam examines body sections from many different angles to build up a three-dimensional picture of the structures.
- Performed with or without contrast dye. Contrast enhances tissue absorption and allows small defects to be seen.
- Purpose: To examine for head, liver, and renal lesions; tumors; abscesses; vascular diseases; stroke; bone destruction; and coronary heart disease. Can be used to find foreign objects within soft tissues (e.g., a bullet lodged in the chest or abdomen, fluid accumulation in the pericardium). New forms of CT can look at the coronary arteries and calculate a calcium score.
- General preparation: If contrast is not used, the CT scan is considered noninvasive.
  - With contrast, patient is NPO (nothing by mouth) for at least 4 hours before the procedure. Patients who are sensitive to iodine or shellfish may be allergic to contrast dye. They may be premedicated with diphenhydramine (Benadryl®) or the test cancelled.
  - Prescribed medications usually given with small amount of water but the patient should otherwise be NPO.
  - CT scanner is tubular with a circular opening. The camera rotates around the table while the patient lies motionless. Patient will hear the camera rotating and clicking.
  - If contrast dye is used, patient may experience warm flush or nausea at the time of injection.
  - If contrast dye is used, instruct patient to increase fluid intake after the scan.
  - Contrast should not be used if the serum creatinine is greater than 1.5 mg/dL, or estimated creatinine clearance below 60 mL/min, or GFR below 60.
- Coronary artery CT can detect calcium, which is present in atherosclerosis. See Figure 12–4.
  - The scan is only sensitive for calcium-laden lesions.
    - Many vulnerable lesions are lipid-laden and will not be detected by this test.
    - Many calcium laden-lesions are older, more stable lesions that are not likely to cause an acute coronary syndrome.
  - The calcium score is reported as a raw number. A score of 0 means no calcium was detected; 1 through 100 indicates an above-average 5-year risk of acute cardiac event; above 1,000 indicates a very high risk of a cardiac event in the near future.
- American Heart Association (AHA) and American College of Cardiology (ACC) recommendations are based on the degree of risk present and symptoms.
  - If symptomatic, the person should undergo other tests that will give more definitive answers, such as cardiac catheterization.

Figure 12–4. CT of the Coronary Artery Identifying Coronary Calcium

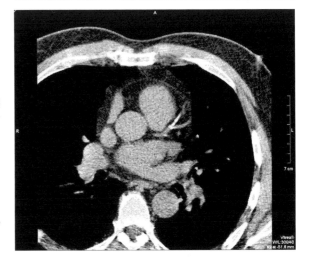

– In asymptomatic patients with intermediate risk, the calcium score will identify people who are at higher risk than previously thought.

– In low-risk, asymptomatic patients, the coronary artery CT test is not recommended because the high rate of false positives.

• CT angiography is the same high-speed CT with intravenous contrast injection. While lesions are identified with this technique, it is not recommended because patients receive a large amount of contrast that can be nephrotoxic, especially if other contrast is needed for subsequent diagnostics such as a cardiac catheterization. There are no recommendations for use of this test at this time. See Figure 12–5.

Magnetic Resonance Imaging (MRI)

• Uses radio waves and a magnetic field to create a computerized image of soft tissue structures. No ionizing radiation is used.

• Purpose: To detect central nervous system lesions, vascular problems, perfusion problems, injury, tumor, or edema.

• General preparation:
  – Remove all metal objects and cosmetics that may contain metallic fragments.
    • People with pacemakers, some metallic heart valves, prosthetic joints, recent surgical clips, etc., may not be candidates for MRI.
    • Remove hearing aids and dentures. Patients with metallic fillings may experience a "tingling" sensation in teeth but fillings will not be pulled out.
  – Contraindicated during pregnancy.
  – Patient must lie still on table within the scanner. Open scanners are available.
  – MRI can disrupt the flow of intravenous fluid.

• Contrast dye may be used with MRI to evaluate problems in the brain and spine. This dye is chemically unrelated to the contrast dye used in CT scan or arteriogram.

• Resuscitation equipment cannot be used in the MRI room.

Electrocardiogram (ECG)

The ECG provides a graphic record of the electrical activity in the heart.

• Cardiac electrical activity is recorded at standard speed (25 mm/sec) on special graph paper. The grid on the paper consists of small and large boxes, both horizontally and vertically.
  – On the horizontal axis, one small box (1 mm) represents 0.04 seconds; on the vertical axis, one small box represents 0.1 mV.
  – On the horizontal axis, one large box (5 mm) represents 0.20 seconds; on the vertical axis, one large box represents 0.5 mV.
  – ECG paper is marked with a vertical line in the top margin at 3-second intervals.

• ECG waves, complexes, and intervals reflect electrical activity within the heart. Normal characteristics have been described for each wave, complex, and interval.
  – P wave represents atrial depolarization. It is normally no taller than 0.25 mV or wider than 0.11 second.
  – PR interval, measured from the beginning of the P wave to the beginning of the QRS complex, represents the time required for the impulse to travel through the atria, AV junction, and Purkinje system. Normal duration is 0.12 to 0.20 second.

Figure 12–5. Coronary Artery CT With Contrast: Lesion in the Left Anterior Descending Coronary Artery

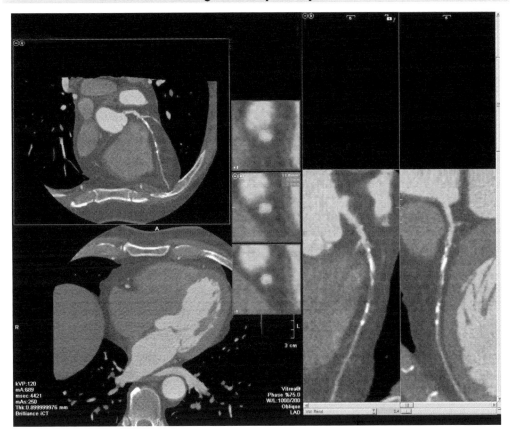

Multiple views of the same lesion are shown. Note the lesion is the brightest white in the vessel.

- QRS complex represents ventricular depolarization. Q is the initial negative deflection from baseline. R is the first positive deflection from baseline. S is a negative deflection that follows an R wave. Normal QRS duration is 0.04 to 0.10 second.
- ST segment represents the time when the ventricles are depolarized. It begins at the end of the QRS and extends to the beginning of the T wave. Normal ST segment should be a flat baseline and gently curve up to the T wave.
- T wave represents ventricular repolarization. It is normally in the same direction as the QRS complex. Normal T waves are not taller than 5 mm in the limb leads or 10 mm in the precordial (chest) leads.
- QT interval represents ventricular depolarization and repolarization. It is measured from the beginning of the QRS complex to the end of the T wave.
  - Duration of the QT interval varies with HR.
  - A nomogram is used to correct the observed QT interval to a rate of 60 bpm (QTc).
    - Normal QTc is 0.42 second for men and 0.43 second for women.
- U wave is a small wave that follows the T wave. It is not always visible.

Table 12–3. Lead Placement for the 12-Lead ECG

Limb leads are placed on each limb as marked	
V1	4th intercostal space at the right sternal border
V2	4th intercostal space at the left sternal border
V3	Halfway between V2 and V4
V4	5th intercostal space at the left midclavicular line
V5	5th intercostal space at the left anterior axillary line
V6	Parallel to V5 at the left midaxillary line

- Heart rate can be determined from an ECG strip.
  - Count the number of R–R intervals in a 6-second strip (two 3-second markers in the top margin) and multiply by 10.
  - If the rhythm is regular, count the number of small boxes between 2 R waves and divide into 1,500.
- Purpose:
  - To detect and evaluate coronary and valvular heart disease
  - To detect cardiac dysrhythmia
  - To identify electrolyte imbalance and drug effect
  - To evaluate effects of antidysrhythmic drugs on ECG intervals
- 12-lead ECG provides 12 standard views of the electrical activity of the heart.
  - Lead placement is defined in Table 12–3.
  - The normal 12-lead ECG appearance (see Figure 12–6)
    - Leads I, aVL, V5-6 provide a view of the lateral wall of the LV. These leads may have a small R wave followed by a tall R wave.
    - Leads II, III, and aVF provide a view of the inferior wall of the LV. These leads have a tall R and small- to medium-size S waves.
    - The precordial leads start with small R waves and deep S waves. The R gradually gets larger and the S wave smaller as you move from V1 to V6. This is called normal R wave progression.
    - Lead aVL normally is negative with inverted P and T waves.
- ECG signs of coronary heart disease:
  - Myocardial ischemia: classic pattern of ischemia is T-wave inversion. T-wave inversion is nonspecific. Other signs of myocardial ischemia include:
    - ST segment depression of 0.5 mm or more below baseline
    - ST segment that remains at baseline longer than 0.12 second
    - ST segment that forms a sharp angle with the upright T wave
    - Tall, wide-based T waves and inverted U waves
  - Myocardial injury is most frequently indicated by ST segment elevation 1 mm or more above the baseline. Other signs of acute injury include:
    - Straightening of the ST segment that slopes up to the peak of the T wave without any time spent at baseline
    - Tall, peaked T waves
    - Symmetric T wave inversion

Figure 12–6. Normal 12-Lead ECG

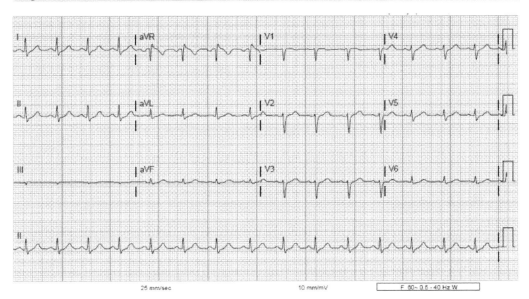

25 mm/sec   10 mm/mV   F 60~ 0.5 - 40 Hz W

- Myocardial infarction: The classic pattern is development of new Q waves in the leads reflecting the affected cardiac surface. See Figure 12–7.
    - Abnormal Q waves are more than 0.03 second wide or more than 25% of the amplitude of the R wave.
    - Other signs include decreased R wave amplitude, ST segment depression, and T wave inversion.
- Left ventricular hypertrophy is commonly associated with valvular heart disease and hypertension. See Figure 12–8.
    - Increased amplitude of R waves in leads I, aVL, V5, and V6
    - Increased amplitude of S waves in leads V1 and V2
    - R plus S wave amplitude in any precordial lead 45 mm or more
- Selected drug and electrolyte effects
    - Digoxin in therapeutic doses can produce sagging (cupping) of the ST segment with flattening of the T waves, shortening of the QT interval, and prolongation of the PR interval.
    - Digoxin toxicity causes conduction disturbances, extrasystoles, and tachycardia.
    - Beta blockers cause sinus bradycardia with slight prolongation of PR interval.
    - Hyperkalemia (serum potassium 5 mEq/L or above)
        - Tall peaked T waves and short QT interval
        - PR interval longer than 0.20 second
        - With severe elevation, QRS becomes broad and bizarre and ventricular fibrillation may occur.
    - Hypokalemia (serum potassium below 3 mEq/L) and hypomagnesemia increase risk of dysrhythmia and digoxin toxicity.

Figure 12–7. Acute Anterior Wall Myocardial Infarction

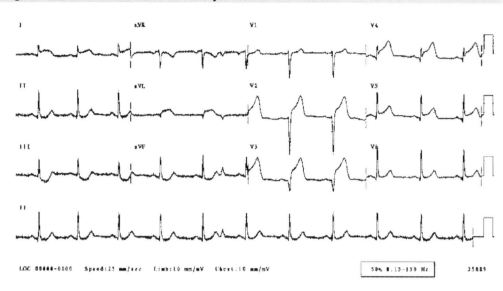

Ambulatory ECG

Ambulatory ECG (Holter monitor) records cardiac electrical activity continuously for a period of time (e.g., 24 hours) during unrestricted activity, rest, and sleep.

- Used in the diagnostic investigation of dizziness, syncope, and palpitations and to monitor effect of antidysrhythmic drugs; can document silent ischemia
- Patients are instructed to mark and describe symptoms occurring during the monitoring period (e.g., palpitations, rapid heart rate, light-headedness).
  - Monitor should not get wet. Avoid bathing and showering while monitoring.
  - Avoid use of electric razor or toothbrush to avoid ECG artifacts.
- An intermittent monitoring device, called an event monitor, may be used.
  - The patient activates the recorder only when he or she experiences symptoms.
  - The recording can be sent over the telephone to the physician's office.

Exercise ECG

Exercise ECG identifies exercise-induced myocardial ischemia and evaluates cardiac dysrhythmia.

- ECG is monitored and recorded while patient exercises under gradually increasing workload.
  - Treadmill or exercise bicycle with predetermined levels of increasing speed, grade, or resistance is used (e.g., the Bruce protocol).
- BP is obtained in the arm for evaluation of cardiovascular exercise response. Expired gases may be collected to evaluate pulmonary function (e.g., screening tool used to evaluate patients before heart transplant).
- Clinicians assess for symptoms and ECG indications to stop the test.
  - Severe angina
  - Marked ST segment depression
  - Ventricular or atrial tachycardia, atrial fibrillation, or high degree A-V block
- Patients exercise to reach capacity for their age and gender. The goal is to exercise at 85% of maximal heart rate for 3 minutes.

Figure 12–8. Left Ventricular Hypertrophy

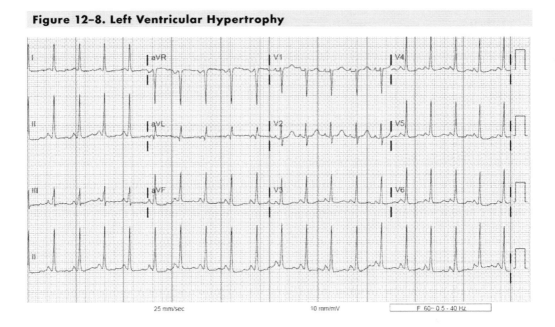

25 mm/sec   10 mm/mV   F 60~ 0.5 - 40 Hz

Head-Up Tilt-Table Test

Head-up tilt-table test is used to evaluate vasodepressor syncope and near-syncope.

• Patient is placed on a table and is tilted to an upright position.

• ECG and BP are monitored to evaluate the relative contribution of bradycardia and hypotension to syncope.

Electron Beam Tomography

Electron beam tomography is a high-speed electron beam that images the heart (and other structures) in three dimensions.

• Calcification of coronary or carotid arteries can be determined and scored.

• This test is used to quantify risk in younger patients (30 through 50 years old) with a family history of early heart disease.

DIAGNOSTIC ULTRASONOGRAPHY

Principles

• High-frequency (above that which can be detected by the human ear) sound waves are sent through body structures by a transducer.
  – Sound waves cannot be heard or felt by the patient.
  – No known damage to tissues from clinical use of sound waves.

• The transducer also receives returning sound waves, which are reflected back as they bounce off bodily structures.

- Sound waves reflected from a moving substance are changed in a predictable way (i.e., Doppler effect). When the substance is moving toward the detector, the frequency increases; when the substance is moving away from the detector, the frequency decreases.
  - In clinical applications, high-frequency sound waves are reflected off red blood cells and transformed into audible sound waves.
  - Color Doppler assigns a different color to the image of the blood in relationship to its speed and direction.
- Ultrasound does not penetrate air or bone.
  - Use coupling gel between transducer and skin
  - Ultrasound techniques are less useful for detecting thoracic than abdominal disease.
- Real-time imaging refers to the use of rapid scanners that are able to display motion.
- Duplex scans use both real-time imaging and Doppler flow imaging.

Echocardiography (ECHO)

ECHO uses high-frequency sound waves and the Doppler effect to evaluate the size, shape, and motion of cardiac structures and the direction and velocity of blood flow through the heart.

- Transthoracic ECHO uses a transducer on the chest wall.
  - Stress ECHO helps identify silent and exercise-induced ischemia. Ventricular wall motion and thickness are evaluated at rest and at peak exercise (just as the patient comes off the treadmill).
    - Exercise (bicycle ergometer or treadmill) or drugs (dobutamine or dipyridamole) are used to stress the cardiovascular system.
    - Used in diagnosis of coronary heart disease, valvular heart disease, cardiomyopathy, and intracardiac masses or clots.
    - Used to calculate left ventricular ejection fraction.
    - Able to assess diastolic function.
- Transesophageal ECHO: A transducer, mounted on a flexible endoscope is introduced into the esophagus and to the stomach to obtain clearer visualization and greater anatomic detail than possible with transthoracic ECHO.
  - This test provides better views of valve structures and often is used to find vegetations of infective endocarditis.
  - Requires sedation and respiratory monitoring during the procedure.

Venous and Arterial Duplex

Uses sound waves and the Doppler principle to determine and evaluate blood flow in specific vascular structures.

- Used to evaluate carotid stenosis in those with cervical bruit or transient ischemic attack (TIA) and to follow up after carotid endarterectomy (CEA).
  - Patients with TIA and more than 70% stenosis or ulcerated plaques are usually advised to have CEA.
- Used to evaluate renal and peripheral artery stenosis
- Venous duplex is a primary tool used to diagnose DVT.
- Arterial duplex is used to rule out pseudoaneurysm of the femoral artery after cardiac catheterization.

Transcranial Doppler

Uses sound waves and the Doppler principle to evaluate blood flow in selected intracranial blood vessels.

- Bone is not penetrated by ultrasound.
- Acoustic windows allow evaluation of the middle cerebral, anterior communicating, posterior communicating, ophthalmic, distal internal carotid, vertebral, and basilar arteries.
- Used to evaluate subarachnoid hemorrhage, vertebrobasilar insufficiency, and collateral circulation in people with internal carotid artery lesions.

DIAGNOSTIC TESTING USING RADIONUCLIDES

Blood Pool Imaging

A scintillation camera obtains images as a bolus of radioactive tracer (technetium 99) mixed with blood passes through the heart.

- Assesses cardiac function (i.e., ejection fraction and wall motion).
- Normal ejection fraction is 55% or more.

Myocardial Perfusion Imaging

A radioactive tracer (thallium 201 or technetium 99m sestamibi) accumulates in the myocardium in proportion to myocardial blood flow and the extraction of the radionuclide by myocardial cells.

- Need viable myocardial cell for tracer to accumulate.
- Areas of scar tissue and areas that are hypoperfused do not take up the tracer.
- Can be combined with exercise to increase sensitivity and specificity of the test
- Dipyridamole and adenosine may be infused intravenously to dilate coronary arteries and increase myocardial blood flow.
  - Severely narrowed coronary arteries do not dilate and blood flow is not increased.

INVASIVE DIAGNOSTIC TESTING

Cardiac catheterization or coronary angiography is an invasive test that delineates coronary anatomy. The test is the "gold standard" to diagnose coronary heart disease.

- Indications include patients with acute coronary syndrome (symptoms and ECG pattern of ischemia or injury) and those who have been evaluated with noninvasive tests that suggest myocardial ischemia.
- Patients may undergo right- or left-heart catheterization or both.
- Right-heart catheterization:
  - In the catheterization lab under fluoroscopy, a specially designed catheter is placed through a peripheral (often the femoral) vein and threaded into the right side of the heart.
  - Sensors on the catheter tip read chamber pressures and monitor blood flow rates.
  - The catheter is floated into the pulmonary artery and pressures reflected from the left side of the heart are assessed.
    - Pulmonary artery pressures and cardiac output are measured
    - Left ventricular end diastolic pressure (pulmonary artery wedge or capillary pressure) is measured.

- Left-heart catheterization:
  - A second catheter is threaded in a retrograde direction from the femoral artery into the left side of the heart.
  - Radio-opaque dye is injected into the coronary arteries to evaluate patency of the arteries and myocardial perfusion.
  - Radio-opaque dye is injected into the left ventricle to assess ventricular function (ejection fraction).
- The patient is on a cardiac monitor throughout the procedure because the catheter or the dye may irritate the heart and cause cardiac dysrhythmia.
- Data recorded from the catheters and from fluoroscopic imaging can provide information about
  - Coronary circulation and areas of stenosis
  - Pressures in each chamber of the heart
  - Cardiac output and ejection fraction
  - Cardiac size and malformations
  - Aortic and mitral valvular stenosis and regurgitation (velocity and flow)
- Postprocedure, patients may be on bed rest and monitored for 1 to 12 hours, depending on the size of the catheters and the type of antiplatelet medicines used.
  - Precautions are taken to prevent bleeding at the arterial puncture site.
    - Angioseals such as Perclose™ may be placed in the catheterization laboratory to establish immediate hemostasis. These patients may be ambulatory after catheterization.
  - Puncture site and distal circulation is assessed frequently.
    - Assess site for visible bleeding, swelling, or tenderness.
    - Monitor circulatory parameters—pulse, limb temperature, capillary refill—distal to the puncture site.
      - Diminished or absent pulse and circulation may signify arterial occlusion.
    - Auscultate the femoral artery puncture site.
      - Presence of a bruit suggests pseudoaneurysm.
      - Arterial duplex confirms pseudoaneurysm.
  - BP is monitored; cardiac rhythm may be monitored.
  - The contrast dye used in the procedure acts as an osmotic diuretic and patients require a large amount of fluids to facilitate excretion of the dye.
    - Encourage patients to drink at least four glasses of water or juice if not contraindicated (e.g., severe cardiomyopathy, renal disease).
    - Monitor urine output for several hours after procedure.
  - Other potential problems after cardiac catheterization include MI, stroke, and heart failure.
  - Patients with poor renal function may be treated with acetylcysteine (Mucomyst®) for 2 days prior to the procedure along with special hydration protocols and $NaHCO_3$ (sodium bicarbonate) in the periprocedural period.
  - Patients on warfarin need to be bridged to heparin so that bleeding can be better reversed during the procedure.
  - Patients on aspirin (ASA) will need to stop taking the drug for 3 to 5 days prior to the cardiac catheterization.

Electrophysiology Studies (EPS)

Used to assess the diagnosis and mechanism of cardiac dysrhythmia.

- Indications: cardiac arrest survivors, differential diagnosis of wide complex tachycardia (ventricular or supraventricular tachycardia), syncope when believed because dysrhythmia, and the diagnosis and treatment of accessory pathways.
- Procedure:
    - Specialty catheters with multiple electrodes are threaded into the heart from the periphery under fluoroscopy.
    - Timing and sequence of cardiac activation is recorded.
    - Attempts are made to induce dysrhythmia and to relate it to clinical symptoms.
    - If the patient is hemodynamically stable in the induced dysrhythmia, attempts are made to find the ectopic site or pathway that corresponds to the ECG signal.
- Therapeutic radio-frequency ablation may be done on fast or slow conduction pathways, atrial flutter zones, the atrial-ventricular node, or dysrhythmogenic foci.
- Postprocedure patients require monitoring of the catheter site for bleeding or compromised distal perfusion as outlined above for patients undergoing cardiac catheterization.
    - Intensive monitoring of cardiac rhythm may be required.
    - Laboratory studies including electrolytes and renal function tests may be required.

Angiograms and Venograms

- Angiograms: x-ray procedure used to examine the arterial supply of a specific region.
    - Contrast medium is injected through a selectively placed catheter.
    - Catheters often are placed under fluoroscopy. Procedure is done in x-ray suite.
    - Angiograms are more sensitive and specific that ultrasound and Doppler studies, but they carry higher risk of harm than noninvasive studies.
- Venograms: x-ray procedure that uses contrast medium to visualize venous system of a region. Procedure is done in x-ray suite. Usually an ambulatory patient procedure.

SUMMARY

This chapter provided an overview of key aspects of obtaining the health history. The history provides the key to understanding what is happening with the patient. Good assessment skills will help the nurse obtain even more valuable data. The chapter also contained a brief overview of many of the cardiac and vascular tests that can be obtained. The next chapter describes common cardiac and vascular disorders and the nurse's role in patient care.

REFERENCES

Bickley, L. S., & Hoekelman, R. A. (2007). *Bates' guide to physical examination and history taking* (9th ed.). Philadelphia: Lippincott.

Crawford, M. H. (2009). *Cardiology: Current diagnosis and treatment.* New York: McGraw Hill.

Estes, M. E. (2010). *Health assessment and physical examination.* Clifton Park, NY: Delmar.

Gary, R., & Davis, L. (2008). Diastolic heart failure. *Heart and Lung, 37,* 405–416.

Greenland, P., Bonow, R. O., Brundage, B. H., Budoff, M. J., Eisenberg, M. J., Grundy SM, ... Society of Cardiovascular Computed Tomography. (2007). ACCF/AHA 2007 clinical expert consensus document on coronary artery calcium scoring by computed tomography in global cardiovascular risk assessment and in evaluation of patients with chest pain: A report of the American College of Cardiology Foundation Clinical Expert Consensus Task Force (ACCF/AHA Writing Committee to Update the 2000 Expert Consensus Document on Electron Beam Computed Tomography) developed in collaboration with the Society of Atherosclerosis Imaging and Prevention and the Society of Cardiovascular Computed Tomography. *Journal of the American College of Cardiology, 49,* 378–402.

Jarvis, C. (2007). *Physical examination and health assessment* (4th ed.). Philadelphia: W. B. Saunders.

Labus, D. (2008). *Cardiovascular care made incredibly easy.* Philadelphia: Springhouse.

LeFever Kee, J. (2009). *Laboratory and diagnostic tests* (8th ed.). Upper Saddle River, NJ: Prentice Hall.

McPhee, S. J., & Hammer, G. D. (2009). *Pathophysiology of disease: An introduction to clinical medicine* (6th ed.). New York: McGraw-Hill.

Moser, D., & Reigel, B. (2008). *Cardiac nursing: A companion to Braunwald's heart disease.* St. Louis, MO: Elsevier-Saunders.

Seller, R. H. (2007). *Differential diagnosis of common complaints* (5th ed.). Philadelphia: W. B. Saunders

Woods, S. L., Sivarajan-Froelicher, E. S., Motzer, S. A., & Bridges, E. J. (2010). *Cardiac nursing* (6th ed). Philadelphia: Lippincott Williams & Wilkins.

Zipes, D. P., Libby, P., Bonow, R. O., & Braunwald, E. (2009). *Braunwald's heart disease: A textbook of cardiovascular medicine* (8th ed.). Philadelphia: Elsevier-Saunders.

13

Cardiac and Vascular Disease Manifestations

This chapter reviews the most common forms of cardiac and vascular disease. These disorders are likely to be on the certification exam. Background regarding each disorder is provided. General assessment and diagnostic testing is included. Nursing care of the patient with each problem is provided. This chapter builds on the previous two chapters, which discussed physiology and assessment, and provides the foundation of care for the patient with cardiac or vascular disease.

ANGINA PECTORIS

Description
Chest pain or discomfort from myocardial ischemia is because of inadequate coronary blood flow to the heart muscle. Angina pectoris is usually transient and reversible.

Etiology
Angina pectoris is usually from an atherosclerotic lesion. Other causes include spasm and anomalies of the coronary artery.

Incidence and Demographics
- Angina pectoris affects approximately 9,800,000 people in the United States.
- More women than men are affected.
- Only 18% of those who have a myocardial infarction have advance warning with a history of angina.

Risk Factors
- Nonmodifiable risk factors for coronary heart disease (CHD) include increasing age, male gender, heredity, and race (Black, Hispanic, and Native American).
- Modifiable risk factors include tobacco smoking, hypertension (HTN), high serum cholesterol with elevated serum low-density lipoprotein cholesterol (LDL-C) and low serum high-density lipoprotein cholesterol (HDL-C), diabetes mellitus, stress, excess alcohol consumption, physical inactivity, and overweight or obesity.

Assessment
- History
  - Typical chest pain is substernal and may radiate to the arm or jaw.
  - Atypical chest pain includes symptoms such as dyspnea, nausea, vomiting, and fatigue.
  - Chronic stable angina from transient myocardial ischemia is stimulated by a predictable amount of physical exertion or fatigue.
  - Unstable angina has a similar pattern of symptoms but the occurrences become more frequent, severe, or prolonged and may not have a specific triggering mechanism.
  - Noncardiac problems such as pleurisy or costochondritis may mimic some of these symptoms.
  - Risk factors for CHD
- Physical findings may be present at rest or only during pain.
  - S4 heart sound
  - Cardiac murmur
  - Dysrhythmia
  - Tachycardia
  - HTN or hypotension
- Diagnostic tests
  - Nitroglycerin test dose to determine if there is relief of symptoms.
  - Electrocardiogram (ECG) may show ST segment depression or T wave inversion during pain.
  - Exercise tolerance test to assess left ventricular function and evidence of ischemia when myocardial oxygen consumption is increased.
  - Echocardiogram to determine if there are ventricular wall motion abnormalities.
  - Nuclear studies to examine perfusion of the myocardium at rest and with exercise.

Management
- Pharmacologic management
  - Aspirin is used as an antiplatelet agent.
  - Beta-adrenergic blockers are used to decrease cardiac workload and myocardial oxygen demand.

  – Cholesterol-lowering drugs are used to slow the progression of atherosclerosis and reduce inflammation in the vessel wall, thus stabilizing the lesion.
  – Nitrates are used for systemic vasodilatation to decrease myocardial preload and coronary artery dilation to increase blood flow. They can be short-acting for acute pain or long-acting for prophylaxis.
  – Calcium channel blockers are used for vasodilation and to reduce myocardial contractility.
  – Beta blockers, nitrates, and calcium channel blockers work by decreasing resting myocardial oxygen consumption and by keeping the heart rate and blood pressure below the ischemic threshold when the person is active.
  – Ranolazine (Ranexa®) is a newer anti-anginal drug that works by slowing the late sodium channels and not by lowering oxygen consumption.
• Patient and family education
  – Teach patients and their families about the etiology, risk factors, and course of CHD.
  – Educate them about risk factor modification including diet, exercise, weight reduction, smoking cessation, stress reduction, and pharmacological interventions including actions, dosage, and side effects of medications.
  – Discuss with them the acute symptoms associated with unstable angina and MI and when to call 911 and seek emergency care.
  – Refer to a cardiac rehabilitation program for monitored exercise and lifestyle modification education.
  – Family members of people with cardiac disease should learn cardiopulmonary resuscitation (CPR) and how to activate the Emergency Medical System (EMS) in the event of cardiac arrest.

Outcomes and Follow-Up
• Patients and their families will be knowledgeable about angina pectoris and its treatment.
• Patients will not experience any complications such as myocardial infarction.
• Patients will follow up as indicated with their healthcare providers after diagnostic testing.
• Patients will reduce risk factors as secondary prevention measures.

MYOCARDIAL INFARCTION (MI)

Description
• Acute coronary syndrome (ACS) includes unstable angina, non-ST elevation MI (NSTEMI), and ST-elevation MI (STEMI).
• ACS involves imbalance between myocardial oxygen supply and demand (myocardial ischemia) that can cause myocardial cellular injury or infarct.
• In unstable angina, the oxygen imbalance resolves within 20 minutes, without permanent damage to myocardium.
• In MI, prolonged myocardial ischemia results in necrosis of myocardial tissue beginning within hours and continuing over the next day. Injury begins at the endocardial layer, which receives blood last and has the highest work load. The wavefront of damage spreads eventually toward the epicardial surface. See Figure 13–1.

Figure 13–1. Wave Front of Necrosis Across the Left Ventricular Wall Moves From Endocardium to Epicardial Surface

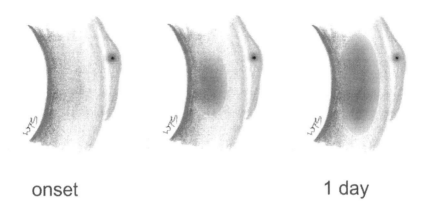

Myocardium Cross-Section Obstruction

onset   1 day

Etiology

- Myocardial ischemia may result from
  - Thrombus formation on preexisting plaque,
  - Coronary vasospasm,
  - Atherosclerotic occlusion in the absence of clot or vasospasm,
  - Inflammation or infection, or
  - Ischemia secondary to decreased oxygen supply (anemia, acute blood loss, or hypoxemia), or secondary to increased demand (metabolic disorders such as thyrotoxicosis).
- The predominant cause of ACS is acute coronary thrombosis resulting from platelet adherence to a disrupted atherosclerotic plaque.
- Plaque rupture is more likely to occur in an unstable, inflamed, lipid-laden lesion with a thin cap that was not hemodynamically significant (60%) before the rupture. After rupture of the plaque, a thin layer of platelets line the erosion and become activated, starting the thrombus formation at the site. Vasospasm can occur because of secretion of thromboxane A from platelets. Total or near-total occlusion results.
  - A total occlusion results in an ST segment elevation form of MI (STEMI).
  - A subtotal occlusion results in a non-ST segment elevation form of MI (NSTEMI). Some tissue infarcts, usually in the subendothelial area.
    - This was once called a non–Q wave MI or subendocardial MI. Early ECG changes include ST depression or T wave inversion.
    - Based on this ECG pattern and pain pattern, the patient is considered a high-risk patient.
  - If the patient has a strong history but normal or nondiagnostic ECG changes, he or she is considered an intermediate/low risk and should be monitored.
  - The American Heart Association includes ACS management in advanced cardiac life support training and this serves as a guideline for practice.

Incidence and Demographics

- Two million Americans are diagnosed with ACS annually; of these, one million will be diagnosed with unstable angina and one million with acute myocardial infarction (AMI).
- Half of the people with AMI will die, about half within the first hour after onset of symptoms, most as a result of ventricular fibrillation. One person has ACS every 25 seconds in the United States and someone dies of it every minute.

Risk Factors

- Presence of modifiable and nonmodifiable risk factors for CHD as discussed in Chapters 7 and 8.
- Family history is a risk factor but at this time there is no specific testing available. Multiple genetic factors influence risk.

Assessment

- History
  - Determine onset of symptoms (time, associated activity or event), location of pain, radiation (arm(s), jaw, or back), duration (constant or intermittent), character (squeezing, sharp, or dull), associated symptoms (fatigue, dyspnea, diaphoresis, nausea, vomiting, confusion, and syncope), relieved by (rest or nitroglycerin), treatments attempted by patient and their effect (rest, nitroglycerin, NSAIDS, or antacids).
  - Presence of modifiable and nonmodifiable risk factors
  - Previous medical history (PMH) such as angina, MI, dysrhythmia (atrial fibrillation, heart block), stroke, transient ischemic attack (TIA), rheumatic heart disease, or diabetes
  - Previous cardiovascular procedures including coronary artery bypass grafting (CABG), angioplasty, stent placement, carotid endarterectomy, pacemaker, or recent surgical procedures
  - Smoking, alcohol, cocaine, or other illicit drug use
- Physical findings
  - S3 and S4 heart sounds
  - Dysrhythmia
  - Tachycardia or bradycardia
  - HTN or hypotension
  - Cardiac murmurs
  - Pericardial friction rub
  - Pulmonary congestion (e.g., crackles and productive cough of pink, frothy sputum)
  - Jugular venous distention
  - Hepatomegaly or splenomegaly
  - Peripheral edema
- Diagnostic tests
  - ECG for patients with ongoing chest pain, and as soon as possible in patients with chest pain consistent with ACS but whose pain has resolved by the time of evaluation. ECG should be compared to previous ECG if available. See Table 13–1 for location of leads and areas of the myocardium, and Table 13–2 for types of ECG changes occurring over time.

Table 13–1. ECG Leads and Associated Area of LV and Coronary Circulation

Area of LV	Leads	Coronary Artery
Anterior wall	V1–V4	Left anterior descending coronary artery
Lateral wall	I, aVL, V5-V6	Left circumflex artery
Inferior wall	II, III, aVF	Right coronary artery
Posterior wall	Mirror image in V1–V4 (ST depression, tall R wave)	Right coronary or left circumflex arteries

- Laboratory tests
  - Creatine kinase (CK) isoenzymes: CK-MB above 3% of total CK is considered positive for MI.
  - Troponin (Tn) and myoglobin: Tn is undetectable in healthy people. Levels above 0.01 ng/mL are considered elevated, levels above 0.1 mg/mL greatly elevated and indicative of high risk of cardiac death.
  - Other tests include a complete blood count (CBC), basic metabolic panel, prothrombin time (PT) with international normalized ratio (INR) and activated partial thromboplastin time (APTT), and blood type and screen. Patients admitted with ACS also should have a lipid profile within the first 24 hours. Brain natriuretic peptide (BNP) may be indicated to assess degree of congestion.
- Chest x-ray to evaluate for pulmonary edema, cardiomegaly, and other noncardiac etiologies for dyspnea or chest pain (pneumonia, rib fractures, etc.)
- Echocardiogram to evaluate left ventricular ejection fraction (EF), cardiac wall motion abnormalities, and to identify pericardial effusions.
- Cardiac catheterization to determine the site of infarct and perform an acute percutaneous coronary intervention (PCI).

Management

- ACS risk categories: The results of history, physical examination, ECG, and cardiac markers are used to assign patients to one of four ACS risk categories.
  - ST-segment elevation. Patients with ST-segment elevation or with left bundle branch block (LBBB) should be treated immediately with either fibrinolytic therapy or primary angioplasty, depending upon time since onset of symptoms as well as relative or absolute contraindications for surgery or fibrinolytics and availability of a cardiac catheterization laboratory. Generally, PCI is the preferred treatment if available. Glycoprotein (GP) IIb/IIIa inhibitors and clopidogrel are recommended for patients undergoing PCI.
    - Door to balloon inflation (PCI) goal is 90 minutes.
    - Door to needle (thrombolytic) goal is 30 minutes.
  - High to intermediate risk: non–ST-segment elevation or unstable angina as identified by patients with continuing ischemic symptoms, elevated cardiac markers, and ST segment depression or elevation of less than 1 mm, or T-wave inversion, should be treated medically with IV nitroglycerin (NTG), beta blockers, and anticoagulants (heparin or bivalirudin, and GP IIb/IIIa inhibitors). ECG should be repeated in 12 hours and enzymes should be repeated (after 6 to 8 hours).

Table 13-2. Sequential ECG Changes With a STEMI

Timing	ECG Change
Acute (onset to days)	ST elevation, followed by development of Q waves
Recent (days to 6 months)	ST segment normalizes, Q waves persist, T wave inverted
Old (> 6 months)	Q waves, ST and T normal

- These patients should not receive thrombolytics because this may actually increase the risk of thrombus formation.
- Early invasive strategy—coronary angiography and PCI—is recommended for the high-risk patient.
    - Low risk: non–ST-segment elevation. Patients with typical or atypical chest pain that is new, intermittent in duration, and with normal ECG or nonspecific ECG changes, and with negative cardiac enzymes, should be admitted for observation and treated medically with NTG (sublingual, nasal spray, or topical paste) and a beta blocker.
- Invasive management
    - PCI with primary angioplasty, with or without placement of a stent.
    - Coronary stenting combined with GP IIb/IIIa inhibitors has been shown to result in better myocardial preservation and reduced need for late revascularization compared to fibrinolysis.
    - Coronary artery bypass surgery is an option for select patients not amenable to PCI.
- Pharmacologic management
    - Aspirin: All patients with ACS should receive aspirin (ASA), 160 to 325 mg p.o., with the first dose chewed and swallowed for immediate antiplatelet effect, followed by daily doses of 75 to 325 mg. ASA is contraindicated for patients with allergy (manifested as asthma); active gastrointestinal, genitourinary, retinal, or other bleeding; or severe untreated HTN. Patients allergic to ASA should receive either clopidogrel or ticlopidine, with clopidogrel preferred.
    - Anticoagulation approaches
        - Unfractionated heparin (UFH): Use an initial bolus of 60 units/kg intravenously (IV), followed by a continuous infusion at 12 units/kg/hour to maintain APTT of 50 to 70 seconds. Assess APTT every 6 hours and adjust infusion rate to achieve an APTT 1.5 to 2.0 times control. After two therapeutic APTT levels have been obtained, the APTT is monitored at least daily.
        - Bivalirudin is an alternative drug and it can be given at 0.1 mg/kg bolus with maintenance of 0.25 mg/kg per hour infusion.
        - Low molecular weight heparin (LMWH or enoxaparin) loading dose of 30 mg IV bolus followed by 1 mg/kg every 12 hours subcutaneously may be used for patients with unstable angina and non–ST-segment elevation MI. Advantages of LMWH over UFH include subcutaneous route of administration and elimination of APTT monitoring. Irreversibility of effect of LMWH is a disadvantage.
    - Fibrinolytics are indicated for ACS with ST-segment elevation if treatment can be administered within 6 to 12 hours of onset of symptoms. Streptokinase and tissue plasminogen activator (tPA) are the most frequently used fibrinolytics. Third-generation fibrinolytics include rPA, lanoteplase (nPA), and TNK-tPA.

- – Beta-adrenergic antagonists (beta blockers): All patients with ACS should receive beta blockers to achieve a heart rate of 60 beats per minute with systolic blood pressure above 90 mm Hg. For patients presenting with AMI, metoprolol 5 mg is given intravenously over 1 to 2 minutes and is repeated every 5 minutes for a total dose of 15 mg IV. Oral metoprolol 25 to 50 mg every 6 hours is started 15 minutes after the last IV dose and is followed by a maintenance dose of 100 mg twice daily.
  - – GP IIb/IIIa inhibitors include abciximab, eptifibatide, and tirofiban.
  - – Nitroglycerin (NTG) sublingual (SL), three doses of 0.4 mg, taken 5 minutes apart, is recommended for relief of angina. NTG may be started IV at a rate of 10 micrograms per minute and titrated to achieve symptom relief, in the absence of hypotension.
  - – Morphine may be administered to patients whose pain is not resolved by three doses of NTG SL, at a dose of 1 to 5 mg IV, and repeated every 5 to 30 minutes, as needed to relieve pain.
  - – Statins (HMG-CoA reductase inhibitors) are recommended for ACS patients.
  - – Angiotensin-converting enzyme (ACE) inhibitors have been shown to reduce morbidity and mortality when given to patients with recent MI. They are of particular benefit to patients with left ventricular dysfunction, diabetes, or with HTN that is not controlled with nitrates and beta blockers.
  - – Antidysrhythmics are used according to the specific rhythm and advanced cardiac life support (ACLS) protocols.
- • Patient and family education
  - – Patients and families should be taught to recognize the symptoms of MI and complications such as dysrhythmias or heart failure.
  - – Family members of people with cardiac disease should learn CPR and how to activate the EMS in the event of cardiac arrest.
  - – Risk factors for CHD should be reviewed with patients and families, and they should be instructed about diet, medications, and lifestyle changes, including weight management, exercise, smoking cessation, and stress management, to promote optimum heart health.
  - – Patients who require invasive cardiovascular interventions should receive specific instruction concerning risks and benefits.
  - – Patients and families should be able to express their emotions triggered by this hospitalization and given support regarding resuming their previous lifestyle.
  - – Patients should be referred to cardiac rehabilitation for continued education, lifestyle change, and monitored exercise.

Outcomes and Follow-Up

- • Patients and their families will be knowledgeable about MI and its treatment.
- • Patients will not experience any complications from this health problem or the associated treatment.
- • Patients will follow up as indicated with their healthcare providers after noninvasive and invasive therapies.
- • Cardiac rehabilitation is recommended for patients after MI, cardiac revascularization, cardiac transplant, and for patients with stable angina and chronic heart failure (HF). Specific exercise recommendations will be based upon age, risk factors, and functional status. Comprehensive cardiac rehabilitation programs include exercise, nutritional counseling, behavioral interventions, and monitoring of drug therapy.

Table 13–3. Valvular Disorders and Associated Heart Murmurs

	Location of Murmur	Timing	Radiation
Mitral Stenosis	5th ICS, MCL	Diastole	Axilla
Mitral Regurgitation	5th ICS, MCL	Systole	Axilla
Aortic Stenosis	2nd ICS, RSB	Systole	Right neck
Aortic Insufficiency	2nd ICS, RSB	Diastole	Right neck

Note. ICS = intercostal space, MCL = midclavicular line, RSB = right sternal border.

VALVULAR HEART DISEASE

Any of the four heart valves can be stenotic or insufficient. Problem with the tricuspid and pulmonic valves are less common in adults and so will not be specifically discussed in the following sections. Pulmonic and tricuspid disorders in adults are often the result of infective endocarditis, especially when the etiology is IV drug abuse. Mitral and aortic valve disorders can arise from congenital disorders or acquired conditions. Acquired etiologies include rheumatic fever, calcification with aging, heart failure with a dilated left ventricle, infective endocarditis, and rupture of the papillary muscles. The four most common forms of valvular dysfunction along with the classic heart murmurs for each are described in Table 13–3.

MITRAL STENOSIS (MS)

Description
MS is the result of fusion of the valve apparatus so that the orifice is constricted or narrowed during diastole.

Etiology
- The most common causes are rheumatic heart disease and infective endocarditis.
- Less frequently occurring causes are congenital defects and systemic diseases such as systemic lupus erythematosus and amyloidosis.
- As the stenosis worsens, the left atrium enlarges. Atrial fibrillation is a common problem in mitral stenosis.

Incidence and Demographics
- 25% of patients with rheumatic heart disease have MS.
- Two-thirds of these patients are female.

Risk Factors
- Infectious processes such as group A streptococcal infection (GAS)
- Congenital heart disease
- Systemic diseases

Assessment

- History
  - Rheumatic heart disease or other associated condition
  - Shortness of breath, dyspnea, or productive cough
  - Chest pain because of right ventricular hypertension, coronary artery atherosclerosis, or both
  - Thromboembolism from atrial fibrillation
- Physical findings
  - Right ventricular lift from pulmonary hypertension
  - Displacement of the left ventricular posteriorly because of right ventricular enlargement
  - Decrescendo–diastolic murmur with accentuated first heart sound and opening snap– may radiate to the axilla or left sternal area
  - Hemoptysis, productive cough, and inspiratory crackles from pulmonary edema, pulmonary infarction, or both
- Diagnostic tests
  - ECG to detect the presence of atrial fibrillation and left atrial enlargement
  - Chest x-ray to detect pulmonary edema and left atrial enlargement
  - Echocardiography to evaluate mitral valve function
  - Angiography

Management

- Invasive management
  - Mitral valve surgery is usually delayed until symptoms become problematic.
    - Closed mitral valvulotomy
    - Open mitral valvulotomy
    - Mitral valve replacement
  - Balloon valvuloplasty
- Pharmacologic management
  - Endocarditis prophylaxis for surgical and dental procedures
  - Diuretics and restriction of sodium intake for symptomatic patients
  - Digitalis to slow the ventricular rate in atrial fibrillation and to treat ventricular failure
  - Antidysrhythmics for the treatment of atrial fibrillation and other dysrhythmia
  - Consider anticoagulant therapy for patients with atrial fibrillation
- Patient and family education
  - Teach patients and their families about the etiology, course of their disease, and preventive care prior to dental and surgical procedures.
  - Educate them about pharmacological interventions to treat this health problem.
  - Discuss with them the symptoms associated with acute mitral valve dysfunction. Family members of people with cardiac disease should learn CPR and how to activate the EMS in the event of cardiac arrest.
  - If surgery is indicated, teach patients about preoperative preparation along with postoperative and discharge care before leaving the hospital.

Outcomes and Follow-Up
- Patients and their families will be knowledgeable about MS and its treatment.
- Patients will not experience any complications from this health problem or its treatment.
- Patients will follow up as indicated with their healthcare providers after noninvasive and invasive therapies.
- Patients will recognize the signs and symptoms associated with uncontrolled atrial fibrillation and seek medical attention.

MITRAL REGURGITATION (MR)

Description
Abnormalities of the mitral valve apparatus, leaflets, chordae tendineae, papillary muscles, and annulus may cause MR because the valve leaflets do not close completely during ventricular systole.

Etiology
- Rheumatic heart disease
- Infectious endocarditis
- Heart failure with dilated left ventricle
- Congenital defect
- Myxomatous degeneration (e.g., mitral valve prolapse, Marfan syndrome)
- Papillary muscle rupture
- Trauma

Incidence and Demographics
- More common in men than in women

Risk Factors
- Infectious process such as GAS
- Congenital heart disease
- Cardiac injury
- CHD
- Heart failure

Assessment
- History
    - Patients may be asymptomatic for years.
    - History of associated diseases or conditions
    - Development of symptoms is longer than in MS.
    - Pulmonary symptoms and embolization occur less frequently than in MS.
- Physical findings
    - Pansystolic murmur best heard at the apex
    - Radiation of murmur to the axilla
    - Thrill palpated at the apex
    - Hemoptysis, inspiratory crackles, productive cough

- Diagnostic tests
  - ECG to identify left ventricular hypertrophy (LVH) and left atrial enlargement
  - Chest x-ray to detect enlarged heart, left atrial hypertrophy, or pulmonary edema
  - Echocardiography to evaluate mitral valve function
  - Angiography

Management
- Invasive management
  - Annuloplasty, reconstruction of the valve, or both
  - Mitral valve replacement
- Pharmacologic management
  - Endocarditis prophylaxis
  - Treatment of heart failure with renin-angiotensin-aldosterone system (RAAS) blockade; vasodilators; and diuretics.
  - Treatment of atrial fibrillation to control the rate or chemically cardiovert.
- Patient and family education
  - Teach patients and their families about the etiology, risk factors, and course of their disease.
  - Educate them about pharmacological interventions including actions, dosages, and side effects of medications.
  - Discuss with them the symptoms associated with acute mitral valve dysfunction. Family members of people with cardiac disease should learn CPR and how to activate the EMS in the event of cardiac arrest.
  - If surgery is indicated, teach patients about preoperative preparation along with postoperative and discharge care before leaving the hospital.

Outcomes and Follow-Up
- Patients and their families will be knowledgeable about MR and its treatment.
- Patients will not experience any complications from this health problem or its treatment.
- Patients will follow up as indicated with their healthcare providers after noninvasive and invasive therapies.
- Patients will recognize the signs and symptoms associated with uncontrolled atrial fibrillation and seek medical attention.

AORTIC STENOSIS (AS)

Description
AS is a valvular defect that results in left ventricular outflow obstruction because the leaflets do not open completely during systole.

Etiology
- Congenital malformations of the aortic valve
- Degenerative calcific AS
- Atherosclerotic AS
- Rheumatic AS results in adhesions and fusions of the commissures and cusps

Incidence and Demographics
- Incidence of AS because of rheumatic fever is decreasing in industrialized countries.
- Older adults have higher frequency of AS than younger adults.
- More men than women develop AS.

Risk Factors
- Atherosclerosis risk factors are diabetes mellitus, hypercholesterolemia, and type II hyperlipoproteinemia.
- Calcified AS (Paget's disease, end-stage renal failure)
- Advancing age

Assessment
- History
  - Most patients become symptomatic in the sixth decade of life because of the long period of latency for this disease.
  - Cardinal manifestations
    - Angina pectoris because of insufficient coronary artery filling because the valve leaflets block the flow into the coronary arteries. Nitrates will not treat this chest pain and only further decrease cardiac output (CO) and increase the risk of syncope.
    - Syncope because of the decreased forward flow of blood through a narrow opening
    - Heart failure because of the enlargement of the left ventricle when the heart tries to eject blood against this increased resistance
- Physical findings
  - Systolic ejection murmur crescendo-decrescendo heard at the base of the heart.
  - Thrill may be present at the base.
  - Radiation to base of heart, occasionally to the apex
  - Inspiratory crackles and productive cough related to pulmonary congestion
- Diagnostic tests
  - ECG shows LVH with ST changes.
  - Chest x-ray shows either normal heart size or LVH.
  - Echocardiography to evaluate aortic valve function and left ventricular ejection fraction.
  - Angiography is done to determine LV pressures and to evaluate the coronary arteries so both problems can be surgically corrected. The systolic pressure gradient is the difference between the left ventricular and aortic systolic pressures. The pressure gradient difference is a measure of the severity of the valve stenosis. At times it can be as great as 100 mm Hg.

Management
- Invasive management
  - Balloon valvuloplasty may be used in older adults with high surgical risk.
  - Aortic valve replacement is the preferred management and is usually performed early so that the left ventricle does not fail.
- Pharmacologic management
  - Endocarditis prophylaxis
  - Cardiac glycosides such as digoxin
  - Diuretics used with caution to avoid hypovolemia
  - Beta blockers used with great caution because of myocardial depression and potential for left ventricular failure
  - Antidysrhythmics for treatment of dysrhythmia such as atrial fibrillation or atrial flutter

- Patient and family education
  - Teach patients and their families about the etiology, risk factors, and course of their disease.
  - Educate them about pharmacological interventions including actions, dosages, and side effects of medications.
  - Discuss with them the symptoms associated with acute aortic valve dysfunction. Family members of people with cardiac disease should learn CPR and how to activate the EMS in the event of cardiac arrest.
  - When surgery is indicated, teach patients about preoperative preparation along with postoperative and discharge care before leaving the hospital.

Outcomes and Follow-Up
- Patients and their families will be knowledgeable about AS and its treatment.
- Patients will not experience any complications from this health problem or its treatment.
- Patients will follow up as indicated with their healthcare providers after noninvasive and invasive therapies.

AORTIC REGURGITATION (AR)

Description
AR may be caused by disease of the valve leaflet, aortic root, or both so the orifice does not close completely during diastole.

Etiology
- Rheumatic heart disease is the most common cause.
- Trauma
- Degeneration
- Infective endocarditis
- Ankylosing spondylitis
- Systemic HTN
- Marfan syndrome
- Rheumatoid arthritis
- Congenital

Incidence and Demographics
- Chronic AR is more frequent with advancing age.

Risk Factors
- Infectious processes such as GAS
- Injury to the heart
- Advancing age
- Systemic diseases

Assessment
- History
    - Most patients are asymptomatic until the forth or fifth decade.
    - Symptoms associated with chronic AR include exertional dyspnea, orthopnea, and paroxysmal nocturnal dyspnea.
- Physical findings
    - De Musset's sign (perceptible head shake with each heartbeat) in chronic severe AR
    - Bisferiens (twice-striking) pulse
    - Widened pulse pressure
    - Decrescendo diastolic murmur
    - Inspiratory crackles, productive cough from pulmonary congestion
- Diagnostic tests
    - ECG may demonstrate LVH and nonspecific ST-segment and T-wave changes.
    - Chest x-ray shows cardiac enlargement and left ventricular enlargement
    - Echocardiography to evaluate valve function
    - Angiography

Management
- Invasive management
    - Aortic valve replacement with acute AR
- Pharmacologic management
    - Cardiac glycosides such as digoxin (Lanoxin®)
    - Afterload reducers such as vasodilators
    - Antidysrhythmic medications to treat dysrhythmia
    - Antihypertensives to treat systolic HTN
        - Avoid using beta-adrenergic blockers
- Patient and family education
    - Teach patients and their families about the etiology, risk factors, and course of their disease.
    - Educate them about pharmacological interventions including actions, dosages, and side effects.
    - Discuss with them the symptoms associated with acute aortic valve dysfunction. Family members of people with cardiac disease should learn CPR and how to activate the EMS in the event of cardiac arrest.
    - If surgery is indicated, teach patients about preoperative preparation along with postoperative and discharge care before leaving the hospital.

Outcomes and Follow-Up
- Patients and their families will be knowledgeable about AR and its treatment.
- Patients will not experience any complications from this health problem or its treatment.
- Patients will follow up with their healthcare providers after noninvasive and invasive therapies.

INFECTIVE ENDOCARDITIS (IE)

Description
IE is the result of an infective process that can damage any of the four valve structures and result in insufficiency or stenosis of the affected valve.

Etiology
- The infective process can be the result of a bacterial, viral, rickettsial, or fungal infection.
  - Bacterial organisms include *Viridans streptococcus, Staphylococcus aureus, coagulase-negative staphylococci, Enterococcus*.
  - Fungal organisms include *Candida albicans* and *Aspergillus*.
  - Consider the most likely entry of the organism to empirically treat the organism prior to confirmation with cultures.
- IE is often described as either an acute or a subacute process.
- Bacteria or other infective agent is introduced into the bloodstream during an invasive procedure, IV injection, or dental procedure.
  - A short-term septicemia is produced and the body mounts a reaction, which is usually successful and complete, to fight the infection.
  - People with a preexisting structural irregularity or damage have a place where the bacteria can cluster, especially on the low pressure side of the valve.
  - The bacteria become encased in a polysaccharide sac in which they can continue to grow.
  - The IE sac is referred to as vegetation; it continues to grow on the valve structure.
  - The infective process also can spread into myocardium and because of proximity to the AV node, the conduction system can be interrupted.
  - Atrial fibrillation is a common problem in mitral valve IE.
- Thrombus can form on the vegetation and the infected thrombus or a piece of the vegetation can break off and form an embolus that can go to the pulmonary or systemic circulation depending on the valve affected.

Incidence and Demographics
- The overall incidence of IE is 2 to 6 per 100,000 person years.
- Two-thirds of these patients are male.
- The incidence of prosthetic heart valves developing IE is 0.1% to 2.3% and this accounts for 15% of the overall IE cases. The mortality in this group has been reported to be as high as 40%.
- The incidence of IE in intravenous drug users is 1% to 5%.

Risk Factors
- Structural valve disorder
- Prosthetic heart valve
- IV drug user
- Dental cleaning or procedures
- Genitourinary (GU) or gastrointestinal (GI) endoscopic procedures
- Placement of a central venous line
- Placement of permanent or temporary pacemaker

Assessment
- History of
  - Fever, chills, shakes
  - Malaise, fatigue
  - Night sweats
  - Weight loss
- Physical findings
  - As found with the affected valve problem
  - Janeway's lesions are small, painless nodules on the palm.
  - Osler's nodes are painful lesions on the palm.
  - Splinter hemorrhages on the nails
- Diagnostic tests
  - ECG to identify the presence of atrial fibrillation or AV blocks
  - Chest x-ray to detect pulmonary edema and left atrial enlargement
  - Echocardiography to evaluate valve function and locate vegetations. A transesophageal echocardiography (TEE) may be needed to adequately view the vegetations.

Management
- Invasive management
  - Not recommended until the infection has been completely treated, about 6 weeks or longer.
  - If needed later, a valve replacement may be done. Approximately 50% of patients will eventually need surgery.
- Pharmacologic management
  - Generally an aggressive approach with two intravenous antimicrobials for 4 to 6 weeks
  - Endocarditis prophylaxis for surgical and dental procedures thereafter
  - Antipyretics for comfort during the acute period
  - Diuretics and restriction of sodium intake for symptomatic patients
  - Digitalis to slow the ventricular rate in atrial fibrillation and to treat ventricular failure
  - Antidysrhythmics for the treatment of atrial fibrillation and other dysrhythmia
  - Consider anticoagulant therapy for patients with atrial fibrillation.
  - A pacemaker may be needed if the AV node is damaged by the infection.
- Patient and family education
  - Teach patients and their families about the etiology, course of IE, and the associated problems related to the affected valve.
  - Teach about prophylactic antibiotics prior to any invasive procedure, dental work, and surgical procedures. The AHA provides current information on IE prophylaxis on its Web site.
  - Educate them about pharmacological interventions to treat this health problem.
  - Prepare the patient and family for home IV therapy or treatment in another appropriate facility.
  - If surgery is indicated, teach patients about preoperative preparation along with postoperative and discharge care before leaving the hospital.

Outcomes and Follow-Up
- Patients and their families will be knowledgeable about IE and its treatment.
- Patients will not experience any complications from this health problem or its treatment.
- Patients will follow up as indicated with their healthcare providers after noninvasive and invasive therapies.

ACUTE PERICARDITIS

Description
Acute pericarditis is an inflammation of the visceral and parietal pericardium.

Etiology
- Acute pericarditis may be idiopathic or caused by viral or bacterial infections, neoplastic disease, autoimmune disorders (e.g., rheumatoid arthritis, systemic lupus erythematosus, rheumatoid arthritis, polyarteritis nodosa), inflammatory disorders (e.g., amyloidosis, sarcoidosis), medications (e.g., hydralazine, procainamide, phenytoin, isoniazid), or trauma (thoracic surgery, pacemaker insertion, cardiovascular diagnostic procedures).
- Postmyocardial infarction (Dressler) syndrome or postpericardiotomy syndrome are forms of acute pericarditis.

Incidence and Demographics
- More common in men than women
- Associated with advancing age

Risk Factors
- Infectious processes (viral, tuberculosis)
- Systemic diseases (uremic pericarditis, neoplastic pericarditis, especially chronic renal failure)
- CHD
- Noninvasive and invasive therapies (thoracic surgery, radiation pericarditis, medications)

Assessment
- History
    - The most frequent symptom is retrosternal chest pain that radiates to the neck. The pain is positional and aggravated by lying down or coughing and relieved by leaning forward.
    - Associated symptoms include dyspnea, cough, and weight loss.
- Physical findings
    - Pericardial friction rub, which is often intermittent or positional
    - Pericardial effusion muffles heart sounds
    - Rales from pulmonary compression
    - Cardiac tamponade results in pulsus paradoxus, hypotension, tachypnea, tachycardia or bradycardia, rales, and jugular venous distention from cardiac compression.
- Diagnostic tests
    - ECG to detect diffuse ST-segment elevations, occasionally PR-segment depression, and may show low voltage in all leads if a large pericardial effusion is present. See Figure 13–2 for an ECG depicting the usual ST segment findings in pericarditis.
    - Chest x-ray to detect enlargement of the cardiac silhouette.
    - Echocardiogram to detect the presence and quantity of pericardial fluid.

Figure 13–2. ECG of Pericarditis

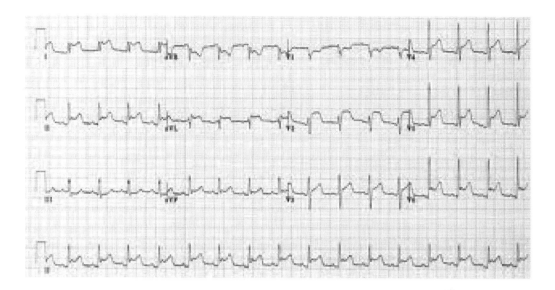

Management
- Invasive management
  - Pericardiocentesis if there is evidence of cardiac compression. A pericardial catheter may be placed for subsequent removal of fluid if the volume is large.
  - Surgery may be needed if other therapies fail in chronic pericarditis. A pericardial window or partial pericardiectomy can be done to prevent fluid from compressing the heart.
- Pharmacologic management
  - Nonsteroidal anti-inflammatory drugs such as aspirin or indomethacin (Indocin®).
  - Corticosteroids, such as prednisone, are used for more severe inflammation.
  - Antibiotics are used for the treatment of purulent pericarditis.
- Patient and family education
  - Teach patients and their families about the etiology, risk factors, and course of their disease.
  - Educate them about pharmacological interventions including actions, dosages, and side effects.
  - Discuss with them the symptoms associated with acute cardiac tamponade and resources for activating emergency care.

Outcomes and Follow-Up
- Patients and their families will be knowledgeable about acute pericarditis and its treatment.
- Patients will not experience any complications from this health problem or its treatment.
- Patients will follow up with their healthcare providers after noninvasive and invasive therapies.

DILATED CONGESTIVE CARDIOMYOPATHY (DCCM)

Description
DCCM is a syndrome that results in cardiac enlargement and systolic dysfunction of one or both ventricles.

Etiology
- Primary (also known as idiopathic) cardiomyopathy is often without a known cause.
- Secondary cardiomyopathy is an end result of a known cause or disease process such as alcohol abuse, viral infection, chemotherapy, or pregnancy.

Incidence and Demographics
- More than 5.4 million patients are treated for heart failure in the United States per year.
- Roughly 35% of heart failure is a result of nonischemic heart disease such as cardiomyopathy.

Risk Factors
- Infectious process
- Genetic predisposition
- Toxic substances such as alcohol or chemotherapeutic agents
- Dysrhythmias, especially atrial fibrillation
- Thyroid-associated

Assessment
- History
  - As cardiac workload increases and exceeds capacity, the patient becomes symptomatic.
  - Cardinal congestive symptoms include fatigue from the low cardiac output and dyspnea (in 75% of patients). Weight gain is a cardinal sign.
  - Noncongestive symptoms include chest pain, palpitations, light-headedness, and syncope.
  - Congestive symptoms may include dyspnea on exertion (DOE), orthopnea, paroxysmal nocturnal dyspnea (PND), chronic cough, cough with recumbency, abdominal fullness or bloating, early satiety, right upper quadrant pain (secondary to hepatic engorgement), and nausea.
  - Rarely, the first presentation may be an embolic event or cardiogenic shock.
- Physical findings
  - Tachypnea and tachycardia
  - Cardiac rhythm is usually sinus early in the disease process, but atrial fibrillation is commonly seen as the heart enlarges. Rhythm disturbances have been attributed to the enlarged myocardium interfering with the normal conduction pathways. Bundle branch block may be seen. See Figure 13–3 for an ECG of left bundle branch block (LBBB).
  - Diminished stroke volume results in a narrowed pulse pressure.
  - Apical impulse (formerly known as the point of maximal impulse or PMI) is displaced inferiorly and laterally, secondary to increased cardiac size.
  - S3 heart sound is present, especially if decompensated.
  - S4 heart sound may be heard and may precede signs of heart failure.

Figure 13–3. ECG Showing a Left Bundle Branch Block

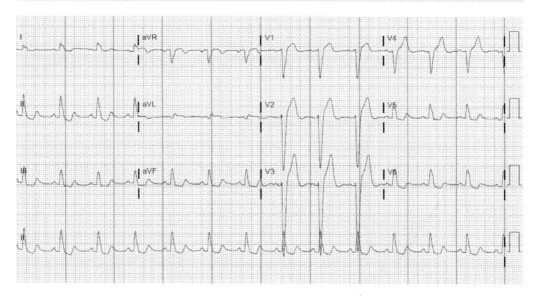

- If valvular disease is also present, systolic murmurs of mitral or tricuspid regurgitation will be heard.
- Jugular vein distention
- Hepatomegaly and liver pulsatility
- Ascites from hepatic congestion is often seen.
- Peripheral edema
- Diagnostic tests
  - ECG may demonstrate low voltage, dysrhythmia such as atrial fibrillation and ventricular ectopy (atrial ectopy is seen less frequently), left ventricular hypertrophy, BBB. and nonspecific ST-T wave changes.
  - Chest x-ray signs include enlarged heart and evidence of pulmonary venous congestion. Acute interstitial edema may be evident by Kerley's B lines and peribronchial cuffing. Pleural effusions may be demonstrated by flattening of the diaphragm with loss of the right or left angle.
  - Echocardiogram signs may be difficult to distinguish DCCM from an ischemic left ventricle. Characteristic findings include:
    - Biventricular dilation in early disease that may include all four cardiac chambers in later disease
    - Decreased EF as a result of the decreased cardiac muscle function
    - Decreased mitral valve opening if the mitral annular opening or papillary muscles have been affected
    - Other findings may include mural thrombus in any chamber, pericardial effusion, and mitral or tricuspid regurgitation

Clinical Course

- Progressive downhill course over a 3- to 5-year period.
- Most patients, especially those over 55 years of age, die within 5 to 10 years of the onset of symptoms.
- Most powerful prognostic factor is the ejection fraction (EF). Those with an EF of less than 20% have a 1-year mortality rate of 50%.
- As symptoms worsen, the patient experiences progressive exercise intolerance, symptoms refractory to treatment, and increasing cardiac size.
- Initially only systolic dysfunction will be present, but as the disease process progresses, diastolic dysfunction may develop also.
- Most patients develop some form of mitral valvular heart disease. As the ventricle enlarges, it dilates the anterior annular ring and displaces the papillary muscles, pulling the leaflets apart and causing functional MR.
- HF results from various mechanisms, including neurohormonal changes leading to ventricular remodeling, and changes in pumping capacity.
- HF is classified by impact on function. Different levels of treatment are indicated for each class. The classification scale used currently is the New York Heart Association Functional Classification Scale. See Table 13–4.
- Sudden death in severe DCCM is most often a result of dysrhythmia. Insertion of an implantable cardioverter defibrillator is usually recommended.

Management

- Invasive management begins with treating an identifiable cause if able (PCI or surgical revascularization). After that a number of options exist.
  - Cardiac valve repair or replacement
  - Implantable defibrillators and permanent pacemakers are useful for patients with malignant or symptomatic dysrhythmias. Biventricular pacing is recommended for those with a BBB to correct septal dyssynchrony.
  - Cardiac transplantation is used for patients who are refractory to medical therapy. The surgical techniques have been refined and with the shortage of cardiac donors, healthcare providers are seeking other treatment options.
  - Studies of implantable ventricular assist devices in end-stage DCCM are ongoing. Initially used as a bridge to transplant, some ventricular assist devices are now available as destination therapies.

Table 13–4. New York Heart Association Functional Classifications of Heart Failure

	Symptoms Occur With	Activities	MET Level
NYHA Class I	High levels of activity	Able to walk and climb stairs with symptoms	> 7
NYHA Class II	Moderate levels of activity	Symptoms with stair climbing or hills	5–7
NYHA Class III	Low levels of activity	Symptoms walking 1–2 blocks	2–4
NYHA Class IV	At rest or with ADLs	Symptoms with any activity	< 2

Note. MET = metabolic equivalents or the multiples of the resting oxygen consumption

- Left ventricular volume reduction for pharmacologically refractory DCCM is increasingly used. This relies on ultrafiltration of the blood to remove large volumes.
  - Left ventriculectomy is a treatment option for a select few candidates.
- Pharmacologic management
  - The goals of therapy are to control symptoms, slow the disease progression, and prevent the complications of thromboembolism, poor organ perfusion, and sudden death. Treatment is based on presenting symptoms, the type of ventricular dysfunction, and comorbid conditions. The initial health history and physical examination establish the baseline data. Most targets for drug therapies are aimed at reducing activation of the RAAS. Most of these drugs become lifelong therapies even if LVEF improves. Treatment is based on careful monitoring for any changes from baseline, daily body weight, and symptom monitoring.
  - Systolic dysfunction treatment to reduce cardiac workload or improve contractility.
    - Diuretics reduce volume overload, which decreases both preload and afterload.
      - Furosemide (Lasix®) is generally used but resistance can develop over time.
      - Switching to torsemide (Demadex®) or bumetanide (Bumex®) may be needed eventually because they are more potent and have a higher bioavailability.
      - When chronic doses of diuretics are increased, there is a reflexive increase in RAAS activation. Thus, there is usually a need for higher doses in one or more of the drugs affecting the RAAS.
    - Vasodilators reduce afterload.
      - Nitrates cause venous dilatation and decrease preload.
      - Hydralazine promotes arterial dilatation and decreases afterload.
    - Inotropes increase cardiac contractility. People with end-stage HF on continuous IV inotropes feel better but have a higher incidence of sudden cardiac death (SCD).
  - ACE inhibitors decrease ventricular remodeling as well as decreasing cardiac workload through vasodilation. Angiotensin receptor blockers can be used if ACE inhibitors are not tolerated. Neither of these can be used in pregnancy.
  - Specific beta blockers (carvedilol, metoprolol, bisoprolol) decrease mortality in DCCM. These drugs decrease the work of the heart and block renin. Current recommendation is for all patients with severe HF to take one of these beta blockers.
  - Spironolactone (Aldactone®) or eplerenone (Inspra®) are recommended as aldosterone antagonists. Care must be taken to prevent hyperkalemia from these drugs.
  - Antidysrhythmics treat dysrhythmia.
- Noninvasive management
  - Eliminate exacerbating factors. Stressors, both emotional and physical, worsen the HF symptoms. Infections increase the metabolic processes, cardiac workload, and symptoms.
  - Other conditions that increase the cardiac workload and worsen symptoms include dysrhythmia, volume overload (nonadherence to low-sodium diets), pulmonary embolism, and coexisting cardiac diseases.
  - Lifestyle modifications that will help the patient control symptoms include:
    - Reduced physical activity and spacing of energy-intense activities.
    - Eating small, frequent meals to decrease the gastric distention if hepatomegaly is present.
    - Elimination of alcohol, which may increase the cardiomyopathy.
- Prognosis
  - Overall prognosis is dependent upon the underlying pathology of the DCCM and the severity of associated HF.

- Patient and family education
    - Teach patients and their families about the etiology, course, and prognosis of their disease.
    - Educate them about pharmacological interventions including actions, dosages, and side effects.
    - Discuss the symptoms associated with acute HF and pulmonary edema. Family members of people with cardiac disease should learn CPR and how to activate the EMS in the event of cardiac arrest.
    - If surgery is indicated, teach patients about preoperative preparation along with postoperative and discharge care before leaving the hospital.
- Palliative care options should be discussed openly prior to the time when these decisions are urgently needed. For the patient with end-stage HF, hospice care is appropriate for symptom management. Hospice staff can help prepare the family for the eventual death of a loved one.

Outcomes and Follow-Up
- Patients and their families will be knowledgeable about DCCM and its treatment.
- Patients will follow up as indicated with their healthcare providers after noninvasive and invasive therapies.
- Patients will adapt to changes in their functional status as their disease progresses.
- Patients will have their end-of-life decisions followed.

HYPERTROPHIC CARDIOMYOPATHY (HCM)

Description
- HCM is a familial Mendelian-linked autosomal dominant disorder that is characterized by idiopathic myocardial hypertrophy and myocyte disarray at the cellular level.
- Obstructive HCM is the presence of idiopathic LVH without dilation of the ventricle, causing abnormal diastolic function and a dynamic subaortic pressure gradient.
- Obstructive HCM most often involves hypertrophy of the ventricular septum, which results in narrowing of the left ventricle (LV) outflow tract. The mitral valve leaflet is pulled into contact with the ventricular septum and creates a subaortic pressure gradient. The degree of gradient varies according to the patient's activity level or after pharmacologic therapy.
- Both forms of HCM have diastolic dysfunction.
    - There is decreased ventricular compliance and incomplete relaxation of the thickened ventricular wall.
    - These factors impede diastolic filling and increase the left ventricular end-diastolic pressure.
    - MR may occur secondary to the anterior motion of the mitral valve during systole.

Etiology
- Idiopathic
- Genetic predisposition

Incidence and Demographics
- Obstructive HCM is estimated to have a prevalence of 1 in 500 (0.2%) of the general population.
- 50% of HCM is because of an autosomal dominant familial disease.
- Patients without a family history of the disease may have a sporadic gene mutation.

Risk Factors
- Abnormalities of myocardial calcium kinetics
- Diastolic dysfunction

Assessment
- History
  - Asymptomatic patients may be identified during screening after a relative has been diagnosed.
  - Symptom severity does not always correlate with the functional severity of the cardiomyopathy.
  - Most frequently seen symptoms are those of congestive HF and are not related to the presence or severity of outflow obstruction.
    - Dyspnea because of increased LV stiffness and diastolic dysfunction
    - Orthopnea and lethargy because of pulmonary congestion and decreased cardiac output
  - Angina and palpitations may be because of impaired coronary flow reserve and myocardial ischemia. Luminal obstruction (stenosis) of the coronary arteries may cause angina.
  - Atrial fibrillation may result from increased left atrial size and MR.
  - Patients often present with sudden death secondary to dysrhythmia that may be ventricular, atrial, or bradycardia in origin. Exercise with its associated peripheral vasodilation and induced myocardial ischemia has also been proposed as a possible cause of sudden death.
- Physical findings
  - The apical impulse (also known as PMI) is displaced inferiorly and laterally because of increased cardiac size.
  - A third (S3), if diastolic failure is present, and fourth (S4) heart sound may be heard.
  - A harsh systolic murmur is heard in those patients with significant outflow gradients.
    - Palpable systolic thrill may be present.
  - Tachypnea, inspiratory crackles, and productive cough
  - Jugular venous distention
  - Hepatosplenomegaly may be present
- Diagnostic tests
  - ECG characterized by nonspecific ST-T wave abnormalities, which have been attributed to the thickened ventricle wall. Pseudo-Q waves (no actual infarct has occurred) may be seen in the anterolateral and inferior leads. Large inverted T waves in the precordial leads in those with apical hypertrophy. As a consequence of MR, atrial fibrillation is seen in 25% of those with HCM.
  - Chest x-ray will be normal unless pulmonary congestion and HF are present.
  - Echocardiogram findings may include LVH, small left ventricular cavity, vigorous posterior wall motion, reduced septal wall movement with or without asymmetrical septal hypertrophy, abnormal systolic anterior motion of the mitral valve leaflets; varying degrees of MR may be seen, and increased left atrial size.
  - Angiography is not routinely done nor is it needed for diagnosis. Two findings often seen are elevated left ventricular diastolic pressure secondary to the decreased ventricular wall compliance and systolic pressure gradient if an obstruction is present.

Management

- Invasive management
  - Treatments are based on the risk for sudden death. Risk stratification is based on the criteria of survival of cardiac arrest with documented ventricular fibrillation, nonsustained ventricular tachycardia, family history of sudden death, or high-risk genetic mutation.
    - If high risk, long-term amiodarone (Cordarone®), an implantable cardioverter-defibrillator (ICD), or permanent dual chamber pacing are the treatments of choice.
    - If not high risk, prognosis is good and no restrictions on work or recreational activities are needed. Pharmacologic agents are used for symptom management.
  - Patients with left ventricular outflow pressure gradients above 50 mm Hg that are refractory to medications have three treatment options.
    - Ventricular septal myotomy-myectomy, known as the Marrow procedure, resects a small amount of the hypertrophic ventricular septum. A resultant reduction if not resolution of the outflow obstruction normalizes the left ventricular pressure and provides symptomatic relief. This procedure is not widely used because of the limited number of HCM patients who are suitable candidates.
    - Transcoronary ablation of the septal hypertrophy is accomplished through the use of an ethanol injection into the left anterior descending artery that precipitates MI to the hypertrophic area. This procedure is associated with a 17% risk of complete atrioventricular block requiring a pacemaker implantation.
    - Dual chamber pacing has been used as an alternative to the septal ablation or the Marrow procedure. A 40% to 50% reduction in the outflow gradient was noted, though the mechanism of this reduction was unclear.
  - Cardiac transplantation is indicated for patients in the dilated phase of cardiomyopathy with HF not responsive to therapy.
- Pharmacologic management
  - Beta blockers reduce the obstructive gradient seen in obstructive HCM. By slowing the heart rate, beta blockers lengthen diastolic filling time, reduce the myocardial oxygen consumption, and reduce the outflow gradient. Beta blockers are used by patients with atrial fibrillation to control ventricular rate and by some patients with paroxysmal atrial fibrillation.
  - Calcium channel blockers have both a negative inotropic and chronotropic effect that lessens the outflow tract pressure gradient, increases ventricular filling, and increases coronary sinus perfusion, thus decreasing myocardial ischemia. Care must be taken in observing for adverse effects of peripheral vasodilation with calcium channel blockers. Patients with high outflow gradients need higher filling pressures to overcome the gradient.
  - Antidysrhythmics are used to treat dysrhythmia. Disopyramide, a class 1A antidysrhythmic, decreases the outflow tract gradient through its actions of negative inotropy and peripheral vasoconstriction. It is the drug of choice in symptomatic obstructive HCM.
  - The risk–benefit ratio of anticoagulation must be evaluated individually. Patients with atrial fibrillation and those with severely depressed ventricular function would most benefit from anticoagulation because of their high risk for an embolic event.

- Prognosis
  - There is wide variability in both the presentation and prognosis of HCM.
  - Sudden death is the major cause of death in both symptomatic and asymptomatic patients.
  - No correlation has been found between the severity of the HCM and the risk for sudden death.
- Patient and family education
  - Teach patients and their families about the etiology, course, and prognosis for their disease.
  - Educate them about pharmacological interventions including actions, dosages, and side effects.
  - Discuss the symptoms associated with acute HF and pulmonary edema along with and how to activate the EMS in the event of cardiac arrest.
  - If surgery is indicated, teach patients about preoperative preparation along with postoperative and discharge care before leaving the hospital.

Outcomes and Follow-Up
- Patients and their families will be knowledgeable about HCM and its treatment.
- Patients will follow up as indicated with their healthcare providers after noninvasive and invasive therapies.
- Patients will adapt to changes in their functional status as their disease progresses.

RESTRICTIVE CARDIOMYOPATHY (RCM)

Description
RCM is characterized by ventricular stiffness classically associated with abnormal diastolic filling. The ventricles become stiff as a result of fibrosis, hypertrophy, or secondary infiltration. The ventricular cavity may become partially obliterated by fibrous tissue and thrombus. Though primarily associated with diastolic dysfunction, systolic dysfunction may develop as the disease progresses.

Etiology
- RCM may be idiopathic or have a primary cause such as endomyocardial fibrosis or eosinophilic endomyocardial disease.
  - Endomyocardial fibrosis is most common in the African and tropical regions.
  - Hypereosinophilic syndrome may be a result of an idiopathic process, a parasitic infection, hypersensitivity to various allergens, connective tissue disease, or autoimmune disorder.
- Secondary causes of RCM include amyloidosis, sarcoidosis, Fabry's disease (glycogen storage disease process), carcinoid, and hemochromatosis. Less common secondary causes are fibroelastosis, tumors, and collagen-vascular diseases.

Incidence and Demographics
- Least common form of the cardiomyopathies

Risk Factors
- Predisposition for endomyocardial fibrosis
- Hypersensitivity to allergens
- Systemic inflammatory disease

Assessment
- History
  - Patients may remain asymptomatic or present with symptoms of increasing exercise intolerance and HF. Exercise intolerance results from limited ventricular filling and inability to increase cardiac output (also known as "fixed cardiac output").
  - The underlying cause of the disease determines the patient's presentation.
    - Patients with endomyocardial fibrosis may present initially with pulmonary and venous congestion.
    - Patients with amyloidosis may present with venous congestion, HF, dysrhythmia, or orthostatic hypotension.
  - RCM presentation may mimic constrictive pericarditis.
- Physical findings
  - S3 or S4 heart sounds, or both
  - Cardiac murmurs
  - Pulmonary rales, hypotension, narrowed pulse pressure
  - Jugular venous distention is persistent as preload and impedance to ventricular filling increases.
  - Dependent edema, ascites, and hepatomegaly result from the persistently elevated venous pressure associated with right ventricular failure.
- Diagnostic tests
  - ECG demonstrates low voltage as a result of the replacement of normal myocardium with fibrotic tissue; left axis deviation as the impulse vector is displaced secondary to the myocardial fibrosis; and pseudo-Q waves often are seen. Atrial dysrhythmia frequently is present.
  - Chest x-ray may show pulmonary vascular redistribution if pulmonary congestion is present. There should be no pericardial calcification unless constrictive pericarditis is present. Cardiomegaly with or without atrial enlargement may be seen.
  - Echocardiogram demonstrates symmetrical thickening of the ventricular walls. Ventricles are normal in size, thus excluding HCM and valvular heart disease. Ventricular volumes and systolic function may be normal or slightly reduced. Early diastolic filling is evident. Diastolic mitral or tricuspid regurgitation is observed in RCM as a physiologic indicator of marked elevation of the ventricular diastolic pressure.
  - Cardiac catheterization results will show decreased cardiac output and elevated right and left ventricular end diastolic filling pressures. Systolic function is well preserved. Pulmonary artery pressures are elevated.
  - Endomyocardial biopsy is a definitive method of diagnosis. Myocyte hypertrophy and interstitial fibrosis are seen in RCM without the evidence of myocardial disarray that would be seen with HCM.

Management
- Invasive management
  - Cardiac transplantation is used in those patients with intractable HF.
- Pharmacologic management
  - A general goal of therapy for all types of RCM is to relieve symptoms of right and left ventricular failure. Specific interventions depend upon the underlying pathology. Each patient has a critical level needed for preload and afterload to maintain adequate ventricular filling and cardiac output.
  - Diuretics are used to relieve fluid overload that is seen in the form of peripheral edema, ascites, and pulmonary congestion.
  - Vasodilators, such as calcium channel blockers, are used cautiously. Aggressive reduction of the preload or afterload will adversely affect the patient's status.
  - ACE inhibitors are used cautiously because they may decrease ventricular filling and cardiac output.
  - Digoxin is not used because it may predispose the patient to dysrhythmia. In amyloidosis, digoxin binds to the amyloid fiber in the heart.
- Prognosis
  - Primary RCM has a 9-year survival from time of early diagnosis and treatment. Once HF occurs, mean survival rate drops to less than 5 years.
  - Prognosis of secondary RCM depends on the etiology of the cardiomyopathy.
- Patient and family education
  - Teach patients and their families about the etiology, course, and prognosis for their disease.
  - Educate them about pharmacological interventions including actions, dosages, and side effects.
  - Discuss the symptoms associated with acute HF and pulmonary edema and how to activate the EMS in the event of cardiac arrest.
  - If surgery is indicated, teach patients about preoperative preparation along with postoperative and discharge care before leaving the hospital.

Outcomes and Follow-Up
- Patients and their families will be knowledgeable about RCM and its treatment.
- Patients will follow up as indicated with their healthcare providers after noninvasive and invasive therapies.
- Patients will adapt to changes in their functional status as their disease progresses.

HEART FAILURE (HF)

Description
HF is a clinical condition characterized by the signs and symptoms of intravascular and interstitial volume overload (shortness of breath, rales, and edema) or signs of inadequate tissue perfusion (cold and cyanotic extremities, narrow pulse pressure, fatigue, and decreased exercise tolerance).

Etiology

- HF has many causes. The left ventricle (LV), right ventricle (RV), or both may be affected, with symptoms reflecting the respective areas of damage.
  - Systolic failure, now called HF with impaired EF (less than 45%). It results from ventricular damage, most often because of ischemia or infarction but it also can be because of dilated cardiomyopathy. The heart is dilated and the cardiac silhouette is enlarged on x-ray.
  - Diastolic failure, now called HF with normal EF (HFNEF) is characterized by a restrictive ventricular filling pattern. It results from concentric LVH, most often because of HTN or AS. The cardiac silhouette appears normal in size. The EF remains normal but cardiac output is reduced. Diastolic failure is responsible for approximately 40% of all cases of HF; however, guidelines have not been established for management of this disorder.
- HF may be acute or chronic. Acute HF may occur in persons with a previously normal cardiovascular system as a result of an acute stressor (e.g., thyrotoxicosis, acute MI, acute hemorrhage) or a reversible valvular dysfunction. Chronic HF ensues over time. Acute exacerbation or acute decompensations occur in chronic HF when another acute factor worsens the chronic condition.
- The AHA has defined stages of heart failure as:
  - Stage A: at-risk person because of HTN or strong family history. Aggressive risk factor control is recommended.
  - Stage B: some structural cardiovascular problem but no HF symptoms. This would include persons after MI and treatment would entail ACE inhibitors and beta blockers to prevent remodeling of the heart.
  - Stage C: symptomatic HF, NYHA Functional Classes I to III. Standard treatment of HF should be undertaken per guidelines.
  - Stage D: end-stage HF. Consider transplant, LV assist device, or palliative care options.

Incidence and Demographics

- HF affects 5.7 million people in the United States.
- There are 550,000 new cases of HF each year.
- HF is a major cause of morbidity, with 438,000 hospital discharges among males and 540,000 among females attributed to HF.
- HF results in 46,980 deaths annually: 17,694 among males (37.7% of total HF deaths) and 29,286 among females (62.3% of total HF deaths). About 20% of patients with HF die within the first year and 80% will die within 8 years of diagnosis.

Risk Factors

- HF results from ischemic and nonischemic causes. CHD causes HF in two-thirds of those with systolic HF. Within 6 years after MI, 22% of males and 46% of females will be disabled as a result of HF.
- Nonischemic causes of HF include HTN, valvular heart disease, cardiomyopathy, congenital heart disease, endocarditis, myocarditis, thyroid disease, and alcohol excess. Three of four HF patients have history of HTN.

Assessment

- History
  - LV failure may present with dyspnea, orthopnea, paroxysmal nocturnal dyspnea, or cough. Other symptoms include activity intolerance, fatigue, weakness, palpitations, diaphoresis, and alteration in sleep or confusion.
  - RV failure may present with weight gain, peripheral edema, abdominal distension, and gastrointestinal complaints.
  - Chest pain may indicate an ischemic cause of HF; however, ischemia may be present without chest pain.
  - History of HTN, MI, valvular or congenital disease, rheumatic heart disease, atrial fibrillation, recent viral illness, thyroid disease, lung disease, treatment with cardiotoxic drugs, or alcohol abuse
  - History of CABG, angioplasty, valvular repair or replacement, or thyroid surgery
- Physical findings
  - Tachycardia may be seen in response to decreased cardiac output.
  - Apical impulse may be displaced laterally as a result of cardiac enlargement.
  - S3 reflects left HF.
  - S4 indicates cardiac ischemia, HTN, or hypertrophy.
  - Cardiac murmurs occur with valvular dysfunction.
  - Elevated jugular venous pressure may be seen with RV failure.
  - Rales (crackles) indicate pulmonary congestion.
  - Pale, cool, diaphoretic skin, with dependent edema
  - Hepatomegaly, splenomegaly, or both because of venous congestion
- Diagnostic tests
  - Chest x-ray may reveal cardiomegaly, pulmonary edema, or pleural effusions.
  - ECG with acute ST or T wave changes indicates myocardial ischemia or infarction. Q waves or bundle branch block may reflect cardiac dysfunction from previous MI. Tachycardia or atrial fibrillation may reflect thyrotoxicosis or increased heart rate to compensate for decreased cardiac output or anemia. Bradycardia secondary to heart block or medications may result in HF. A low-voltage ECG or electrical alternans may reveal pericardial effusion. Left ventricular hypertrophy may reflect diastolic dysfunction. A bundle branch block pattern often results in septal wall dyssynchrony, which worsens the LVEF. Figure 13–3 shows an ECG with LBBB.
  - Echocardiogram is used to assess ventricular EF and to differentiate systolic from diastolic failure, detect ventricular enlargement or hypertrophy, valvular dysfunction, congenital heart disorder, and hypokinesis or akinesis secondary to ischemia or infarction.
  - Radionuclide ventriculogram permits more precise measurement of EF than echocardiogram, particularly of RVEF.
  - Laboratory tests include CBC to detect anemia or infection, electrolytes, serum creatinine and BUN to identify electrolyte imbalances secondary to volume overload or diuretic treatment and renal impairment, serum albumin (increased extravascular volume because of hypoalbuminemia), T4 and TSH for patients over age 65 or with evidence of thyroid disease or atrial fibrillation, and urinalysis to detect renal dysfunction.

- Right heart catheterization can measure cardiac output, as well as right and left ventricular filling pressures, permitting assessment and treatment of hemodynamically unstable patients. See Table 13–5 for a listing of information obtained with a right heart catheterization.
- A quick assessment can be done to determine if the patient is warm or cold, wet or dry, based on your assessment. This information provides a quick reference that can aid in managing the patient. Figure 13–4 defines the quick assessment that was first developed by Lynne Warner Stevenson.

Table 13–5. Pressures Obtained During a Right Ventricular Heart Catheterization (in mm Hg)

	Normal	Hypervolemia	Hypovolemia
Mean Right Atrium	0–8	> 10	0
Right Ventricle (Systolic/Diastolic)	15–25/0–8	> 25/10	< 15/0–4
Pulmonary Artery (Systolic/Diastolic)	15–30/0–8	> 30/10	< 15/0–4
Mean Pulmonary Artery	9–17	> 18	< 8
Pulmonary Artery Occlusive Pressure	5–15	> 16	0–5

Pulmonary artery occlusive pressure reflects left ventricular end diastolic pressure, an indication of LV preload.

Note: Numbers vary slightly by source.

Figure 13–4. Assessing the Patient With Heart Failure: The Warner-Stevenson Model of Assessing Perfusion and Congestion

Congestion Present: Dry or Wet
Signs of congestion: S3, systolic murmur, DOE, orthopnea, edema, jugular venous distention

Warm and Dry Normal No treatment	**Warm and Wet** Hypervolemic Give diuretics
Cold and Dry Hypoperfusion Inotropes, vasodilators	**Cold and Wet** Hypoperfused and hypervolemic Careful mix of treatments

Perfusion at Rest: Warm or Cold
Signs of poor perfusion: cold, narrow pulse pressure, hypotension, cyanosis, low serum sodium, renal dysfunction.

Management

- Invasive management
  - Cardiac surgery may be indicated to repair AS or other valvular dysfunction.
  - After MI, there may be viable stunned or hibernating myocardial tissue surrounding infarcted tissue that can be salvaged by revascularization, preventing HF.
  - Patients with acutely decompensated HF may require a left ventricular assist device (LVAD). These devices are used for patients with profound hemodynamic instability resulting from MI and to support the circulation while awaiting cardiac transplant. Now destination therapy is available for life-long management in end-stage HF.
  - Continuous ultrafiltration or, less frequently, arteriovenous hemofiltration (CAVH), can be used to reduce fluid overload in acutely decompensated HF.
  - Patients with symptomatic dysrhythmia may need a pacemaker or an implanted cardioverter-defibrillator. Sudden death secondary to dysrhythmia is a major cause of death in patients with HF.
  - Cardiac transplantation should be considered for patients with HF who have severe limitations or require frequent hospitalizations secondary to HF, in whom aggressive medical therapy fails and surgical revascularization is not appropriate.
- Pharmacologic management
  - ACE inhibitors are recommended for all patients with systolic dysfunction. They have been shown to improve symptoms and prolong life. Angiotensin II receptor blockers (ARBs) are an alternative to ACE inhibitors, and may be used for patients intolerant of ACE inhibitors because of angioedema or intractable cough, but they have not been proven to be equal to or better than ACE inhibitors.
  - Combined therapy with hydralazine and isosorbide dinitrate may be used for patients unable to tolerate ACE inhibitors or ARBs because of angioedema, intractable cough, hypotension, or renal insufficiency. Neither drug taken alone is recommended for HF.
  - Beta blockers are recommended for patients in HF. Beta blockers are indicated for long-term management of HF, but should not be used in acutely decompensated HF requiring hospitalization for aggressive diuresis or intravenous therapy, nor for patients with symptomatic bradycardia, hypotension, or advanced heart block. A pacemaker may be needed to support the heart rate.
  - Spironolactone reduces morbidity and mortality in patients with recurrent dyspnea on other therapies.
  - Diuretics are recommended for all symptomatic patients, with dosage as needed to control symptoms. Loop diuretics (furosemide, bumetanide, torsemide) are the most potent diuretics. A thiazide diuretic such as metolazone may be added to potentiate diuresis.
  - Digoxin is a positive inotrope and negative chronotrope recommended to improve the clinical status of patients who remain symptomatic despite treatment with ACE inhibitors, beta blockers, diuretics, and spironolactone.
  - Most calcium channel blockers (CCBs) are not recommended for treatment of HF. Amlodipine and felodipine have been shown to not affect survival adversely in HF; however, clinical evidence is lacking to support CCBs in treatment of HF and they may worsen fluid retention. There are instances when CCBs are helpful in persons with a history of HTN and HFNEF.

Heart Failure with Normal EF

- Dysrhythmia is a frequent cause of death for patients with HF. Class I antidysrhythmic agents (quinidine, procainamide, flecainide, encainide) should not be used in HF, except in treatment of refractory life-threatening dysrhythmia. Class II antidysrhythmics (beta blockers) are recommended for patients with HF, as previously discussed. Class III antidysrhythmics (sotalol, amiodarone) are preferred over Class I antidysrhythmics in the treatment of atrial dysrhythmias in patients with HF. Amiodarone also is recommended for treatment of ventricular tachycardia and ventricular fibrillation.
- IV medications used for inpatient management of acutely decompensated HF include positive inotropes such as dopamine, dobutamine, and phosphodiesterase inhibitors (milrinone, amrinone), which enhance cardiac contractility and increase renal blood flow (promoting diuresis). These drugs provide short-term improvement in symptoms, but long-term use is associated with increased mortality.
- Patient and family education
  - The AHA, American Association of Heart Failure Nurses (AAHFN), and Heart Failure Society of America (HFSA) list the following topics for patient, family, and caregiver education.
    - Information should be provided about HF, its causes, symptoms, self-monitoring with daily weights, and what to do if symptoms worsen. Smoking cessation should be emphasized. Patients should be encouraged to obtain influenza and pneumococcal vaccinations.
    - Patients and family should be informed about their prognosis (life expectancy), and advance directives and end-of-life choices should be discussed.
    - Work, recreation, sex, and other exercise recommendations should be based upon the patient's age, comorbidities, and exercise stress test results. Cardiac rehabilitation improves symptoms and functional capacity, and reduces morbidity and mortality related to HF. HF Action study showed an increase quality of life and no risk to participation in cardiac rehabilitation.
    - A low-sodium diet (less than 2 g Na+) is generally recommended for HF patients. Fluid restrictions may be required. Moderation or abstinence in intake of alcohol is recommended (two or fewer drinks per day for men and one for women).
    - Patients should be instructed about their medications: their benefits, possible side effects and what to do if they occur, actions, dosages, and timing of medications.
    - Patients should be advised about the importance of compliance with the treatment plan, and should receive counseling about qualified support groups and HF management programs.

Outcomes and Follow-Up
- Patients and their families will be knowledgeable about HF and its treatment.
- Patients will follow up as indicated with their healthcare providers after noninvasive and invasive therapies.
- Patients will adapt to changes in their functional status as their disease progresses.
- Patients will have their end-of-life decisions followed.

ATRIAL FIBRILLATION

Description
- A-fib is a cardiac dysrhythmia characterized by absent P waves, irregularly irregular R-R intervals, and baseline undulations of variable shape and amplitude (f waves). A-fib can occur in chronic or paroxysmal forms. Chronic A-fib often is well-tolerated; however, it carries the risk of developing mural thrombi within the atria, thromboembolism, and the need for long-term anticoagulation therapy. Acute presentations of A-fib often are not well-tolerated, because the body has not had time to adjust to the loss of atrial kick, which decreases the cardiac output by 10% to 15%. ECG manifestations of A-fib are
  - P-R interval: unable to measure, no P waves
  - QRS duration: 0.04 to 0.12 seconds
  - Rate: atrial rate estimated to be 400 to 600 impulses per minute, ventricular rate ranges from normal to a rapid ventricular response.
  - Regularity: irregularly irregular R-R intervals

Etiology
- A-fib is caused by multiple ectopic foci and reentry circuits that lead to chaotic depolarization of the atria. Many conditions that lead to stretching or inflammation of the atrial tissue, decreased velocity of conduction through the atria, or ischemia can trigger the dysrhythmia.

Incidence and Demographics
- A-fib is the most frequently occurring dysrhythmia; incidence increases with age.
- A-fib occurs in 9% of people over 70 years of age and in 20% to 30% of patients undergoing coronary artery bypass graft surgery.

Risk Factors
- Pulmonary diseases
- Valvular disease
- Congenital heart disease
- Coronary artery bypass surgery
- Congestive heart disease
- Atherosclerosis
- MI
- Rheumatic heart disease
- Thyrotoxicosis

Figure 13–5. Atrial Fibrillation

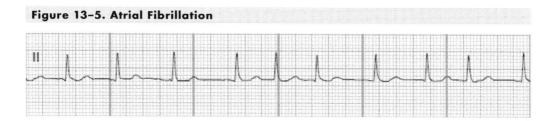

Assessment

A-fib causes loss of atrial kick, which is responsible for 10% to 25% of cardiac output. It is important to determine when the symptoms started to estimate the length of time in A-fib, and whether it is chronic or intermittent.

- History
  - Fatigue, dizziness, activity intolerance, inability to perform activities of daily living, palpitations, shortness of breath
- Physical findings
  - Rapid or irregular heart rate
  - Varying intensity of S1
  - Hypotension
- Diagnostic tests
  - ECG to confirm rhythm and differentiate from atrial flutter
  - Echocardiogram to evaluate cardiac structure and function, and assess for presence of mural thrombi that would impact treatment.
  - Thyroid function studies to detect and correct hyperthyroidism, because it interferes with treatment success.

Management

Treatment is aimed at restoring sinus rhythm, controlling ventricular response, and preventing thromboembolism by identifying and treating the cause of the dysrhythmia.

- Electrical management
  - Synchronized electrical cardioversion is indicated for hemodynamic instability, to restore sinus rhythm in acute onset, and for conversion to sinus rhythm after anticoagulation in chronic cases.
    - Length of time in A-fib should be less than 48 hours for acute onset
    - Confirmation of the absence of mural thrombus by echocardiogram prior to cardioversion to prevent thromboembolism
  - Permanent atrial pacemaker can be implanted to pace the atria at a set rate.
- Pharmacologic management
  - Medications are used to slow the ventricular rate if it is above 100 beats per minute.
    - Calcium channel blockers
    - Beta blockers
    - Digitalis
  - Antidysrhythmic agents are used to convert to sinus rhythm.
    - Type 1A agents: quinidine, procainamide
      - May speed conduction at the atrioventricular node
      - An agent to slow ventricular response is used before attempting to convert.
    - Type IC agents: flecainide, propafenone
    - Type III agents: amiodarone, sotalol, ibutilide

Table 13-6. CHADS Score for Determining Anticoagulation Need to Prevent Stroke in the Patient With Atrial Fibrillation

Step 1. Count the points on this chart.

	Condition	Points
C	Congestive heart failure	1
H	Hypertension (treated or uncontrolled)	1
A	Age > 75 years	1
D	Diabetes	1
S_2	Prior stroke or TIA	2

Step 2. Determine the risk for CVA based on CHADS Score.

CHADS Score	Stroke Risk	95% Confidence Interval
0	1.9%	1.2%–3.0%
1	2.8%	2.0%–3.8%
2	4.0%	3.1%–5.1%
3	5.9%	4.6%–7.3%
4	8.5%	6.3%–11.1%
5	12.5%	8.2%–17.5%
6	18.2%	10.5%–27.4%

Step 3. Determine recommendation for anticoagulation.

CHAD Score	Risk	Anticoagulation Therapy	Considerations
0	Low	Aspirin	ASA 81–325 mg daily
1	Moderate	Aspirin	ASA daily or raise INR to 2–3 depending upon such factors as patient preference
2+	High	Warfarin	Raise INR to 2.0–3.0 unless contraindicated (bleeding or fall risk, noncompliance with monitoring)

– Anticoagulants are used to reduce the risk of thromboembolism (see Table 13–6).
  • Heparin is used acutely in the inpatient setting until the INR is therapeutic on warfarin (Coumadin).
  • Warfarin is used before cardioversion is performed and the patient must be at therapeutic INR for a minimum of 3 weeks prior to cardioversion and for 4-6 weeks after successful rhythm change. If cardioversion is unsuccessful, then long-term warfarin therapy is indicated.
    – Two genetic factors have been identified that help explain the wide variation in dosing needed to reaching therapeutic INR levels. This is explained in Chapter 15.
    – Bolus doses should not be used when starting warfarin.
    – Routine monitoring of INR must be done at a minimum of monthly and even weekly during times of dose adjustment.
    – If warfarin needs to be stopped for a surgery or procedure, some patients may need to be bridged with LMW heparin.
– Ablation procedures may correct A-fib and are performed in the electrophysiology lab.
– The Maze surgical procedure is used for the treatment of A-fib and may be recommended for some patients.
• Patient and family education
  – Patients and their families should learn the signs and symptoms of A-fib and report them to their healthcare provider. They should also be instructed on the signs and symptoms of stroke.
  – Patients on warfarin should learn to self-monitor for signs of bleeding and to avoid situations that will put them at risk for bleeding (e.g., falls, vigorous activities, shaving with a straight razor). Medications that interact with warfarin should be identified and avoided. The list is extensive and includes antibiotics and herbals. The dietary intake of vitamin K must remain constant.
  – Family members of people with cardiac disease should learn CPR and how to activate the EMS in the event of cardiac arrest. They should also know how to control bleeding.

Outcomes and Follow-Up

• Approximately, 50% of patients treated for A-fib with antidysrhythmic agents remain free from further recurrence at 12 months.
• Patients receiving antidysrhythmic drugs should be monitored carefully with blood levels and physical examination on a regular basis.
• Healthcare providers should treat the underlying disease or condition that caused the A-fib.

ATRIAL FLUTTER

Description

• AF is a regular reentry dysrhythmia characterized by identical sawtooth F waves at rapid rates and varying ventricular responses. Conduction ratios between the atria and ventricles usually occur at even intervals (e.g., 2:1, 4:1, 6:1) but also can vary. Like A-fib, AF can occur acutely or chronically. The acute presentation may cause the patient to be unstable because of loss of atrial kick, and chronic manifestations may include mural thrombus that could lead to thromboembolism. AF can occur in combination with A-fib.

Figure 13-6. Atrial Flutter

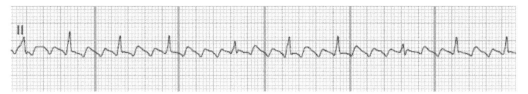

- ECG manifestations of AF
  - P-R interval: unable to measure
  - QRS duration: Normal
  - Rate: Atrial rate between 250 and 450, ventricular rate varies as the AV node blocks most of the impulses. It usually presents with an atrial rate of 300 and a ventricular rate of 150 beats per minute (bpm). Ventricular rates below 100 bpm are considered controlled, and rates above 100 bpm are considered a rapid ventricular response.
  - Regularity: regular F waves with varying ventricular response; can be regular or irregular depending on the AV node.

Etiology
- AF arises from a reentry circuit in the right atrium, which achieves depolarization rates between 250 and 450 times per minute in rapid identical waves. There are two types of AF; type 1 results in an atrial rate of 300 and type 2 is responsible for much faster rates, averaging 400 to 450 per minute. Underlying cardiac and pulmonary conditions predispose patients to AF.

Incidence and Demographics
- AF is less common than A-fib and the two often occur concomitantly. AF can be intermittent or sustained, and is more common in adults than in children. AF used to be considered a transient rhythm; it is now understood to be chronic in some patients.

Risk Factors
- Pulmonary diseases
- Valvular heart disease
- Congenital heart disease
- Coronary artery bypass surgery
- Congestive heart disease
- Atherosclerosis
- MI
- Rheumatic heart disease
- Thyrotoxicosis

Assessment

AF causes loss of atrial kick, which is responsible for 10% to 15% of cardiac output. It is important to determine when the symptoms started to estimate the length of time in AF, and whether it is chronic or intermittent.

- History
  - Fatigue, dizziness, activity intolerance
  - Inability to perform activities of daily living
  - Palpitations, shortness of breath
- Physical findings
  - Rapid or irregular heart rate, depending on the conduction ratio through the AV node
  - Varying intensity of S1 with irregular conduction ratios
  - Hypotension
- Diagnostic tests
  - ECG to confirm rhythm and differentiate from A-fib
  - Echocardiogram to evaluate cardiac structure and function, and assess for formation of mural thrombi, which would impact treatment
  - Thyroid function studies to detect and correct hyperthyroidism, which interferes with treatment success
  - Electrophysiology studies (EPS) to identify reentry circuits

Management

The choice of treatment for the patient will depend on hemodynamic stability and how long they have been in AF.

- Invasive management
  - Radiofrequency ablation of reentry circuits can be done in an electrophysiology lab to prevent recurrence.
  - Rapid atrial pacing is used to overdrive the reentry circuit with the sinus node.
  - Electrical cardioversion may convert AF to sinus rhythm. The amount of time the patient has been in AF should be assessed, and if longer than 48 hours, an echocardiogram should be done to assess for a thrombus prior to converting the rhythm.
- Pharmacologic management
  - Medications are used to slow the ventricular rate if it is above 100 beats per minute.
    - Calcium channel blockers
    - Beta blockers
    - Digitalis
  - Antidysrhythmic agents are used to convert to sinus rhythm.
    - Type 1A agents: quinidine, procainamide
    - Type IC agents: flecainide, propafenone
    - Type III agents: amiodarone, sotalol, ibutilide
  - Anticoagulants to reduce thromboembolism
    - Heparin is used acutely in the inpatient setting until the INR is therapeutic on warfarin.
    - Warfarin is used for 4 weeks before cardioversion. If cardioversion is unsuccessful, then long-term warfarin therapy is indicated.

- Patient and family education
  - Patients and their families should learn the signs and symptoms of AF and report them to their healthcare provider. They should be instructed on the signs and symptoms of stroke also.
  - Patients on warfarin should learn to self-monitor for signs of bleeding and to avoid situations that will put them at risk for bleeding (e.g., falls, vigorous activities, shaving with a straight razor). Medications that interact with warfarin should be identified and avoided.
  - Family members of people with cardiac disease should learn CPR and how to activate the EMS in the event of cardiac arrest.

Outcomes and Follow-Up
- The goal of treatment is to restore sinus rhythm.
- Patients receiving antidysrhythmic drugs should be monitored carefully with blood levels and physical examination on a regular basis.
- Healthcare providers should treat the underlying disease or condition that caused the AF.

FIRST-DEGREE ATRIOVENTRICULAR BLOCK (1°AVB)

Description
- A delay in the conduction of impulses from the SA node to the AV node, seen on ECG as a prolonged P-R interval. It is usually asymptomatic.
- ECG manifestations of 1°AVB
  - P-R interval: prolonged more than 0.20 second
  - QRS duration: normal
  - Rate: normal or often bradycardic
  - Regularity: regular P-P and R-R intervals

Figure 13–7. First-Degree Atrioventribular Block

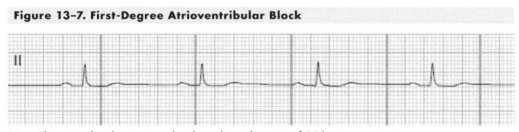

Note: This strip also depicts sinus bradycardia with a rate of 50 beats per minute.

Etiology

- Normal impulse from the SA node with prolonged relative refractory period in the AV node leads to a delay in ventricular response.
- Causes for this delay include:
  - Ischemia, MI, CHD
  - Scarring of atrial tissue in the area of the internodal pathways
  - Infiltration by amyloid, sarcoid, Lyme carditis, endocarditis
  - Degenerative diseases
  - Rheumatic heart disease
  - Electrolyte imbalances
  - Atrial stretch
  - Increased vagal tone
  - Inflammatory diseases
  - Cardiac medications such as digoxin, calcium channel blockers, beta blockers
- Prolonged P-R interval can occur as a normal variant in some people.

Incidence and Demographics

- 1°AVB can occur in people of all ages and may go undiagnosed because of its benign nature and multitude of common etiologic factors.

Risk Factors

- People with known cardiac disease or any of the condition listed above are at higher risk for developing 1°AVB.
- Cardiac medications are often the cause of intermittent 1°AVB, requiring dose adjustments with telemetry monitoring.

Assessment

- History
  - 1°AVB is often asymptomatic and discovered during ECG monitoring as an incidental finding.
  - Activity intolerance or shortness of breath is often associated with higher degrees of AV block.
- Physical findings
  - There may be no findings on physical examination to indicate 1°AVB, unless the patient is bradycardic (heart rate less than 60 bpm).
  - There may be findings consistent with an underlying disease state such as a murmur from rheumatic heart disease.
- Diagnostic tests
  - ECG to diagnose 1°AVB.
  - Laboratory studies including cardiac markers, electrolytes, blood gases, and drug levels may identify underlying conditions that cause 1°AVB.

Management

- Invasive management
  - There are no recommended invasive procedures for 1°AVB. Cardiac pacing may be implemented for higher degrees of AV block.
- Pharmacologic management
  - Atropine may be used if the patient is bradycardic and symptomatic because of increased vagal tone.
  - More commonly, current cardiac medications are held or doses reduced during episodes of 1°AVB until it resolves.
- Patient and family education
  - Medication education is extremely important for patients and their families when cardiac medications are prescribed. Schedules, food–drug, and drug–drug interactions should be discussed.
  - Instruct patients to report signs and symptoms of drug overdose and adverse reactions to their healthcare providers.

Outcomes and Follow-Up

- Patients will keep scheduled appointments with their healthcare providers to monitor response to medications and for diagnostic testing, if indicated.
- Patients will adhere to medication schedules.

SECOND-DEGREE ATRIOVENTRICULAR BLOCK (2°AVB) TYPE I (WENCKEBACH, MOBITZ I)

Description

- Progressively lengthening P-R intervals until a P wave occurs that is not followed by a QRS complex, and then the pattern begins again. This dysrhythmia is usually asymptomatic.
- ECG manifestations of 2°AVB type I
  - P-R interval: gradually increasing until a QRS is dropped
  - QRS duration: usually normal
  - Rate: normal, with atrial rate faster than ventricular rate because of dropped QRS complexes
  - Regularity: regularly irregular pattern with grouped beating and progressively lengthening P-R intervals. Cycles range from two to eight beats.

Figure 13–8. Second-Degree Atrioventricular Block (2°AVB) Type I (Wenckebach, Mobitz I)

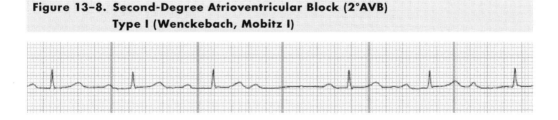

Etiology
- Excessive parasympathetic tone or medications that slow conduction through the AV node.
- Conditions that lead to increased parasympathetic tone include:
  - Inferior MI
  - CHD
  - Aortic and mitral valve disease
  - Atrial septal defects
  - Medications (e.g., digitalis, beta blockers, calcium channel blockers)

Incidence and Demographics
- 2°AVB type I occurs primarily in adults, and may be asymptomatic if the ventricular rate is fast enough to support cardiac output.
- It occurs most often with inferior wall ischemia or MI.
- It can be a normal variant in some people.

Risk Factors
- CHD, medications that slow conduction through the AV node, and the conditions listed above predispose patients to this type of heart block.
- Conditions that impair cardiac perfusion and stimulate parasympathetic tone.

Assessment
- History
  - Symptoms of decreased cardiac output: light-headedness, activity intolerance, shortness of breath, chest pain, and syncope
- Physical findings
  - There may be detectable pauses in pulse if the delay is long enough.
  - Hypotension
- Diagnostic tests
  - ECG is diagnostic for 2°AVB type I.
  - Holter monitor may capture the dysrhythmia during normal activity if it occurs intermittently.
  - Electrolytes and drug levels should be measured to identify contributing factors.

Management
- Invasive management
  - In symptomatic patients with impaired cardiac output, a pacemaker may be indicated. Usually no invasive treatment is necessary.
- Pharmacologic management
  - Atropine can be used to decrease vagal tone and increase heart rate in symptomatic patients.
  - Cardiac medications including digoxin and antidysrhythmic agents may need to be held and doses readjusted.
- Patient and family education
  - Patients and their families should be instructed to identify symptoms of impaired cardiac output such as syncope, activity intolerance, and shortness of breath, and report them to their healthcare provider right away, or seek treatment in an emergency room.

Figure 13–9. Second-Degree Atrioventricular Block (2°AVB) Type II, Mobitz II

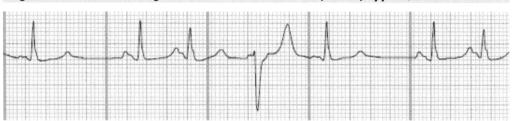

Note. PACs and ventricular escape beats are also evident on this strip.

- Patients should be instructed on the medications that are prescribed, including actions, side effects, dosing schedule, and monitoring tests.
- Family members of people with cardiac disease should learn CPR and how to activate the EMS in the event of cardiac arrest.

Outcomes and Follow-Up
- 2°AVB type I is often benign and requires no immediate treatment. If it is the result of medications, holding them and readjusting doses resolves the block. Resolution of the underlying cause is the best way to achieve the goal of returning to sinus rhythm.
- Patients will keep scheduled appointments with their healthcare providers to monitor response to medications and for diagnostic testing, if indicated.
- Adherence to medication schedules should be emphasized.

SECOND-DEGREE ATRIOVENTRICULAR BLOCK (2°AVB) TYPE II (MOBITZ II)

Description
- 2°AVB type II is an intermittent failure of conduction of impulses below the AV node, resulting in dropped QRS complexes with consistent P-R intervals. Location of the block within the AV node effects QRS duration.
- ECG manifestations of 2°AVB type II
  - P-R interval: normal, consistent when beats are conducted, may be > 0.20
  - QRS duration: If the block is in the bundle of His, the QRS duration can be less than 0.12 second. If the block is lower in the bundle branches, the QRS duration can be longer than 0.12 second.
  - Rate: normal, atrial rate greater than ventricular rate because of dropped QRS complexes. This rhythm may be associated with a bradycardia.
  - Regularity: Atrial rhythm is regular, ventricular is irregular; can occur in varying conduction ratios.

Etiology

- 2°AVB type II is often associated with His-Purkinje system cardiac disease, which can progress to complete heart block or ventricular asystole from bilateral bundle branch blocks.
- Conditions that cause this type of block include:
  - Anterior wall MI
  - Rheumatic heart disease
  - Congestive heart disease
  - Coronary artery disease
  - Primary diseases of the conduction system

Incidence

- 2°AVB type II occurs most often in adults and is associated with a high mortality rate when it occurs in the setting of an anterior wall MI.

Risk Factors

- The most common risk factor for 2°AVB type II is anterior wall MI.
- Conditions that impair the conduction system, such as those mentioned above, will also put a patient at risk for developing this type of block.

Assessment

- History
  - Symptoms of activity intolerance, syncope, shortness of breath, chest pain, and nausea
- Physical findings
  - Hypotension
  - Diaphoresis
  - Pauses in pulse may indicate heart block of this degree, which causes decreased cardiac output.
- Diagnostic tests
  - ECG is diagnostic for 2°AVB type II.
  - Electrolyte and medication levels should be monitored to identify contributing factors.
  - Electrophysiology studies may be helpful in identifying high-degree blocks.

Management

- Invasive management
  - Cardiac pacing may be indicated because this type of block often is permanent and can progress to complete heart block.
  - If the patient becomes symptomatic, transcutaneous pacing can be used in the acute setting until a transvenous or permanent pacemaker is placed.
- Pharmacologic management
  - Atropine is not indicated for high-degree AV blocks because it can further challenge the impaired conduction system, enhancing the progression to complete heart block.
  - Isoproterenol and dopamine can be used to achieve hemodynamic stability in an acutely symptomatic patient if a pacemaker is not readily available.
- Patient and family education
  - Patients and their families should be instructed to activate the EMS (call 911) and seek immediate care for signs of MI, shortness of breath, and syncope related to 2°AVB type II. Because this is a higher degree of block, patients will be much more symptomatic than with previously mentioned blocks.

- Pacemaker education, routine checks, and battery changes should be discussed with patients and their families.
- Family members of people with cardiac disease should learn CPR and how to activate the EMS in the event of cardiac arrest.

Outcomes and Follow-Up
- Goal of treatment is to restore sinus rhythm or maintain cardiac output using a pacemaker.
- Patients will keep scheduled appointments with their healthcare providers to monitor response to medications and for diagnostic testing, if indicated.
- Patients will adhere to medication schedules.

THIRD-DEGREE ATRIOVENTRICULAR BLOCK (3°AVB), COMPLETE HEART BLOCK

Description
- 3°AVB is the complete dissociation of impulses between the atria and ventricles. The sinus node controls the atria and either a nodal (junctional) or a ventricular escape pacemaker controls the ventricles. The result is a series of P waves and QRS complexes that do not relate to each other. This dysrhythmia is not well-tolerated because of the loss of atrial kick and bradycardia, and patients usually seek treatment.
- ECG manifestations of 3°AVB
  - P-R interval: no consistent P-R interval, no relationship between P and QRS complexes
  - QRS duration: less than 0.12 second if controlled by a junctional pacemaker; longer than 0.12 second if controlled by a ventricular pacemaker
  - Rate: Atrial rate is normal; ventricular rate is slow, that of either junctional or ventricular escape pacemaker.
  - Regularity: Both atrial and ventricular activity are regular, but independent of each other.

Etiology
- 3°AVB can be caused by rate-reducing cardiac medications. It also can arise from advanced structural heart disease that completely prevents impulses from traveling from the atria to the ventricles. Cardiac ischemia and infarction can result in 3°AVB. It can also be congenital, diagnosed as an incidental finding.

Figure 13–10. Third-Degree Atrioventricular Block (3°AVB), Complete Heart Block

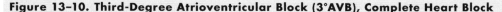
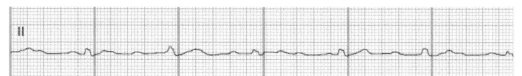

Note: Also wide QRS.

- 3°AVB can occur secondary to the following conditions:
  - CHD
  - MI
  - Cardiac surgery
  - Lev and Lenègre disease
  - Congenital heart disease

Incidence and Demographics
- 3°AVB is more common in adults than children; however, it can occur in congenital heart disease. It can occur intermittently or persistently, depending on the etiology.

Risk Factors
- A history of cardiac disease such as those mentioned above
- Patients with 2°AVB type II have a great risk of progressing to complete heart block, as do patients who are hyperkalemic or have digitalis toxicity.

Assessment
- History
  - Symptoms of activity intolerance, syncope, shortness of breath, chest pain, diaphoresis, and nausea
- Physical findings
  - Bradycardia
  - Hypotension and poor perfusion
- Diagnostic tests
  - ECG is diagnostic for complete heart block.
  - Digitalis level and electrolytes should be measured to identify contributing factors.
  - Echocardiogram may be indicated to assess cardiac function.
  - Electrophysiology studies may be used also to assess conduction.

Management
- Invasive management
  - A cardiac pacemaker should be inserted for complete heart block if the patient is symptomatic. Transcutaneous and transvenous pacemakers can be used in the acute management phase until a permanent pacemaker is inserted.
- Pharmacologic management
  - Atropine is not indicated for 3°AVB because this block is often unresponsive to it.
  - Medications used to maintain hemodynamic stability and cardiac output, such as dopamine and isoproterenol, can be used for acute management.
  - Medications that slow conduction through the AV node, such as digoxin and antidysrhythmic agents, should be held, and often the heart block will resolve.
- Patient and family education
  - Patients and their families should be instructed to activate EMS and seek immediate care for signs of MI, shortness of breath, and syncope related to 3°AVB. Because this is a higher degree of block, patients will be much more symptomatic than with previously mentioned blocks.
  - Pacemaker education, routine checks, and battery changes should be discussed with patients and their families.

Outcomes and Follow-Up

- Goal of treatment is to restore sinus rhythm or maintain cardiac output using a pacemaker.
- Patients will keep scheduled appointments with their healthcare providers to monitor response to medications and for diagnostic testing, if indicated.
- Patients will adhere to medication schedules.

VENTRICULAR TACHYCARDIA (VT)

Description

- VT is a rapid, regular, wide QRS complex tachycardia with dissociation between atria and ventricles. QRS complexes in VT are often in the opposite direction of the QRS complexes of the sinus rhythm. VT that originates in the right ventricular outflow track will have the same QRS deflection as the sinus rhythm. VT that lasts longer than 30 seconds is called sustained, and VT that lasts less than 30 seconds is called nonsustained. QRS complexes that look identical come from the same ectopic focus, and are called monomorphic VT. QRS complexes that come from different ectopic foci have different shapes and are called polymorphic. Polymorphic VT has a worse prognosis than monomorphic VT.
- ECG manifestations of VT
  - P-R interval: Unable to measure; often no evidence of atrial activity, or a sporadic dissociated P wave
  - QRS duration: longer than 0.12 second
  - Rate: fast, ranging from 120 to 300 beats per minute
  - Regularity: usually regular, often paroxysmal in short runs

Etiology

- VT can be caused by a reentry circuit in the ventricles, and irritable ectopic foci that propagate impulses from cell to cell instead of through the conduction system.
- Causes of VT
  - Hypoxia
  - Myocardial ischemia, MI, cardiac surgery
  - Hypokalemia, hypomagnesemia, acidosis
  - Increased catecholamines
  - Exercise
  - Digitalis toxicity
  - Caffeine, nicotine, cocaine, and other sympathomimetic agents

Figure 13–11. Ventricular Tachycardia (VT)

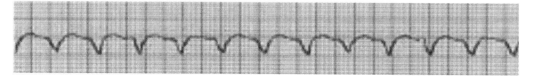

Incidence and Demographics
- VT occurs often in asymptomatic, nonsustained runs.
- Conditions that cause VT occur equally in men and women, young and old, and across all races.
- The majority of adult cardiac arrests are because of lethal dysrhythmia, which include VT and ventricular fibrillation (VF). VT often precedes VF in cardiac arrest.

Risk Factors
- Untreated premature ventricular complexes (PVC) can be a risk factor for developing VT.
- Ischemia or electrolyte imbalances

Assessment
- History
  - Syncope, fainting, palpitations, chest pain or pressure, shortness of breath
  - History of MI, cardiac surgery, structural heart disease, HF, or cardiomyopathy
  - Social history including alcohol abuse and drug use
  - History of renal failure could cause electrolyte imbalances and metabolic disturbances.
- Physical findings
  - May have a pulse or be pulseless and in full cardiac arrest
  - Rapid heart rate, either sustained or intermittent
  - Hypotension
  - S3 with concurrent HF
  - Inspiratory crackles and productive cough from pulmonary edema
- Diagnostic tests
  - ECG to diagnose and distinguish from supraventricular tachycardia with aberrant conduction
  - Laboratory studies of electrolytes, arterial blood gases (ABG), magnesium, and drug levels to identify contributing factors

Management
- Invasive management
  - Synchronized electrical cardioversion for sustained VT with a pulse; electrical defibrillation for pulseless VT
  - Overdrive pacing may be indicated and is a protocol in many implanted cardioverter defibrillators.
  - Radiofrequency ablation can be done to obliterate a reentry circuit or excitable ectopic foci.
  - Implantable cardioverter defibrillators (ICD) are indicated for patients with recurrent episodes of VT, inducible clinically significant VT, or hypotensive VT. See the AHA guidelines on who should have a permanent ICD.
  - In some cases, the life vest may be used to provide for immediate defibrillation for the person who is being closely monitored for ventricular dysrhythmias or awaiting an ICD implant.
- Pharmacologic management (ACLS protocols)
  - Pulseless VT is treated with epinephrine or vasopressin as a choice of catecholamines, followed by either amiodarone or lidocaine as an antidysrhythmic agent. Magnesium also can be used.
  - VT with a pulse is treated with amiodarone or synchronized cardioversion. Provide sedation if needed for the cardioversion.

- Patient and family education
  - Teach the signs and symptoms of cardiac arrest and the procedure for activating the EMS if needed.
  - Medication indications, actions, doses, schedules, interactions, and side effects also should be taught.
  - Family members should learn basic life support skills in the event of cardiac arrest.
  - ICD education, routine checks, and battery changes should be discussed with patients and their families.

Outcomes and Follow-Up
- The goal of treatment is to restore and maintain sinus rhythm. This may be accomplished by correcting reversible causes of VT or by long-term antidysrhythmic therapy and ICD.
- Patients will keep scheduled appointments with their healthcare providers to monitor response to medications and for diagnostic testing, if indicated.
- Patients will adhere to medication schedules and ICD check schedules.

VENTRICULAR FIBRILLATION (VF)

Description
- A rapid, chaotic dysrhythmia with no organized atrial or ventricular activity. VF can be classified as coarse or fine, depending on the amplitude of the electrical activity. Coarse VF is more responsive to treatment. This is a life-threatening dysrhythmia that does not support circulation.
- ECG manifestations of VF
  - P-R interval: none
  - QRS duration: no measurable QRS complex
  - Rate: rapid, more than 300 fibrillations per minute, uncoordinated
  - Regularity: irregular, chaotic

Etiology
- VF is caused by an interruption of the normal electrical activity at a point during depolarization when the cells are half polarized and half depolarized. The positive and negative ions are in a state of chaos and lose the ability to either complete depolarization or complete repolarization. The result is ineffective quivering of the ventricles. Another cause of VF is multiple ectopic foci firing at the same time.
- Causes of VF
  - CHD
  - MI
  - Electrolyte imbalance, hypomagnesemia
  - Blunt trauma to the chest
  - Hypoxemia
  - Structural heart disease
  - Prolonged QT syndromes
  - Acidosis
  - Drug toxicity: poisons, tricyclic antidepressants
  - Electrocution

Incidence
- Sudden cardiac death often is attributed to a VF arrest in people with CHD.
- VF can occur at any age, equally in men and women as a result of the causes listed above. VF is rare in children.

Risk Factors
- The major risk factor for a VF arrest is CHD.
- All of the conditions listed above can predispose to VF.

Assessment
- History
  - A history may be obtained from bystanders who were present when the patient arrested, because the patient will not be able to give a history. Determine the victim's condition prior to the arrest including illnesses, complaints of chest pain, discomfort, trauma, and activity. A complete health history should be obtained from those who know the victim well and from the victim if he or she survives the arrest.
  - Risk factors associated with VF
- Physical findings
  - Apnea
  - Pulselessness
  - Unresponsive
- Diagnostic tests
  - Immediate cardiac monitoring to analyze the patient's rhythm.
  - Laboratory tests include ABG, electrolytes, magnesium, cardiac markers, drug levels, and toxicity screening to identify contributing factors.

Management
- Invasive management
  - Immediate CPR and defibrillation within 4 to 6 minutes for the best chance of survival.
  - EPS after successful resuscitation
  - An ICD is usually indicated after EPS unless the situation was due to a treatable condition.
- Pharmacologic management (ACLS protocols) alternates with defibrillation and continued CPR.
  - Epinephrine or vasopressin should be given initially, followed by an antidysrhythmic agent such as amiodarone or lidocaine during subsequent CPR cycles.
  - Magnesium also may be given.
- Patient and family education
  - Patients and their families should be taught to activate the EMS (call 911) with complaints of chest pain or unresponsiveness.
  - Family members should learn basic life support skills.

Outcomes and Follow-Up Care
- Mortality rate is high for VF arrests unless defibrillation takes place within minutes, and reversible causes are identified and treated.
- Evaluation in an electrophysiology lab for ICD placement may be indicated for patients surviving a VF arrest.
- Patients will keep scheduled appointments with their healthcare providers to monitor response to medications and for diagnostic testing, if indicated.
- Adherence to medication schedules should be emphasized.
- ICD education, routine checks, and battery changes should be discussed with patients and their families.

SUDDEN CARDIAC DEATH (SCD)

Description
SCD is the syndrome of death from cardiac causes within 60 minutes of the onset of acute symptoms. The time and form of death are unexpected and the preexisting heart condition may or may not have been known.

Etiology
- There are multiple causes of SCD. This syndrome results in lethal dysrhythmia (VT, VF, bradydysrhythmia, or asystole) or circulatory failure.
- Causes of SCD
  - Coronary atherosclerosis
  - Abnormalities of the coronary arteries
  - HF
  - Myocarditis
  - Valvular heart disease
  - Congenital heart disease
  - VT
  - VF
  - Prolonged QT syndrome
  - Dissecting aortic aneurysm
  - Cardiac tamponade
  - Acute pulmonary embolism
  - Systemic diseases such as sarcoidosis, progressive systemic sclerosis, amyloidosis, hemochromatosis
  - Electrolyte disturbance

Incidence and Demographics
- Average age for SCD is 60 years.
- In 90% of the adult victims, two or more coronary arteries were narrowed from atherosclerosis.
- Two-thirds of the people who experienced SCD had previous MIs.

Risk Factors

The risk factors associated with SCD are the causes of this syndrome.

Assessment

- History
  - History of conditions associated with SCD
  - Symptoms prior to the terminal event such as chest pain, dyspnea, or palpitations
  - Before SCD, many people have an acute change in their condition such as dysrhythmia, hypotension, chest pain, or dyspnea.
- Physical findings
  - Loss of cardiac function
  - Loss of consciousness
- Diagnostic tests
  - ECG to detect cardiac rhythm if present

Management

- Invasive management
  - Immediate assessment that the collapse is because of cardiac arrest
  - Once confirmed, start CPR.
  - Initiate ACLS protocol based on the cardiac rhythm or cause of the arrest
- Pharmacologic management
  - ACLS protocol for medications
- Patient and family education
  - Teach the signs and symptoms of cardiac arrest and the procedure for activating the EMS if needed.
  - Patients with conditions contributing to SCD should be taught about the medications and treatments for these health problems.
  - Family members should learn CPR and how to activate EMS in the event of SCD.

Outcomes and Follow-Up

- SCD is associated with high mortality unless treatment is initiated promptly.
- Patients should adhere to their medication regimen, especially if antidysrhythmics are indicated.
- Patients may need further diagnostic testing to determine the contributing cause of this syndrome.

PULMONARY ARTERY HYPERTENSION (PAH)

Description
Pulmonary hypertension is present if the pulmonary artery mean pressure is above 25 mm Hg at rest or above 30 mm Hg with exercise.

Etiology
- The etiology of primary pulmonary hypertension (PPH) is unknown.
- Causes of secondary pulmonary hypertension
  - Cardiac disease: AS, CHD, cardiomyopathy, MS, MR
  - Lung disease: chronic obstructive pulmonary disease, restrictive lung disease, interstitial lung disease, chest wall abnormalities
  - Pulmonary vascular disease: congenital heart disease, atrial septal defect, patent foramen ovale
  - Pulmonary vascular obstruction: thromboembolic pulmonary hypertension, tumor embolization, mediastinal fibrosis
- The classification of PAH has been recommended. See Table 13–7.

Table 13–7. Pulmonary Hypertension Classification (World Health Organization)

WHO Group I: Pulmonary arterial hypertension (PAH)
• Idiopathic (IPAH)
• Familial (FPAH)
• Associated with other diseases (APAH): collagen vascular disease (e.g., scleroderma), congenital shunts between the systemic and pulmonary circulation, portal hypertension, HIV infection, drugs, toxins, or other diseases or disorders
• Associated with venous or capillary disease
WHO Group II: Pulmonary hypertension associated with left heart disease
• Atrial or ventricular disease
• Valvular disease (e.g., mitral stenosis)
WHO Group III: Pulmonary hypertension associated with lung diseases, hypoxemia, or both
• Chronic obstructive pulmonary disease (COPD), interstitial lung disease (ILD)
• Sleep-disordered breathing, alveolar hypoventilation
• Chronic exposure to high altitude
• Developmental lung abnormalities
WHO Group IV: Pulmonary hypertension because of chronic thrombotic or embolic disease or both
• Pulmonary embolism in the proximal or distal pulmonary arteries
• Embolization of other matter, such as tumor cells or parasites
WHO Group V: Miscellaneous

- Pathology starts with risk factors and susceptibility (abnormal BMPR-2 gene), which leads to vascular injury.
  - Vascular injury leads to endothelial dysfunction.
    - Decreased nitric oxide synthesis
    - Decreased prostacyclin production (potent vasodilator substance)
    - Increased thromboxane production (potent vasoconstrictor substance)
    - Increased endothelin-1 production
  - Vascular smooth muscle hypertrophies
  - Plexiform lesions develop in the pulmonary artery, further impairing blood flow.

Incidence and Demographics
- More than 100,000 are diagnosed with the disorder.
- It is thought that the numbers with PH are probably higher as the disorder is probably under diagnosed.
- Higher incidence in women than men

Risk Factors
- Portal hypertension
- HIV infection
- Systemic infection
- Pulmonary veno-occlusive disease
- Pulmonary capillary hemangiomatosis
- Family history of PPH
- Collagen vascular disorders
- Sickle cell anemia

Assessment
- History
  - Symptoms of dyspnea, fatigue, or syncope
- Physical findings
  - Right ventricular heave
  - Split S2 with a loud P2-pulmonic component
  - S4 heart sound
  - Midsystolic ejection murmur
  - Hepatomegaly
  - Ascites
  - Peripheral edema
- Diagnostic tests
  - ECG to identify right atrial and ventricular enlargement
  - Chest x-ray to detect enlargement of the pulmonary arteries
  - Echocardiography to evaluate right atrial and ventricular enlargement and dimensions
  - Right heart catheterization to measure pressures
  - Pulmonary angiography
  - Lung scintigraphy to identify perfusion abnormalities
  - 6-minute walk test to evaluate functional level and monitor progress with drug therapies. This is usually done at each office visit to the specialist.

Management
- Invasive management
  - Heart-lung and lung transplant
- Pharmacologic management
  - Cardiac glycosides to improve myocardial contractility
  - Diuretic therapy to decrease venous congestion
  - Calcium channel blockers are a first-line drug but effect is usually suboptimal.
  - Endothelin receptor antagonists include oral bosentan or ambrisentan.
  - Phospodiesterase-5 inhibitor is sildenafil. A low-dose daily version is marketed as Revatio®.
  - Prostanoids include epoprostenol, treprostinil, and inhaled iloprost.
  - Warfarin therapy is recommended because of the high risk of thrombus development.
- Patient and family education
  - Teach patients and their families about the etiology, risk factors, and course of their disease.
  - Educate them about pharmacological interventions including actions, dosages, and side effects.
  - Discuss with them the symptoms associated with acute HF and how to activate the EMS in the event of cardiac arrest.

Outcomes and Follow-Up
- Patients and their families will be knowledgeable about pulmonary hypertension and its treatment.
- Patients will not experience any complications from this health problem or its treatment.
- Patients will follow up with their healthcare providers after noninvasive and invasive therapies.
- Patients will improve the 6-minute walk distance and quality of life.

CAROTID ARTERY OCCLUSIVE DISEASE (CAOD)

Description
CAOD, caused by atherosclerosis, may be either asymptomatic or symptomatic. In asymptomatic carotid stenosis, atherosclerotic disease develops slowly and the course is unpredictable. In symptomatic carotid stenosis, patients experience symptoms as the vascular flow through the affected carotid artery becomes increasingly diminished. Symptoms depend upon the area of the brain that suffers ischemia.

Etiology
- Most atherosclerotic lesions develop at branch points or in areas where the artery is curved.
  - The most frequently occurring site is the common carotid bifurcation that includes the internal and external carotid arteries.

Incidence and Demographics
- CAOD is associated with advancing age.
- Major risk factor for the development of stroke (see Table 13–8 for all etiologies of stroke).

Table 13-8. Etiology of CVA

Etiology	Percentage of Overall CVAs	Pathophysiology	CT Findings
Thrombotic	53%	New thrombus appearing at the site of atherosclerotic lesion	Initial noncontrast CT will appear normal
Embolic	31%	Clot or substance formed in another area of the body lodges in a cerebral blood vessel. May occur with atrial fibrillation and mural thrombus, valve disease or replacement, atrial septal defect, patent foramen ovale, septic clot, fat emboli, air emboli.	Initial noncontrast CT will appear normal
Hemorrhagic Intracerebral Subarachnoid	10% 6%	Rupture of a cerebral aneurysm or congenital arterial-venous malformation, or trauma. Blood compresses and injures brain tissue.	Immediate appearance of blood on a noncontrast CT
Lacunar	Unable to determine	May be asymptomatic because size of brain area affected is very small.	Often only diagnosed when CT performed for other reason; 5 mm area of hypo density on CT

Risk Factors

- Risk factors for the development of CAOD are similar to those of other vascular problems associated with atherosclerosis such as hypercholesterolemia, cigarette smoking, and HTN. See Chapters 7 and 8.
- Concomitant conditions that increase risk are diabetes mellitus, obesity, hyper-triglyceridemia, and a family history of cardiovascular disease.

Assessment

- History
  - Symptomatic patients may manifest focal, global, or vertebrobasilar symptoms.
  - Focal symptoms
    - Transient ischemia attack (TIA): Symptoms last less than 24 hours and result in complete recovery. Left carotid TIAs may present as motor dysfunction (dysarthria, weakness, or paralysis of face, right extremities, or both), loss of vision in the left eye (amaurosis fugax), sensory disturbances (numbness or paraesthesia of the face, right extremities, or both) and aphasia. Right carotid TIAs may present with similar symptoms on the opposite side except that the aphasia occurs only when the right hemisphere is dominant for speech.

- Reversible ischemic neurologic deficit (RIND): hemiparesis, monoparesis, and aphasia that last more than 24 but less than 72 hours and result in complete recovery.
- Cerebrovascular accident (CVA): hemiparesis, monoparesis, and aphasia that result in permanent deficits.
  - Global symptoms
    - CVA: Neurological symptoms are related to the area of injury, resulting in permanent deficits that may demonstrate some improvement.
  - Vertebrobasilar symptoms
    - Dysarthria, aphasia, vertigo, syncope, cognitive deficits, and diplopia. The symptoms last for less than 24 hours and there is complete recovery.
- Physical findings
  - Vascular
    - Carotid bruits, although the absence does not exclude CAOD
    - Diminished or absent carotid pulses
    - Blood pressure difference between arms of more than 10 mm Hg
  - Neurologic deficits according to the area of injury
- Diagnostic tests
  - Doppler ultrasonography for physiological information of flow velocities
  - Carotid duplex scan to detect morphologic and hemodynamic abnormalities
  - CT scan or MRI study to identify abnormalities of the carotid artery
  - Arteriography to diagnose CAOD and evaluate carotid artery anatomy

Management

- Invasive management
  - Indications for carotid endarterectomy (CEA)
    - Proven benefit for symptomatic patients (TIA or mild stroke) with 70% or greater stenosis
    - Acceptable benefit for symptomatic patients with 50% to 69% stenosis
    - Proven benefit for asymptomatic patients with 60% or greater stenosis
  - Carotid interventions and stenting depend on location and size of the lesion
- Pharmacologic management
  - Antiplatelet therapy: Aspirin has resulted in a decrease in the percentage of strokes but does not change the progression of COAD.
  - Warfarin is used to prevent clot formation in selected conditions.
- Patient and family education
  - Education of patients and their families should focus on medications and related laboratory testing depending on the type of pharmacologic management.
  - Teach them about risk factor modification including diet, exercise, weight reduction, smoking cessation, and stress reduction.
  - Patients and families should be taught the symptoms associated with TIA, RIND, and CVA and how to activate the EMS if needed.
  - Patients electing to undergo CEA should have preoperative teaching before the procedure and postoperative and discharge education before leaving the hospital.

ACUTE MANAGEMENT OF THROMBOTIC CVA

If treatment is instituted within 3 hours of hours of onset of symptoms, tissue damage may be prevented or minimized if it is a thrombotic CVA. Window of time to treatment is extended to 4.5 hours in certain situations.

- Upon arrival to the hospital or EMS arrival at the scene with carryover to ED
    - Determine time of onset of symptoms.
    - Rule out other causes of neurologic deficit: hypoglycemia, seizure, metabolic or toxic condition, tumor.
    - Obtain history and initial assessment.
    - Determine if there are any contraindications to administering a thrombolytic (TPA).
- For any suspected CVA within the window of time, obtain a stat noncontrast CT of the head to rule out a bleed.
- If there is no evidence of bleeding and symptoms have not resolved (as might happen with a TIA), continue with thrombolytic therapy.
- Observe and monitor for neurologic improvement, bleeding, seizure, hemorrhagic conversion, and signs of cerebral edema.

Outcomes and Follow-Up

- Patients will be knowledgeable about CAOD and its treatment.
- Patients will not experience any neurological sequelae as a result of CAOD and related invasive and pharmacological interventions.
- Follow-up care should include monitoring asymptomatic patients for evidence of disease progression and monitoring of all patients for adverse outcomes such as TIA, RIND, or CVA.

ABDOMINAL AORTIC ANEURYSM (AAA)

Description

- Aneurysms are areas in the arterial wall that have dilated as a result of weakening and defects.
- True aneurysms involve the intima, media, and adventitia arterial layers.
    - Fusiform aneurysm is dilation of the entire circumference of a segment of the aorta.
    - Saccular aneurysm is an outpouching of one side of the aorta.
- Dissecting aneurysm occurs when the intima opens and blood separates the intima and some of the media from the adventitia. This process results in a false and true lumen for the vessel.

Etiology

- Degenerative atherosclerotic lesions weaken the arterial wall.
- Inflammation secondary to infectious arteritis from bacterial or fungal infections or from autoimmune diseases
- Mechanical trauma that disrupts the integrity of the aortic wall
- Congenital weakness at the bifurcations because of connective tissue disorders such as Marfan or Ehlers-Danlos syndromes

Incidence and Demographics
- Aortic aneurysms affect approximately 1% to 5% of the U.S. population.
- AAA is associated with advancing age, HTN, family history, and male gender.
- An aneurysm enlarges approximately 10% a year.
- Risk for rupture increases with the diameter of the aneurysm.

Risk Factors
- Risk factors for the development of AAA are similar to those for other vascular problems associated with atherosclerosis such as hypercholesterolemia, cigarette smoking, and HTN.
- Concomitant conditions that increase risk are diabetes mellitus, peripheral vascular disease, presence of other aneurysms, and a family history of cardiovascular or genetic diseases.

Assessment
- History
  - May be asymptomatic
  - Symptomatic
    - Abdominal pain, either persistent or intermittent
    - Back pain that is dull or aching
    - Patients report pulsations, especially when recumbent.
    - Weight loss and nausea from abdominal involvement
- Physical findings
  - Palpable, pulsatile mass in the upper abdomen
  - Bruit heard over the aneurysm
  - HTN
- Diagnostic tests
  - Abdominal x-ray to detect calcifications of the aorta
  - Ultrasound to identify and monitor the size of the aneurysm
  - Abdominal CT or MRI study to identify and monitor the size of the aneurysm
  - Aortography to visualize the aneurysm and the aorta

Management
- Invasive management
  - AAA repair with a graft for symptomatic aneurysms, rapidly enlarging aneurysms, and infrarenal aneurysm 5 cm or larger. Repair may be surgical or endovascular depending on the size and location of the defect.
  - Aneurysms smaller than 4 cm and with asymptomatic patients are monitored every 6 months for size.
- Pharmacologic management
  - Agents for risk factor management such as antihypertensives, lipid-lowering drugs, and glucose-lowering drugs.
- Patient and family education
  - Teach patients and their families about the etiology of the disease, risk factors, and course of the disease.
  - Teach them about risk factor modification including diet, exercise, weight reduction, smoking cessation, and stress reduction.
  - Discuss symptoms associated with leaking or rupture of the aneurysm and how to activate the EMS if needed.
  - If surgery is indicated, teach the patient about preoperative preparation along with postoperative and discharge care before leaving the hospital.

Outcomes and Follow-Up
- Patients and their families will be knowledgeable about aortic aneurysm and its treatment.
- Patients will not experience any complications from the aortic aneurysm or its related treatment.
- Patients with aneurysms smaller than 4 cm will follow up with their healthcare providers for routine monitoring.

UPPER EXTREMITY ARTERIAL OCCLUSIVE DISEASE (AOD)

Description
Stenosis of the arteries of the upper extremities from atherosclerosis and other conditions can result in diminished blood flow to the arms and hands.

Etiology
- Upper extremity AOD may be the result of multiple factors including atherosclerosis, particularly of the proximal left and right subclavian arteries.
- Embolization from thrombi (A-fib, MI), atherosclerotic plaques, or other substances (platelet products, particulate matter) may lodge in the subclavian, axillary, and brachial arteries. Other arteries that may be affected include the ulnar and radial arteries.
- Trauma from penetrating and blunt injuries. Other factors include radial artery cannulation and hemodialysis cannulation sites in the arm that can contribute to hand ischemia.
- Immune arteritis, an inflammatory process, results in damage to the intima of the affected arteries leading to stenosis and occlusion. Numerous conditions are associated with this pathology including polyarteritis nodosa and Raynaud's phenomenon.
- Thoracic outlet syndrome as a congenital abnormality or because of trauma results in atherosclerotic changes and plaque formation. This process results in aneurysm formation, thrombosis, and distal embolization. It is more common in women because of the smaller opening for the artery and easier entrapment by the surrounding bony structures.

Incidence and Demographics
- Approximately 10% of all embolic events involve the upper extremities.
- Upper extremity AOD increases with advancing age.
- Women are affected more often than men by thoracic outlet syndrome and Raynaud's phenomenon.

Risk Factors
- Risk factors for the development of upper extremity AOD are similar to those of other vascular problems associated with atherosclerosis such as hypercholesterolemia, cigarette smoking, and HTN.
- Concomitant conditions that increase risk are diabetes mellitus, obesity, hypertriglyceridemia, and a family history of cardiovascular disease.

Assessment
- History
  - Presence of atherosclerosis risk factors
  - Coexisting health problems that may precipitate embolic events (e.g., A-fib, MI, ventricular aneurysm)
  - Recent invasive procedures (such as arterial cannulation) or presence of hemodialysis access site
  - Acute injury to the artery from trauma
  - Chronic injury from repetitive occupational stress
- Physical findings
  - Diminished or absent pulses in the affected artery
  - Color changes in the upper extremity such as erythema, pallor, purplish rubor, and cyanosis. Other changes may include muscle atrophy, edema, and gangrene.
  - Bruits in area of arterial stenosis
  - Adson maneuver is used to detect compression of the subclavian artery at the thoracic outlet. Have the patient sit with hands on thighs. Palpate both radials while patient takes a deep breath, holds it, and turns the head and neck to the affected side. If the pulse is diminished on the affected side, the test is positive for thoracic outlet syndrome.
  - Allen Test to evaluate radial and ulnar artery patency was described in Chapter 12.
- Diagnostic tests
  - Doppler ultrasound to detect decreased blood flow
  - CT or MRI study to detect upper extremity abnormalities
  - Arteriography to diagnose upper extremity occlusive disease

Management
- Invasive management
  - Embolectomy for acute occlusions because of emboli
  - Repair of lacerations or intimal injuries from trauma
  - Arterial bypass procedures with either autologous (e.g., saphenous vein) or prosthetic graft material for proximal arterial lesions
  - Endarterectomy to remove atherosclerotic plaque
  - Percutaneous angioplasty with or without a stent for arterial stenosis
  - Surgical removal of a rib for thoracic outlet syndrome
- Pharmacologic management
  - Fibrinolytic therapy
  - Anticoagulation with heparin or warfarin to prevent emboli
  - Treatment of vasospasm using calcium channel blockers
- Patient and family education
  - Teach patients and their families about the etiology, risk factors, and course of their disease.
  - Discuss symptoms associated with acute occlusion of the artery and how to activate the EMS if needed.
  - If surgery is indicated, teach the patient about preoperative preparation along with postoperative and discharge care before leaving the hospital.

Outcomes and Follow-Up
- Patients and their families will be knowledgeable about upper extremity occlusive disease and its treatment.
- Patients will protect the upper extremity from further injury by keeping it warm, stopping occupational trauma, and avoiding undue pressure or constriction of the affected limb.
- Patients will follow up as indicated with their healthcare providers after noninvasive and invasive therapies.

LOWER EXTREMITY AOD

Description
- Lower extremity AOD is because of stenosis of the iliac arteries or the infrainguinal vessels (femoral, popliteal, tibial, and pedal arteries) that results in diminished blood flow.
- Lower extremity AOD may be acute or chronic.

Etiology
- Acute lower extremity AOD is caused by embolization, thrombosis, or trauma.
- Chronic lower extremity AOD is usually because of atherosclerosis.

Incidence and Demographics
- Lower extremity AOD occurs more frequently than upper extremity AOD.

Risk Factors
- Embolism, thrombosis, and trauma are the most frequent causes of acute AOD. Other causes include compartment syndrome and low-flow states such as circulatory shock or HF.
- Atherosclerosis is the most common cause of chronic lower extremity AOD.
- Risk factors for atherosclerosis include advancing age, male gender, diabetes mellitus, cigarette smoking, HTN, increased lipid levels, and family history of cardiovascular disease.

Assessment
- History
  - Acute lower extremity AOD
    - Sudden onset of symptoms with loss of circulation from embolism or trauma
      - Symptoms occur distal to the site of the blockage and include pain, color changes, and coolness.
      - There is evidence for the source of the embolism such as A-fib, valvular heart disease, or MI.
    - Gradual onset of changes with thrombosis, with some symptoms similar to chronic lower extremity AOD
  - Chronic lower extremity AOD
    - Progressive decrease in arterial flow resulting in pain with activity and color changes in the affected extremity

- Physical findings
  - Acute lower extremity AOD
    - Pain at rest
    - Absent or diminished pulses
    - Paresthesia
    - Tissue necrosis and gangrene
    - Paralysis is an indicator of irreversible ischemia.
  - Chronic lower extremity AOD
    - Intermittent claudication is cramping pain of the lower extremity muscles that occurs with activity or exercise and resolves with rest. The affected arterial segment is proximal to the muscle groups experiencing the symptoms (i.e., the superficial femoral artery causes calf pain; external iliac artery causes thigh pain, aortic disease causes buttock pain).
    - Rest pain is pain that results from progressive AOD, increases with elevating the foot, and is relieved by placing the extremity in a dependent position.
    - Color changes from dependent rubor (dusky, purple color) to pallor on elevation.
    - Diminished or absent pulses
    - Cooler temperature in the affected extremity
    - Tissue necrosis from ischemia
    - Arterial ulcers (toe, heel, or dorsum of foot; ulcer is pale with eschar and perhaps gangrene; associated with moderate to severe pain)
    - Gangrene from tissue death
- Diagnostic tests
  - Ankle–brachial index to detect arterial stenosis
  - Doppler ultrasound to detect changes in vascular flow
  - Arteriography to diagnose lower extremity AOD

Management

- Invasive management
  - Acute AOD
    - Embolectomy to remove the embolus
    - Arterial bypass procedure if the cause is thrombosis
    - Arterial reconstructive procedure for conditions related to trauma
    - Amputation for gangrene, failed revascularization, or muscle necrosis
  - Chronic AOD
    - Percutaneous transluminal balloon angioplasty and stenting are acceptable therapies for stenosis of the iliac artery and other more distant sites.
    - Surgical procedures may be indicated to either remove the obstruction (endarterectomy) or bypass the obstruction to open the artery. Examples of bypass procedures include the axillopopliteal bypass, infrapopliteal bypass, femoropopliteal bypass, and obturator foramen bypass. Graft materials for these surgical interventions include autologous (e.g., saphenous vein, cephalic vein, basilic vein) and prosthetic grafts.
    - Amputation for gangrene, failed revascularization, or muscle necrosis

- Pharmacologic management
  - Thrombolytic therapy
  - Antiplatelet therapy
  - Drugs for risk factor management such as antihypertensives, lipid, and glucose-lowering agents.
- Patient and family education
  - Teach patients and their families about the etiology, contributing conditions, and risk factor modification.
  - Educate them about risk factor modification including diet, exercise, weight reduction, smoking cessation, and stress reduction.
  - Discuss with them the symptoms associated with acute occlusion of the artery and how to activate the EMS if needed.
  - If surgery is indicated, teach patients about preoperative preparation along with postoperative and discharge care before leaving the hospital.

Outcomes and Follow-Up
- Patients and their families will be knowledgeable about lower extremity occlusive disease and its treatment.
- Patients will adhere to strategies for risk factor reduction such as exercise therapy to develop collateral circulation.
- Patients will follow up as indicated with their healthcare providers after noninvasive and invasive therapies.

DEEP VEIN THROMBOSIS (DVT)

Description
DVT is caused by thrombosis of the deep veins. This syndrome may affect veins of the upper and lower extremities.

Etiology
The risk factors for DVT are stasis, hypercoagulability, and endothelial injury (Virchow triad).

Incidence and Demographics
Venous thrombosis is more common in the lower than the upper extremities.

Risk Factors
- Endothelial injury to the intima of the veins from trauma, intravenous catheters, or parenteral medications
- Stasis of blood flow from immobility, age, and HF
- Hypercoagulability because of coagulation disorders, pregnancy, oral contraceptives, and certain malignancies

Assessment
- History
  - Presence of risk factors for the development of DVT
  - Recent symptoms such as pain, swelling, and increased temperature of the affected extremity
- Physical findings
  - Color changes from pallor to red to deep purple
  - Edema of the affected leg
  - Asymmetry of the legs
  - Positive Homans sign (not very sensitive finding; only found in 40% of DVTs)
- Diagnostic tests
  - Venous duplex scan to visualize thrombosis
  - Plethysmography to identify venous obstruction (rarely used)
  - Venography to visualize obstructions in the venous circulation
  - Serum coagulation tests such as partial thromboplastin time, prothrombin time, INR, fibrin, and antithrombin III levels

Management
- Invasive management
  - Thrombectomy
  - Insertion of an inferior vena cava filter
- Pharmacologic management
  - Anticoagulation with heparin or low molecular weight heparin and warfarin for 3 months
  - Fibrinolytic therapy may be used acutely
- Patient and family education
  - Educate patients and their families about the etiology, risk factors, and course of their disease.
  - Teach them about pharmacologic and therapeutic interventions such as compression devices (stockings and pneumatic boots), heat, and elevation of affected extremity.
  - Discuss with patients and their families the symptoms associated with pulmonary embolism and how to activate the EMS if needed.

Outcomes and Follow-Up
- Patients and their families will be knowledgeable about DVT and its treatment.
- Patients will not experience any complications from this health problem and its related treatment.
- Patients will follow up as indicated with their healthcare providers after noninvasive and invasive therapies.

CHRONIC VENOUS INSUFFICIENCY (CVI)

Description
CVI results from disruption of the venous system that may be congenital or acquired. It usually affects the iliac and femoral veins, and less commonly, the saphenous veins.

Etiology
- Venous obstruction from compression of veins by tumor, retroperitoneal fibrosis, or infection
- Venous valvular insufficiency from congenital or acquired valve incompetence from venous valve prolapse and varicose veins
- Calf muscle pump malfunction from muscle wasting disease (paraplegia, trauma, disuse syndromes) and muscular fibrosis (multiple sclerosis)

Incidence and Demographics
CVI is more common than acute venous thrombosis.

Risk Factors
- Family history of CVI
- Advancing age
- Female gender
- Occupation
- Obesity
- History of DVT

Assessment
- History
  - Presence of risk factors for CVI
  - Symptoms such as pain or changes in superficial and deeper veins
- Physical findings
  - Telangiectasias or spider veins often are associated with varicose veins.
  - Distended, tortuous, palpable vessels or varicose veins
  - Hyperpigmentation of feet and ankles
  - Lipodermatosclerosis
  - Venous stasis ulcers (medial distal leg, mild pain, ulcer is pink, and surrounding tissue with stasis dermatitis)
- Diagnostic tests
  - Ambulatory venous pressure measurements to identify venous insufficiency
  - Duplex scan to detect venous abnormalities
  - Plethysmography to detect valve incompetency or calf muscle pump dysfunction
  - Venography

Management
- Invasive management
  - Stripping of superficial varicosities associated with varicose veins. This usually involves ligation of the greater saphenous vein and vein avulsion.
  - Venous bypass (e.g., cross-femoral venous bypass, saphenofemoral venous bypass, saphenopopliteal bypass) has been used to go around obstructed segments of the targeted vein using either autologous vessels or prosthetic grafts.

- Sclerotherapy involves injecting caustic substances into veins to promote scar tissue formation and eliminate the venous lesions.
- Noninvasive management
  - Compression stockings
  - Activity restrictions such as avoiding prolonged standing, elevating legs when seated or recumbent, and wearing loose, nonconstricting clothes.
  - Treatment of venous stasis ulcers such as Unna boot and dressing changes
- Patient and family education
  - Educate patients and their families about the etiology, risk factors, and course of the disease.
  - Discuss with them the symptoms associated with infection of venous stasis ulcers.
  - If surgery is indicated, teach the patient about preoperative preparation along with postoperative and discharge care before leaving the hospital.

Outcomes and Follow-Up
- Patients and their families will be knowledgeable about the disease and its treatment.
- Patients will not experience any complications as a result of this health problem.
- Patients will follow up as indicated with their healthcare providers during noninvasive and invasive therapies.

SUMMARY

This chapter provided an overview of the most common cardiac, valvular, inflammatory, and dysrhythmic disorders. Heart failure, the various forms of cardiomyopathy, and common vascular disorders also were presented. The next chapter focuses on the invasive management of common cardiovascular disorders.

REFERENCES

Abdel-Latif, A., & Moliterna, D. J. (2009). Antiplatelet polypharmacy in primary percutaneous coronary intervention: Trying to understand when more is better. *Circulation, 119*, 3168–3170.

Adams, R. J., Albers, G., Alberts, M. J., Benavente, O., Furie, K., Goldstein, L. B., ... American Stroke Association. (2008). Update to the AHA/ASA recommendations for the prevention of stroke in patients with stroke and transient ischemic attack. *Stroke, 39*(5), 1647–1652.

Barkley, T. W., & Myers, C. M. (2008). *Practice guidelines for acute care nurse practitioners* (2nd ed.). St. Louis, MO: Elsevier Saunders.

Beynon, R. P., Bahl, V. K., & Prendergast, B. D. (2006). Infective endocarditis. *British Medical Journal, 333*, 334–339.

Chen, K. Y., Rha, S. W., Podder, K. L., Jin, Z., Minami, Y., Wang, L., ... Korea Acute Myocardial Infarction Registry Investigators. (2009). Triple versus dial antiplatelet therapy in patients with acute ST segment elevation myocardial infarction undergoing primary percutaneous coronary intervention. *Circulation, 119*, 3207–3214.

Crawford, M. H. (2009). *Cardiology: Current diagnosis and treatment.* New York: McGraw Hill.

Date, M. (2007). Protect your patients from venous thromboembolism. *American Nurse Today, 2*(11), 25–27.

Dunagan, W. C., Littenberg, B., Ewald, G. A., Jones, C. A., Emery, V. B., Waterman, B. M., ... Rogers, J. G. (2005). *Journal of Cardiac Failure, 11*(5), 358–364.

Frey, B. J. (2009) Varicose veins: Today's treatment tools. *Advance for Nurse Practitioners, June*, 49–51.

Gary, R., & Davis, L. (2008). Diastolic heart failure. *Heart and Lung, 37*, 405–416.

Hill, K. M. (2009). Mitral valve repair: A new choice. *American Nurse Today, 4*(5), 8–10.

Hirsch, J., Guyatt, G., Albers, G. W., Harrington, R., & Schunemann, H. J. (2008). Antithrombotic and thrombolytic therapy: Executive summary. *Chest, 133*, 71S–109S.

Kozik, T. M., & Wung, S. F. (2009). Cardiac arrest from acquired long QT syndrome: A case report. *Heart and Lung, 38*, 238–242.

Labus, D. (2008). *Cardiovascular care made incredibly easy.* Philadelphia: Springhouse.

LeFever Kee, J. (2009). *Laboratory and diagnostic tests* (8th ed.). Upper Saddle River, NJ: Prentice Hall.

Martinez, C. A., Carmeli, E., Barak, S., & Stopka, C. B. (2009). Changes in pain free walking based on time in accommodating pain free exercise therapy for peripheral arterial disease. *Journal of Vascular Nursing, 27*(1), 2–7.

McCaffrey, R., & Blum, C. (2009). Venothrombotic events: Evidence-based risk assessment, prophylaxis, diagnosis, and treatment. *Journal for Nurse Practitioners, 5*(5), 325–333.

McPhee, S. J., & Hammer, G. D. (2009). *Pathophysiology of disease: An introduction to clinical medicine* (6th ed.). New York: McGraw-Hill.

Moser, D., & Reigel, B. (2008). *Cardiac nursing: A companion to Braunwald's heart disease.* St. Louis, MO: Elsevier-Saunders.

Prudente, L. A. (2008). Quelling atrial chaos: Current approaches to managing atrial fibrillation. *American Nurse Today, 3*(8), 21–25.

Sandau, K. E., & Smith, M. (2009). Continuous ST segment monitoring: Protocol for practice. *Critical Care Nurse, 29*(4), 39–49.

Serruys, P. W., Morice, M. C., Kappetein, P., Colombo, A., Holmes, D. R., Mack, M. J., ... SYNTAX Investigators. (2009). Percutaneous coronary interventions versus coronary artery bypass grafting for severe coronary disease. *New England Journal of Medicine, 360*, 961–972.

Shoulders-Odom, B. (2008). Management of patients after percutaneous coronary interventions. *Critical Care Nurse, 28*(5), 26–43.

Soat, M. (2009). Aortic aneurysm: Causes, clues, and treatment options. *American Nurse Today,* *4*(7), 7–9.

Stout, K. K., & Verrier, E. D. (2009). Acute valvular regurgitation. *Circulation, 119,* 3232–3241.

Whitten, S. E. (2008). Systolic heart failure in a patient with hypertrophic obstructive cardiomyopathy: A potentially life-threatening complication. *Critical Care Nurse, 28*(5), 44–52.

Woods, S. L., Sivarajan-Froelicher, E. S., Motzer, S. A., & Bridges, E. J. (2010). *Cardiac nursing* (6th ed). Philadelphia: Lippincott Williams Wilken.

Zipes, D. P., Libby, P., Bonow, R. O., & Braunwald, E. (2009). *Braunwald's heart disease: A textbook of cardiovascular medicine* (8th ed.). Philadelphia: Elsevier-Saunders.

Invasive Management of Cardiac and Vascular Disease

Percutaneous balloon angioplasty interventions are widely used in the treatment of vascular disease in the coronary arteries, the carotid arteries, and peripheral arteries. This chapter reviews the care of those patients undergoing various forms of this intervention. Another adaptation of this procedure is the balloon valvuloplasty for certain stenotic heart valves. Care of the patient undergoing implantation of a permanent pacemaker or implantable cardiac defibrillator also is presented. Finally, the common surgical procedures used in the treatment of persons with cardiac and vascular disease are presented.

PERCUTANEOUS CORONARY INTERVENTION (PCI)

Description
- PCI is a mechanical procedure in which the narrowed portion of an artery can be enlarged selectively.
- Balloon pressure is applied to an area of atherosclerotic stenosis and causes plaque rupture, endothelial disruption, and stretching and thinning of the medial wall. The desired outcome is increased blood flow.

- PCI can be performed at the time of a diagnostic coronary catheterization, electively some time after catheterization, or urgently in the setting of unstable angina or an acute myocardial infarction (MI).
- Conscious sedation and local anesthetic are used.
- Most PCI procedures also deploy a metallic stent.
    - Stents provide more stability to the intimal wall of the vessel.
    - Stents may be uncoated (bare metal) or have a drug-eluting coating (DES). The drugs on the stents are either paclitaxel or sirolimus, to reduce inflammation and prevent intimal wall cell proliferation.
    - Acute stent thrombosis can occur in the first 24 hours after placement. Care is taken to provide multiple drugs to prevent thrombus formation.
    - Postprocedure management may vary based on the type of stent placed.
- Restenosis occurs most often 3 to 12 months after PCI because of hyperplasia of the intima or remodeling of the vessel (only occurs with nonstented PCI).

Procedure

- A guide catheter is introduced through a femoral, brachial, or radial artery sheath into the ostium of the diseased coronary artery. (See Figure 14–1.)
- The guide wire is advanced through the central lumen of the balloon catheter into the diseased artery and across the stenosis.
- The balloon is positioned across the lesion and inflated to variable pressure and for variable duration to achieve optimal results, which are assessed angiographically.

Figure 14–1. Percutaneous Coronary Intervention

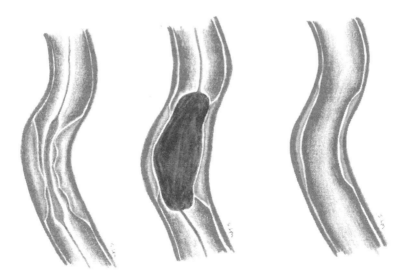

- Stents are deployed after vessels are dilated with the balloon catheter. (See Figure 14–2.)
  - Balloon-expandable stents are ones in which the stent fits over the balloon. After the lesion is crossed, the balloon is inflated and the stent is deployed.
  - Self-expanding stents are covered by a retaining sheath that, when removed, allows the stent to expand. Dilatation of the stent continues until equilibrium is reached between the circumference of the vessel and the dilating force of the stent. To achieve optimal coronary dilatation, balloon expansion of the device may be performed.
- Periprocedural medications include:
  - Antiplatelet drugs
    - Loading doses of clopidogrel are given preprocedure and continued post.
    - Prasugrel (Effient®) may be used in place of clopidogrel. This newer drug has reduced cardiac events but slightly increases risk of bleeding.
    - Glycoprotein IIb/IIIa receptor inhibitors are a new class of antiplatelet agents that often are used during stent procedures and continued up to 12 hours post-PCI.
    - Ticlopidine and persantine are other antiplatelet drugs that are used rarely in the acute setting.
  - Anticoagulants
    - Heparin is used routinely during the procedure.
    - Bivalirudin (Angiomax®) is a thrombin inhibitor that is gaining in clinical use and does not cause heparin-induced thrombocytopenia.

Indications
- Angina refractory to medical therapy
- Unstable angina
- Objective evidence of ischemia such as an abnormal stress test (exercise echocardiogram, dipyridamole, sestamibi, exercise thallium)
- Acute MI with an obstructed or severely stenosed infarct-related coronary artery
- Angina pectoris after coronary artery bypass surgery (CABG)
- Unsuitable coronary anatomy for CABG
- Restenosis after successful PCI and in-stent restenosis
- Longer lesions may be treated by tandem procedures.
- Multivessel disease may be treated by staged procedures over a number of days to weeks to prevent large doses of contrast material that could lead to contrast-associated nephropathy. Furthermore, staged procedures eliminate the complication of acute multisite closures that could cause extensive myocardial damage.

Figure 14–2. Stent Placement in a Coronary Artery

Preinflation

Inflation of balloon with deployment of stent

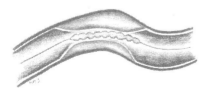
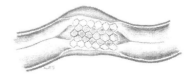

Contraindications

- High-risk coronary anatomy, such as unprotected left main disease, that could lead to hemodynamic compromise.
- Severe, extensive, diffuse coronary artery disease (CAD) may be better treated surgically.
- Bifurcating lesions at difficult-to-reach sites.
- Bleeding disorder
- Multiple PCI restenosis
- A person at very high risk of bleeding who could not undergo the antiplatelet and anticoagulation regimen required for the procedure

Complications

- Abrupt closure of the coronary artery
  - Risk factors for abrupt closure include female gender; unstable angina; diffuse (more than 10 mm), eccentric, calcified, or branched lesions; intracoronary thrombus before intervention; and extensive procedural dissection.
- Periprocedural MI (3% to 5%)
- Emergency CABG (less than 5%)
- Coronary restenosis
- Bleeding or hematoma at the vascular access site
- Contrast-associated nephropathy
- Arterial embolus (1% to 2%)
- Pseudoaneurysm of the vessel
- Retroperitoneal bleeding
- Death (less than 1%)

Nursing Implications

- Preprocedure
  - Obtain baseline vital signs, including 12-lead electrocardiogram (ECG).
  - Complete nursing history and physical assessment.
  - Screen the patient for potential problems, including:
    - History of contrast allergy or bleeding disorder
    - Medications taken day of procedure include insulin, hypoglycemic and antihypertensive agents, warfarin, clopidogrel, and ticlopidine.
      - Metformin should be held the day before the procedure and 48 hours post because of a risk of metabolic acidosis. Insulin may be needed to prevent hyperglycemia.
      - Warfarin is usually stopped 2 days prior to the procedure and the patient is placed on low molecular weight heparin (LMWH) for those days preprocedure and followed postprocedure, because the warfarin is more difficult to reverse if needed during the procedure.
      - Aspirin (ASA) is stopped several days preprocedure because it has an irreversible effect on the platelets.
    - Prothrombin time longer than 16 seconds or International Normalized Ratio (INR) above 1.5
    - Potassium below 3.0 mEq or above 6.0 mEq
    - Hematocrit below 30%

- Creatinine above 1.4 mg/dL or glomerular filtration rate (GFR) below 60
  - These measures identify a person at high risk for contrast-associated nephropathy (CAN) because of osmotic effect of the dye.
  - The most effective way to prevent CAN is to provide adequate hydration before, during, and after the procedure.
  - Acetylcysteine (Mucomyst®) has been used as a prophylactic for renal protection, but studies do not provide strong support for this practice. If used, it is given p.o. in twice-daily dosing for 1 to 2 days preprocedure and up to a day postprocedure.
  - Sodium bicarbonate intravenously (IV) also has been used, although support is weak for this practice.
  - Monitor postprocedure renal function closely.
  - Verify that informed consent is obtained and documented. Provisional consent for CABG usually is obtained at the same time.
  - Insert a saline lock in a vein of the patient's arm.
  - Have the patient void when called to the catheterization laboratory.
  - Patient should have nothing by mouth (NPO) for 4 to 6 hours preprocedure, except medications as ordered. Aspirin may be restarted just before the procedure.
- During PCI (i.e., in the cardiac catheterization laboratory)
  - Anticoagulation with intravenous heparin is usually maintained throughout the procedure and activated clotting time (ACT) is monitored. An alternative is to use bivalirudin (Angiomax®) to prevent heparin-induced thrombocytopenia.
  - Nitroglycerin is frequently administered into the coronary artery to dilate the artery and prevent coronary artery spasm.
  - If acute thrombus is present, intracoronary thrombolytic agent may be given.
  - A glycoprotein (GP) IIb/IIIa receptor inhibitor (e.g., abciximab, eptifibatide, tirofiban) is given and continued into the early postprocedure period.
- Measure and record vital signs and ECG.
  - Connect patient to bedside ECG monitor and select the ST segment monitoring option.
  - Vital signs should be measured every 15 minutes for the first hour or until stable, every 30 minutes twice, hourly four times, and then routinely.
  - Perform a complete physical assessment, including vascular access. Monitor distal limb perfusion and complications of bleeding or hematoma formation. The patient may return with sheaths in place or the access site may be closed with an arterial closure device.
    - Protocols for sheath removal by trained nursing staff can be used.
    - The period of bed rest varies by institution, but the puncture site must be stable prior to getting out of bed.
  - Evaluate the patient for cardiac ischemic pain.
  - Review the procedure summary in the clinical record. Note the type of intervention, target lesions, last ACT, and plan for sheath removal.
  - Sheaths usually are removed 2 to 4 hours after the heparin is stopped and can be removed if the ACT is less than 150 seconds or at ordered value. Most hospitals have specific protocols to follow and these should be used.
  - Patients usually are discharged the day after the procedure. Laboratory data are obtained in the morning and may include renal panel, hematocrit, cardiac enzymes, and ECG.

- Be alert to the signs and symptoms associated with retroperitoneal bleeding.
    - Excessive back or flank pain
    - Feeling like the bladder is full or the patient needs to have a bowel movement
    - Drop in blood pressure and increase in heart rate
    - Drop in hemoglobin or hematocrit
    - Retroperitoneal bleeding is an emergency and requires prompt medical attention.
    - Rarely is there a sign of bleeding, but if present, the ecchymosed areas will be the back and flank on the side of the arterial puncture.

Patient and Family Education
- Preprocedure
    - Review planned procedure including conscious sedation, preparation of the vascular access site, and the catheterization environment. Use sensory preparatory teaching to prepare the patient for what might be heard, felt, and seen during the procedure.
    - Review informed consent and advance directives.
    - Explain the estimated length of the procedure.
- Postprocedure
    - Instruct patient to report symptoms including chest pain, back pain, or discomfort at arterial access site. Teach patient and family how to activate the emergency medical service (EMS) if needed.
    - Discharge instructions include giving to the patient and family pictures or diagrams of the lesion or lesions before and after the procedure.
    - Discuss all medications that the patient is to be taking and give written instructions. All patients are to take aspirin (unless allergic) plus another antiplatelet therapy. Additional medications may include a beta blocking agent, antihypertensive agents, antilipid therapy (statin), and nitrate products.
    - Assess the patient for atherosclerosis risk factors, including hyperlipidemia, smoking history, hypertension, and activity level. Discuss resources for further interventions, which may include nutritional consultation, use of a statin as an antilipid agent, smoking cessation programs, and cardiac rehabilitation.
    - Review prescribed activity level and when patient can return to normal activities or work.

Follow-Up Care
- Follow-up appointment should be made within the first few weeks after intervention.
- Cardiac stress testing usually is performed 2 to 6 months after PCI.

CORONARY ATHERECTOMY

Description
- Atherectomy catheters remove atherosclerotic plaque, debulking, and smoothing the vessel wall.
- Atherectomy minimizes the degree of arterial wall stretch and controls vascular injury.
- Three atherectomy devices are available that have specific applications, dependent on the coronary anatomy and lesion morphology.
- Atherectomy may be done in combination with PCI and stent placement.

Procedure

- Vascular access is similar to PCI.
- Directional coronary atherectomy (DCA). This device consists of a catheter-mounted cutter housing unit, with a flexible nose cone collection chamber, window and cup-shaped cutter, support balloon, and a battery-operated motor drive unit. The catheter is placed at the stenotic lesion and the balloon is inflated at low pressure against one wall of the vessel, resulting in the plaque being pushed into the cutter housing. The cutter can be moved manually and the atheroma excised with the cutter rotating at 2,000 rpm by the motor drive unit. The excised atheroma is stored in the nose-cone collection chamber.
- Rotational atherectomy. This catheter-based device uses a high-speed (140,000 to 180,000 rpm) rotating elliptical metal burr coated with diamond chips that abrade atheromatous plaque into fine microparticles.
- Transluminal extraction atherectomy (TEA). The system consists of a conical cutting head with two stainless-steel blades at the distal end of a hollow flexible tube. Attached to the proximal end of the hollow lumen are suction bottles that collect excised material. The TEA increases the luminal dimensions of the coronary artery by cutting plaque and aspirating it.

Indications

- Directional coronary atherectomy
  - Bifurcation lesions
  - Ostial lesions, particularly for lesions in the left anterior descending coronary artery
  - Eccentric lesion
- Rotational atherectomy
  - Calcified lesions
  - Ostial lesions
  - Lesion length; rotational atherectomy shows a 92% success rate for lesions 15 mm to 25 mm in length.
  - In-stent restenosis
- Transluminal extraction atherectomy
  - Lesions in which thrombus or debris has to be removed from the artery. This includes patients with acute ischemic syndromes such as unstable angina, acute MI, and after failed thrombolytic therapy. TEA has been used in degenerated saphenous vein grafts.

Contraindications

- Similar to those for PCI
- Each device has specific indications, thus contraindicating other uses.

Complications

- Similar to those for PCI
- Vascular spasm at or distal to the treated site
- Distal embolization in those with acute coronary syndrome and in interventions on saphenous vein grafts
- Vessel perforation (0.5%)

Nursing Implications
Same as for PCI and stents

Patient and Family Education
Same as for PCI and stents

Follow-Up Care
Same as for PCI and stents

PERCUTANEOUS TRANSLUMINAL ANGIOPLASTY (PTA) OF THE LOWER EXTREMITY

Description
PTA is an alternative to surgical intervention for patients with peripheral artery disease. As in coronary balloon angioplasty, the balloon pressure applied to an area of atherosclerotic plaque causes dilation of the artery and increases the arterial lumen diameter and blood flow. Peripheral endovascular therapy includes stents, use of thrombolytic therapy, and atherectomy procedures also.

Procedure
- Iliac PTA and stenting
  - Vascular access is achieved using either a retrograde approach or an iliac crossover approach. If necessary, PTA can be performed from an axillary or brachial artery.
  - After the lesion is crossed with a guide wire, the balloon is inflated. Balloon size is usually 6 mm to 10 mm.
  - If the patient has an acute or subacute occlusion of an iliac artery, intra-arterial thrombolytic therapy may be needed before PTA or stenting.
  - Stenting of the iliac artery provides a larger lumen than PTA alone does, preventing or treating dissection, inhibiting elastic recoil, and thus decreasing restenosis of the artery.
- Femoropopliteal PTA
  - Vascular access is achieved using an antegrade femoral approach or femoral crossover approach.
  - After the lesion is crossed with a guide wire, the balloon is inflated. Balloon size ranges from 4 mm to 6 mm.
  - The role of stents in the femoral and popliteal arteries is being studied.
- Tibioperoneal PTA
  - PTA below the knee in tibioperoneal vessels is reserved most often for patients who have limb-threatening ischemia.
  - Vascular access is achieved in an antegrade fashion. Heparin is administered and nitroglycerin often is given intra-arterial to prevent vessel spasm. Smaller balloons, 2 mm to 4 mm, are used.
  - Rotational atherectomy can be used in heavily calcified lesions of these vessels. Experience with stenting is limited.

Indications
- Symptoms of claudication that are severe or lifestyle-limiting.
- Critical limb ischemia in which patient may have rest pain, nonhealing ulcer, or gangrene.
- PTA may be performed in conjunction with surgical bypass surgery.

Contraindications
- Medically unstable
- Long arterial occlusions, usually more than 15 mm
- Poor distal runoff
- Patients with diabetes, although not absolutely contraindicated to PTA, have shown consistently negative outcomes.

Complications
- Vasospasm
- Thrombus formation
- Arterial dissection
- Vessel perforation (1%)
- Compartment syndrome
- Arterial dissection
- Restenosis
- Death (less than 0.5%)

Nursing Implications
- Preprocedure
    - Similar to those for PCI and stents
    - Assess and document peripheral pulse quality, skin color and temperature of the feet, and severity of rest pain.
- Postprocedure
    - Similar to the care of patient undergoing PCI and stent placement
    - Evaluate the patient for peripheral ischemic pain including severity of pain, quality of peripheral pulses, sensory and motor function of the extremities, skin color and temperature, and capillary refill.
    - Clinical manifestations of circulatory compromise should be reported immediately.

Patient and Family Education
- Preprocedure similar to PCI and stent placement
- Postprocedure
    - Similar to PCI and stent placement
    - Discuss prescribed medications and give written instructions. Patients will be on long-term aspirin therapy and will receive at least 30 days of the antiplatelet drug clopidogrel. Vasodilators and other antihypertensive agents may be prescribed. Emphasize the importance of blood pressure control.

 – Atherosclerosis risk factors should be assessed and managed. Refer to self-help clinics such as smoking cessation, weight management, and exercise programs. Promote tight glycemic control for patients with diabetes and aggressive lipid management for those with dyslipidemia.
 – Foot care is an important aspect of care for the patient with peripheral vascular disease. Daily hygiene, inspection and lubrication of the skin, care of toenails, proper footwear, safety precautions, and activity are topics to be addressed.
 – Review activity level and when patient can anticipate return to normal activities or work.

Follow-Up Care
• Follow-up appointment should be made within the first few weeks after intervention.
• Foot-care specialist (e.g., podiatrist) may be needed to address the issues of footwear and nail care, particularly in the patient with diabetes.

PERCUTANEOUS TRANSLUMINAL ANGIOPLASTY (PTA) OF THE CAROTID ARTERY

Description
PTA is a nonsurgical approach to open a narrowed carotid artery for patients with hemodynamically significant impairment of the cerebral circulation. Stenting is used along with PTA. The type of stent used for carotid placement is self-expandable, flexible, and noncollapsing because the stent needs to adapt to arteries of different endoluminal diameters. The procedure is carried out under conscious sedation and local anesthesia.

Procedure
• The usual vascular approach to the internal carotid artery (ICA) is via the femoral artery. Alternative approaches are from the brachial or axillary artery.
• The guide wire is advanced into the distal ICA close to the skull base across the lesion. The stenosis usually is predilated, most often with a 4 mm coronary balloon.
• A stent then is deployed and post-dilated with a 5 to 6 mm balloon.

Indications
• Stenosis of the ICA exceeding 70% in a symptomatic patient
• High degree of stenosis in patients with recurring transient ischemic attacks (TIA), and if infarcted, area is small
• Bilateral carotid stenosis and contralateral carotid artery occlusion
• Postoperative recurrent carotid artery stenosis
• Patients who have had previous neck irradiation or radical neck dissection
• Patients with increased operative risk (e.g., severe coronary artery disease)
• Symptomatic restenosis after conventional carotid endarterectomy

Contraindications
• Major thrombus formation
• Thick circular or semicircular stenosis

Complications
- TIA
- Stroke (major and minor)
- Cerebral hemorrhage
- Amaurosis fugax (loss of vision in one eye because of retinal ischemia)
- In-stent restenosis
- Cranial nerve injury
- Death (less than 0.4%)

Nursing Implications
- Preprocedure
  - Similar to the care of the patient undergoing PCI and stent placement
  - Assess and document the baseline neurological status.
  - Before the procedure, the patient is heparinized and given 5 mg of nifedipine. Patients are premedicated with 0.5 mg to 1.0 mg of atropine, depending on the heart rate, to prevent severe bradycardia as a result of carotid body stimulation during balloon dilatation.
- Postprocedure
  - Similar to the care of the patient undergoing PCI and stent placement
  - Assess the patient's neurological function including level of consciousness, reflexes, motor strength, level of sensation, and pupillary size and reaction to light.
  - Assess puncture site for bleeding, hematoma, tracheal shift.
  - Patients usually remain on heparin therapy for 24 to 48 hours and begin clopidogrel along with aspirin immediately after the procedure.

Patient and Family Education
- Similar to the care of the patients undergoing PCI and stent placement both pre- and postprocedure.
- Discuss prescribed medications and give written instructions. Patients will be on long-term aspirin therapy and on clopidogrel daily for 4 to 8 weeks postprocedure.
- Atherosclerosis risk factors should be assessed and managed.
- Review activity level and when patient can anticipate return to normal activities or work. Also review signs and symptoms patient should report to his or her healthcare provider.

Follow-Up Care
- Follow-up appointment is made within the first week postprocedure.
- A complete neurological exam is performed.
- Doppler ultrasound surveillance is performed every 3 to 6 months initially and then on an annual basis. MRI of the head may be done 3 months postprocedure.

PERCUTANEOUS TRANSLUMINAL ANGIOPLASTY (PTA) OF THE RENAL ARTERY

Description
PTA is a nonsurgical approach to open a narrowed renal artery, which may alleviate renovascular hypertension or improve renal function. Stenting usually is accomplished along with PTA in patients with atherosclerotic lesions, whereas PTA alone can be used in fibromuscular dysplasia.

Procedure
- Vascular access is either by the femoral or brachial approach. The patient is pretreated with aspirin and heparin is given. The lesion is crossed with a guide wire and an appropriate size balloon is used (4 mm to 8 mm).
- The predominant cause of renal artery stenosis is atherosclerotic plaque. The lesion is usually ostial in location and caused by the plaque in the aorta, which encroaches on the lumen of the renal artery. PTA alone may not be successful and renal stenting is used.
- Renal artery narrowing in the younger patient is fibromuscular dysplasia and responds well to PTA.

Indications
- Renovascular hypertension caused by atherosclerotic or fibromuscular narrowing of a renal artery after failed medical therapy
- Renal transplant artery stenosis
- Renal artery or vein bypass graft stenosis
- Renal insufficiency with more than 50% renal artery stenosis

Contraindications
- Borderline lesion (less than 50% or no pressure gradient)
- Long segment (more than 2 cm) of total occlusion
- Aortic plaque extending into the renal artery
- Unstable medical condition

Complications
- Complications involving the vascular access site are similar to those for PCI.
- Worsening renal failure
- Thrombus (1%)
- Nonocclusive dissection (2% to 4%)
- Embolus to peripheral artery (1.5% to 2.0%) or to distal renal artery (2%)
- Rupture of artery (1%)
- Death (1%)

Nursing Implications
- Similar to the care of patients having PCI and stent regarding puncture site assessment
- Careful measurement of urine output, daily serum creatinine levels, and assessment and management of hypotension or hypertension
- Discuss prescribed medications and give written instructions. Most patients will be on aspirin, and those with stents will receive at least 30 days of clopidogrel in addition to the aspirin.

Patient and Family Education
- Similar to PCI
- Education regarding hypertension management including antihypertensive medication use, monitoring of blood pressure at home, diet, and activity
- Assess for other risk factors including smoking, diabetes, and hyperlipidemia and discuss resources for further intervention.

Follow-Up Care
- Follow-up appointment should be made within the first week following the procedure.
- Management of hypertension and careful monitoring of renal function is indicated.
- Renal vascular ultrasound is used to monitor renal blood flow over time.

PERCUTANEOUS BALLOON VALVULOPLASTY

Description
Percutaneous technique is an alternative to surgical intervention for the treatment of valvular disease. The procedure is performed in the cardiac catheterization laboratory.

Procedures
- Percutaneous balloon mitral valvuloplasty (PBMV)
  - Vascular access is the same as for PCI.
  - Transeptal catheterization is performed in which one or two catheters are advanced into the right atrium, through the atrial septum into the left atrium, and across the mitral valve.
  - A large balloon catheter is placed over the guide wire and positioned with the balloon across the mitral valve. The balloon is inflated, increasing the size of the valve orifice. When two balloons are used, they are inflated simultaneously.
- Percutaneous balloon aortic valvuloplasty (PBAV)
  - Before PBAV, an evaluation for coronary artery disease and peripheral vascular disease is indicated.
  - Vascular access is the same for PCI.
  - A transeptal approach is used as described above. A balloon-tipped catheter is advanced in a retrograde fashion across the stenotic valve. After the balloon is positioned, it is inflated.

Indications
- Mitral valve
  - Symptomatic mitral valve stenosis, isolated or combined with mixed valvular disease with less than moderate mitral regurgitation
  - Patients who are not surgical candidates and are symptomatic with immobile, severely thickened and fused valves or those with severe calcification
- Aortic valve
  - As a short-term palliative procedure, patient selection is limited to
    - Symptomatic patients who are not candidates for valve surgery
    - Patients with poor left ventricular function, as a bridge to surgery
    - Symptomatic patients who are scheduled to undergo major noncardiac surgery

Contraindications
- Presence of atrial thrombus
- Severely calcified, thickened or immobile, fused valve leaflets are negative predictors for success.
- Severe left main coronary artery disease
- Aortic regurgitation greater than 2+ because the amount of regurgitation may increase after PBAV

Complications
- Similar to those of PCI regarding the puncture site (thrombus, hematoma, retroperitoneal bleed)
- Hemopericardium or tamponade (less than 2%)
- Mitral regurgitation (MR) is noted in all patients postprocedure, with increases in 20% to 50% of patients. Significantly increased MR occurs in 8% to 10%, and severe MR that requires valve replacement occurs in 0.9% to 3%.
- Atrial septal defects, which are usually so small that they are not of hemodynamic significance
- Restenosis, which occurs in approximately half of the patients within 6 months, is a major problem in PBAV.
- Precipitation of severe aortic regurgitation (less than 2%)
- Mortality (0% to 2%)

Nursing Implications
- Pre- and postprocedure care is similar to that for PCI.
- Carefully assess and document heart sounds, particularly noting a change in the nature of a murmur, and evaluate for any evidence of heart failure.

Patient and Family Education
- Similar to those for PCI both pre- and postprocedure
- Discuss prescribed medications and give written instructions. Patients are instructed to take an aspirin daily and to use antibiotics prophylactically before all dental or surgical interventions.

Follow-Up Care
- Follow-up appointment should be made within the first week after intervention.
- Transthoracic or transesophageal echocardiogram is usually performed in the 3 to 6 months after procedure, and may be repeated annually or biannually.
- If symptoms or signs of progressive dyspnea, chest pain, palpitations, or syncope occur, these should be reported to the provider.

PACEMAKERS

Description

Cardiac pacemakers provide an artificial electrical stimulus to the heart muscle when the intrinsic heart rate (HR) fails to provide a cardiac output adequate to meet physiologic demands, or to stimulate the heart in an effort to terminate tachyarrhythmias. The pacing system consists of a pulse generator and a unipolar or bipolar lead, which is placed in the right atrium or right ventricle in contact with the endocardium.

- Permanent pacemaker (PPM)
  - Implanted under local anesthesia in the cardiac catheterization laboratory or operating room
  - The pulse generator is placed in a subcutaneous pocket in the pectoral area. The cephalic vein is located and cannulated. Less commonly, the internal or external jugular vein is used. Under fluoroscopy, the pacing lead is placed into the right ventricular apex (single lead). If a dual-chamber pacemaker is used, a second lead is placed in the right atrial appendage.
  - Many permanent pacemakers now have additional monitoring information that is useful for patient care.
    - Heart rhythm can be monitored for occurrence of atrial fibrillation and ventricular arrhythmias.
    - Heart rate variability can be monitored. A decrease in variability can be a sign of heart failure worsening.
    - Measure of fluid using impedance or right ventricular pressure can be used to assess for fluid overload.
- Temporary pacemaker
  - Transvenous pacing
    - A temporary transvenous pacemaker can be placed under fluoroscopy in a cardiac catheterization laboratory or at the bedside. Venous access is established by percutaneous puncture of the internal jugular, subclavian, antecubital, or femoral vein, or by venous cutdown in an antecubital vein. A bipolar, transvenous pacing lead usually is placed and attached to an external pulse generator, which is kept at the bedside.
  - Transcutaneous pacing
    - Noninvasive method of pacing that uses large surface-adhesive electrodes, which are attached to the anterior and posterior chest wall and connected to an external pulse generator. This method of pacing is used temporarily in emergency situations until a transvenous or permanent pacing system can be established.
  - Epicardial pacing
    - Pacing leads are loosely sutured on the epicardial surface of the atria, ventricles, or both during cardiac surgery. The proximal end of the lead exits through the chest wall and is attached to an external pulse generator.
  - Transthoracic pacing
    - Temporary method of pacing that is used in extreme cardiac emergencies. A long needle is inserted subxiphoid and the pacing lead is threaded through the needle to the right ventricle. The proximal end of the lead is attached to an external pulse generator.

- Single-chamber pacing
  - The pacing system allows either the atria or the ventricles, but not both, to be paced.
- Dual-chamber pacing
  - The pacing system allows the atria, the ventricles, or both to be paced.
  - Most pacing systems implanted are dual chamber with option to program specific type of pacing used.
- Rate-modulated pacing
  - Also referred to as rate-responsive pacing
  - This mode of pacing uses a physiologic sensor that responds and helps a patient adapt to physiologic stress with an increased HR. The most common sensors used are motion and minute ventilation sensors. Body movement and muscle motion activate the motion sensor. Minute ventilation sensor is a respiration sensor that measures transthoracic impedance and increases the pacing rate when the respiratory rate is increased, for example, in response to exercise.
  - The upper pacing rate is typically twice the lower limit of pacing.
  - The time over which the rate of pacing increases can be programmed to meet the activity tolerance needs of the patient. It can be a slow and gradual increase for the less fit person and more rapid increase for the person who exercises routinely.
- Atrial overdrive pacing
  - In an attempt to terminate atrial tachydysrhythmias such as atrial tachycardia and atrial flutter, atrial pacing rates of 200 to 500 impulses per minute can be used.
  - The short burst of high-rate pacing captures the heart's electrical conduction system.
  - When pacing is stopped, the rhythm should return to the normal sinus conduction.
- Antitachycardia pacing
  - One to several paced impulses are delivered to the heart to interrupt tachycardia. This is done most frequently to terminate ventricular tachycardia.
  - This feature is incorporated into implantable cardioverter defibrillators (ICD) and used prior to delivering a shock.
- Pacemaker code
  - Pacemakers are classified using a five-letter code, which describes the various types of pacemakers and their programmed function. Position 1 describes the chamber(s) being paced. Position 2 describes the chamber(s) being sensed. Position 3 describes the device's response to sensing. An "I" indicates an inhibited mode in which a sensed event inhibits pacing. This is the most common form of sensing. "T" indicates a triggered response in which the pacemaker senses an event and triggers a pacing stimulus. Position 4 describes the programmability and rate modulation function. Position 5 is restricted to antitachycardia functions and rarely is used. (Table 14–1 shows the pacemaker code.)
  - The most common pacing modes are VVI and DDD. In the VVI mode, the pacing lead both senses and paces the ventricle. The pacemaker inhibits its output when it senses intrinsic ventricular depolarization. In the DDD mode, pacing leads are able to pace and sense in both the atrium and the ventricle. The pacemaker will either trigger or inhibit its output in response to sensed intrinsic activity.

Table 14–1. The Generic Pacemaker Code

Position Category	1 Chamber(s) Paced	2 Chamber(s) Sensed	3 Response to Sensing	4 Program mability	5 Antitachy cardia
Manufacturers' Designation	O = None	O = None	O = None	O = None	O = None
	A = Atrium	A = Atrium	T = Triggered	P = Simple	P = Pacing
	V = Ventricle	V =Ventricle	I = Inhibited	M = Multiprogram	S = Shock
	D = Dual (A+V)	D = Dual (A+V)	D = Dual (T+I)	C = Communicating	D = Dual (P+S)
		S = Single (A or V)			

- Operational settings
  - Rate: The number of times per minute that the pacemaker will fire when patient's own rate drops to less than the set rate.
  - Output: Intensity of the electrical current used to depolarize the myocardium, measured in milliamperes (mA)
  - Sensitivity: The ability of the pacemaker to detect patient's own intrinsic HR measured in millivolts (mV). The lower the number, the more sensitive the pacemaker is set and will inhibit pacing.

Indications
- Permanent pacing
  - Class I indications for pacing are conditions under which implantation of a permanent pacemaker is considered necessary and acceptable. (Table 14–2 lists the Class I indications for permanent pacing.)
  - The need for additional monitoring of electrical events and fluid overload indicators may be warranted in some patients.
- Temporary pacing
  - Symptomatic bradycardia after acute MI or associated hyperkalemia, drug toxicity (e.g., digitalis)
  - A bridge method before permanent pacing in symptomatic patients
  - Bradycardia not responsive to atropine or isoproterenol
  - Transient, new bifascicular (RBBB plus either the anterior or posterior left bundle) bundle branch block or alternating bundle branch block in the setting of an acute MI
  - Transient right bundle branch block occurring during cardiac catheterization
  - After cardiac surgery, to treat or prevent symptomatic bradycardia and to have available the ability to use atrial overdrive pacing

Table 14–2. Indications for Permanent Pacing in Adults

Pacing for Acquired Atrioventricular (AV) Block • Third-degree AV block • Second-degree AV block with symptomatic bradycardia
Pacing for Chronic Bifascicular and Trifascicular Block • Intermittent third-degree block • Type II second-degree AV block
Pacing in Sinus Node Dysfunction • Sinus node dysfunction with documented symptomatic bradycardia, including frequent sinus pauses • Symptomatic chronotropic incompetence
Pacing for AV Block Associated With Acute Myocardial Infarction • Persistent second-degree AV block with bilateral bundle branch or third-degree heart block • Persistent and symptomatic second- or third-degree AV block • Transient advanced second- or third-degree infranodal AV block and associated bundle-branch block
Pacing to Prevent Tachycardia • Sustained, pause-dependent ventricular tachycardia, with or without prolonged QT, for which the efficacy of pacing is documented
Pacing for Hypertrophic Cardiomyopathy or Dilated Cardiomyopathy • Sinus node dysfunction or AV block as previously described
Pacing in Hypersensitive Carotid Sinus Syndrome and Neurally Mediated Syncope • Recurrent syncope caused by carotid sinus stimulation
Pacemakers That Automatically Detect and Pace to Terminate Tachycardia • Symptomatic recurrent supraventricular tachycardia that is reproducibly terminated by pacing after drugs and catheter ablation fail to control the arrhythmia

Contraindications

Pacing not recommended for

- First-degree atrioventricular (AV) block, asymptomatic Mobitz I second-degree block, transient AV block
- AV block because of inferior wall MI
- Asymptomatic sinus node dysfunction, including athletes with high vagal tone
- Suppression of ventricular tachycardia (unless an ICD is inserted)

Complications

- Permanent pacing
  - Related to venous access
    - Pneumothorax or hemothorax, because of inadvertent bleeding from the vein or entry into an artery
  - Related to lead placement
    - Perforation of heart or vein, damage to heart valve, damage to lead

- Related to pulse generator
  - Inadequate or improper connection of leads
  - Pain, erosion, infection in pacemaker pocket, migration
- Related to lead function
  - Intravascular thrombus or constriction (i.e., superior vena cava obstruction)
  - Brady- or tachydysrhythmias
  - Infection causing endocarditis; perforation causing pericarditis
  - Lead failure because of insulation failure
- Patient-related
  - "Twiddler's syndrome" in which the patient manipulated the pulse generator in its pocket, often twisting the pacing wires with possible disruption of pacing
  - Skin erosion from manipulation
- Temporary pacing
  - Transvenous pacing
    - Malfunction of the pacing system manifested as inconsistent pacing or sensing occurs in 14% to 43% of patients. The causes are multifactorial and include catheter dislodgment or perforation, local myocardial necrosis or fibrosis, hypoxia, acidosis, lead fracture, and electrocautery or cardioversion damaging the lead.
    - Ventricular tachycardia during catheter manipulation
    - Thromboembolic events
    - Clinical infection or phlebitis (3% to 5%)
  - Transcutaneous pacing
    - Failure to capture
    - Pain during pacing
  - Epicardial pacing
    - Failure to capture or sense appropriately
    - Infection
  - Transthoracic pacing
    - Pneumothorax or hemothorax
    - Laceration of the right atrium, ventricles, coronary arteries, venae cavae, great vessels, liver, or lung
    - Hemopericardium and cardiac tamponade

Nursing Implications

- For all types of pacemakers, the nurse should have a working knowledge of pacemakers that includes:
  - Understanding how the pacemaker is programmed (e.g., VVI, DDD), the minimum rate of the pacemaker, and any other programmable feature.
  - Ability to evaluate appropriate pacemaker function by interpreting ECG or rhythm strips
  - Ability to intervene appropriately with corrective measures
    - Loss of stimulation is lack of a pacing spike when it should have appeared. Most commonly this is because of battery failure, accidentally turning off the device, or lead malfunction.
    - Loss of capture is seen as a pacing spike that does not have either a P or QRS complex following it. This is because of an output that is insufficient to result in ventricular depolarization. It is fixed by increasing the mA voltage.

- Over-sensing is characterized by a lack of pacing spikes when they should occur. This results when electrical current other than the heart is sensed and the pacemaker is inhibited from firing. In this case, the sensitivity needs to be reset so extraneous current is not detected and the unit inhibits only when the intrinsic heart activity is detected.
- Under-sensing is seen as inappropriately placed pacing spikes because the unit did not sense the heart's electrical activity. In this case the sensitivity needs to be set to a lower number so the conduction system is recognized by the pacing unit. This will increase the sensitivity or ability to detect the intrinsic electrical activity.
- Permanent pacemaker
  - Preprocedure
    - Similar to PCI including baseline vital signs, history and physical, screening of the patient for potential problems, informed consent, IV access, and NPO status.
    - Obtain posteroanterior chest X-ray.
    - Patients on oral anticoagulants are converted to intravenous heparin, which can be stopped 4 to 6 hours before implant. Heparin can be restarted 8 to 12 hours after the procedure and warfarin restarted the day of the procedure.
    - Antibiotic prophylaxis is usually given intravenously before the procedure.
    - Nasal cultures may be done preoperatively and nasal topical antibiotics given to those who are chronic carriers of methicillin-resistant Staphylococcus aureus (MRSA).
  - Postprocedure
    - Obtain baseline vital signs, including ECG. A postprocedure chest x-ray should be done.
    - Perform a complete physical assessment and evaluate the pacemaker site for evidence of hematoma or infection. A sling to immobilize the arm on the side of the pacemaker generator implant may be used until the day of discharge, which is usually the day after the procedure.
- Temporary pacemakers
  - Maintaining a clean insertion site is important to prevent infection. Guidelines for the care of central venous catheters and dressings should be followed.
  - Epicardial wires are placed during cardiac surgery. Either one or two atrial and ventricular wires exit through the skin and this area should be cleaned with liquid iodine daily and covered with a dressing.
    - The wires should be insulated to prevent dysrhythmia from extraneous current.
    - Wires are removed by specially trained nurses with the patient in bed.
    - Post removal, monitor for dysrhythmias or a sudden change in voltage.
    - Post procedure, assess for the rare complication of cardiac tamponade which would be evident by Beck's triad: muffled heart sounds, increased jugular pressure, and hypotension.
  - Electrical safety is of key importance because the wire provides a direct pathway for stray electrical current to reach the heart. Care includes:
    - Wear gloves when handling pacing wires.
    - Insulate the exposed metal ends of pacing wires that are not in use.
    - Keep the dressing dry.

- Be sure electrical equipment in the room is properly grounded.
- Maintain normal humidity to prevent static electricity from developing.
- If static electricity is generated (by walking across carpet, for example), discharge it by touching metal before touching the patient.

Patient and Family Education

- Preprocedure
  - Review planned procedure, including conscious sedation and estimated length of procedure.
  - Review informed consent and advance directives.
- Postprocedure
  - Instruct patient about symptoms to report, including discomfort over chest wall incision site.
  - Discharge instructions include information about pacemaker function, how to check the pulse, and importance of follow-up visits. The patient should monitor the incision site and body temperature for signs of infection.
  - Medications usually include a broad-spectrum antibiotic to be taken orally for 3 to 5 days.
  - Patients should be instructed to carry the pacemaker identification card with them at all times. They should advise all their healthcare providers of their pacemaker.
    - They do not need antibiotic prophylaxis for dental work, and can safely use cellular phones and microwaves.
    - If the person is pacemaker-dependent, he or she should be cautious if exposed to high-strength fields of radiation such as magnetic resonance imaging (MRI) because if sensed, he or she may inhibit the pacemaker from firing.
    - If the patient is to undergo surgery where electrocautery is to be used, the physician familiar with the patient and patient's pacemaker should be consulted.
    - Follow the device interrogation schedule to help fine-tune settings to maintain battery life and prevent over- or under-sensing problems. The information obtained during interrogation also can provide monitoring of some aspects of heart function.
    - If a patient is having an increase in heart failure symptoms, the PPM should be interrogated to obtain current data and compare to baseline. Patients need to keep their cardiologists and electrophysiologists informed of symptoms.
  - Review activity level and when patient can anticipate return to normal activities or work.

Follow-Up Care

- Follow-up appointments usually are made 1 week after permanent pacemaker implantation for wound care check-up and in 2 to 3 months for checking the device's threshold(s) and programming chronic output setting(s). Further programming also can be performed. The patient then should be followed on a semiannual basis.
- Transtelephonic monitoring is telephone transmission of a rhythm strip that allows the pacemaker battery status to be measured. This method is used by many pacemaker clinics. The interrogation also can include more information that will guide care as previously described.

IMPLANTABLE CARDIOVERTER DEFIBRILLATOR (ICD)

Description
The ICD is an electronic device that is used to automatically treat life-threatening dysrhythmia. The device consists of a pulse generator and a lead system similar to those of a pacemaker. Leads are available for sensing, pacing, and shocking.

Procedure
- Implanted under local anesthesia in the cardiac catheterization laboratory, electrophysiology (EP) laboratory, or operating room.
- The pulse generator is implanted subcutaneously in the patient's subclavian area or abdomen.
- Similar to pacemaker implantation, the transvenous lead system is inserted into the right ventricle and then tunneled and connected to the pulse generator. One ventricular patch also is connected to the pulse generator. Some systems have two leads and two ventricular patches.
- Programmability includes defibrillation, cardioversion, antitachycardia pacing, and antibradycardia pacing.

Indications
- Candidates for an ICD are evaluated by a cardiac electrophysiologist.
- Types of patients include:
  - Victims of cardiac arrest caused by ventricular fibrillation (VF) or ventricular tachycardia (VT), not a transient cause
  - People with sustained VT
  - People with a history of undetermined syncope and a positive EP study for inducible VT or VF
  - People with nonsustained, inducible VT that is not suppressed by drug therapy
  - People with an inherited or familial condition including prolonged QT syndrome or hypertrophic cardiomyopathy with high risk for sudden cardiac death
  - People with a low ejection fraction (less than 30%) who are at least one month post-MI or 3 months post cardiac surgery

Contraindications
- Reversible cause of the cardiac arrest such as acute myocardial ischemia or electrolyte abnormalities
- Terminal illness with a life expectancy of less than 6 months
- VF or VT resulting from dysrhythmia that is amenable to ablation therapy (e.g., Wolff-Parkinson-White syndrome, right ventricular outflow tract and fascicular tachycardia)
- An alternative system to an ICD is the external defibrillator vest that may be worn while waiting for approval or meeting the timelines prior to implant in a high-risk patient.

Complications
- Similar to permanent pacemakers
- Acceleration of the dysrhythmia

Nursing Implications

- Similar to pre- and postprocedures for permanent pacemaker implantation in regard to pain management and site assessment and care.
- Consideration of the patient's and family's emotional response is an important aspect of nursing care, and counseling either pre- or postprocedure may be indicated.

Patient and Family Education

- Pre- and postprocedure care is similar to the permanent pacemaker (PPM) care.
- Discharge instructions include what to do if the device discharges, when to notify the provider, and the importance of carrying proper identification that allows medical personnel to quickly check the ICD.
- Provide information about support groups and encourage attendance at cardiopulmonary resuscitation (CPR) courses by family members.
- For the patient and family members who have ongoing emotional concerns, professional counseling may be indicated.
- Review activity level and when the patient can anticipate return to normal activities or work. Driving may be restricted for 6 months, and the provider should give approval prior to resumption.
- Some patients who undergo a shock may need to continue antidysrhythmia medications.

Follow-Up Care

- Initial follow-up appointment is usually within one week. Patients then are seen every 3 to 6 months to review stored data that provide information for any treated episodes of dysrhythmia. Chest x-ray may be done annually to evaluate the ICD.
- If the ICD discharges, the patient should notify the physician or clinic. If the device discharges and the patient does not feel well, or the device discharges twice or more, EMS should be activated.
- Interrogation of the ICD will reveal appropriateness of the shock and a history of the rhythm around the event.

CORONARY ARTERY BYPASS GRAFT SURGERY (CABG)

Description

CABG is a surgical revascularization of ischemic areas of the heart using a graft from the aortic root to a point distal to the ischemic lesion. (See Figure 14–3.) The internal mammary artery (IMA) and the saphenous vein graft are the most commonly used conduits. The gastroepiploic artery (infrequent) and radial artery (increasingly frequent) also can be used. CABG is performed with the patient under general anesthesia. Minimally invasive approaches, robotics, and off-pump procedures are gaining in use.

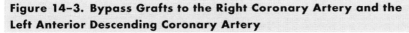

Figure 14–3. Bypass Grafts to the Right Coronary Artery and the Left Anterior Descending Coronary Artery

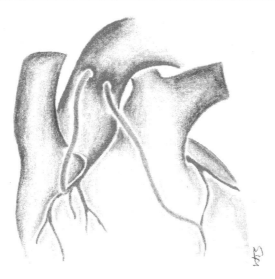

Procedure

- In standard cardiac surgery, a median sternotomy incision is made, the heart is arrested, and circulation is maintained by placing the patient on cardiopulmonary bypass (CPB). Cardioplegia is infused to arrest the heart and provide a motionless, bloodless field as well as to protect the ischemic heart during surgery. Hypothermia, usually 82.4° F to 89.6° F (28° C to 32° C), is maintained during the procedure. Deep hypothermia at 18° C with CPB stopped is done if circulatory arrest with interruption of circulation through the ascending aorta is needed in surgery involving the ascending aorta and aortic arch.
- Minimally invasive direct coronary artery bypass (MIDCAB) is done through a small left anterior thoracotomy, a short parasternal incision, or other small incision using port access and video-assisted technology. Because of the small incisions, this approach is usually limited to proximal disease of the right coronary artery or the left anterior descending coronary artery with IMA grafts to these sites. Surgery is performed on the beating heart. Pharmacological agents (e.g., adenosine, beta blockers) are used to slow or temporarily stop the heart. CPB is on standby during the procedure to facilitate emergent conversion to standard median sternotomy if necessary. Robotic surgery can be performed with this approach.
- Off-pump CABG is done through median sternotomy, but without the use of CPB. Like MIDCAB, grafts are done on the beating heart. Avoidance of CPB and aortic cross-clamping may be necessary for patients with severe aortic arteriosclerosis or poor left ventricular function.

Indications
- Angina refractory to drugs and PCI
- Significant left main disease (greater than 50%)
- Triple vessel diffuse coronary artery disease
- Acute MI (emergent or delayed)
- Left ventricular failure related to cardiogenic shock or congestive heart failure
- Complications from or unsuccessful PCI

Contraindications
Relative contraindications include:
- Lack of adequate conduit
- Small (1.5 mm or less) coronary arteries distal to the stenosis
- Severe aortic sclerosis
- Severe left ventricular failure and coexisting peripheral vascular, renal, and pulmonary disease increase the risk of surgery.

Complications
- Postoperative bleeding and hematologic conditions, which may include:
  - Heparin-induced thrombocytopenia
  - Disseminated intravascular coagulopathy
  - Dilutional anemia
- Myocardial depression
- Cardiac tamponade
- Perioperative MI
- Dysrhythmia, including atrial tachydysrhythmia (e.g., atrial fibrillation), which can occur in 20% to 40% of patients. Ventricular dysrhythmia requiring medical treatment occurs in 9% to 24% of patients.
- Pulmonary complications, including pulmonary edema, atelectasis, or pneumothorax
- Renal impairment ranging from mild renal impairment to acute renal failure (0.1% to 0.7%)
- Gastrointestinal problems such as abdominal distention, ileus, hepatic dysfunction, and mesenteric ischemia
- Neuropsychological problems may include the following:
  - Cerebral ischemia, infarction, or emboli
  - Postcardiotomy delirium, which usually occurs within the first few days postoperatively
  - Peripheral neurological deficits, which include brachial plexus injury and ulnar nerve injury
- Postpericardiotomy syndrome occurs when traumatized tissue in the pericardial cavity stimulates an autoimmune response, resulting in inflammation of the pleura and pericardium, causing pericardial and pleural pain.
- Stress-related hyperglycemia
- Wound infection; includes superficial infection, sternal dehiscence, and mediastinitis. All sternal wound drainage must be reported.
- Death

Nursing Implications

- Preoperative
  - Obtain baseline vital signs, including 12-lead ECG, and labs including blood type and cross-match, electrolytes, renal function, glucose, and hematology.
  - Complete nursing history and physical examination.
  - Screen patient for potential problems and comorbid medical conditions including bleeding disorder, diabetes mellitus, lung disease, peripheral vascular disease, liver disease, and underlying neurological conditions. A carotid duplex Doppler may be done to evaluate carotid stenosis before surgery. Pulmonary function tests may be done to assess pulmonary status.
  - Assess patient and family learning needs as well as the patient's functional level, coping mechanisms, and support systems. Fear and anxiety surrounding anticipated CABG are common and many issues need to be addressed, including knowledge and understanding of the procedure, postoperative course, and long-term rehabilitation.
  - A prophylactic amiodarone protocol may be used to reduce the incidence of postoperative atrial fibrillation.
  - Nasal cultures are obtained to identify MRSA carriers, who are then treated with mupirocin nasal swabs to reduce the risk of sternal wound infection.
- Postoperative: Immediate postoperative care is provided in the intensive care or recovery unit. Patients are transferred to stepdown units when hemodynamically stable and after extubation for subsequent care. The following parameters should be assessed:
  - Cardiac status, including HR and rhythm, heart sounds, peripheral pulses, BP, and pacemaker status and function. Desirable parameters include the following:
    - Resting HR above 60 beats per minute and below 120 bpm without pacing
    - Systolic BP above 90 mm Hg and below 160 mm Hg
    - Guidelines for management of atrial fibrillation are often part of post-CABG protocol and may include beta blockers and amiodarone. Calcium channel blockers (e.g., diltiazem) may be used for rate control if beta blockers are ineffective or contraindicated. Electrical cardioversion is an alternative. Patients who remain in atrial fibrillation for 48 hours or longer, or who have multiple sustained episodes, should be started on warfarin.
    - Nitrates or diltiazem may be used to prevent vasospasm for patients in whom the radial artery was used as a conduit.
  - Respiratory status, including respiratory rate, breath sounds, effective cough and airway clearance, and arterial oxygen saturation (SaO_2)
    - Desirable parameters include respiratory rate of 10 to 20 per minute and SaO_2 above 92%.
    - Monitoring of incentive spirometry volume to demonstrate improvement
  - Neurological status, including level of consciousness, reflexes, motor strength, sensation, and pupil size and reaction to light
  - Renal function, with urine output and daily serum blood urea nitrogen and creatinine levels
    - Desirable parameter is urine output of 30 cc or more per hour.

- Fluid and electrolyte status, including intake and output, potassium, magnesium, and calcium levels
- Peripheral vascular status, including peripheral pulses, skin color and temperature, capillary refill, edema, and condition of invasive lines and dressings. Paresthesia may be experienced by patients who have had an IMA graft because of ulnar nerve compression on the same side of the body as the graft.
- Normal blood glucose is desired to prevent complication including sternal wound infection in patients with or without diabetes. Insulin are drips often needed in the ICU; after transfer to the step-down unit, nurse must be aggressive in assessing blood sugar and using the insulin protocol to manage hyperglycemia without producing hypoglycemia.
- Gastrointestinal status including bowel sounds, fluid and nutritional intake. Patients who had the gastroepiploic artery used as a conduit may experience abdominal incision pain and prolonged paralytic ileus.
- Pain status, including the nature, type, location, duration, radiation, and associated symptoms. It is important to differentiate between incision pain, cardiac ischemic pain, and pericarditis.
- Complications as described above should be identified and action taken to reverse their progression.
- Psychosocial status, including anxiety, fear, and knowledge deficits
- Progressively increase activity and ambulation. Inpatient phase I exercise programs provide a structured approach to ensure this occurs.

Patient and Family Education
- Provide verbal and written instructions including the following:
  - Activity progression and exercise (should include enrollment in a cardiac rehabilitation program)
    - Phase II cardiac rehabilitation occurs after hospital discharge and consists of supervised, individualized exercise training, along with teaching and counseling about lifestyle modification and risk factor reduction.
    - Phase III focuses on maintaining long-term conditioning and cardiovascular stability and is usually self-directed, although supervised programs are available.
  - Diet, which includes low-sodium, low-cholesterol
  - Medication regimen, which should include a statin, beta blocker, and angiotensin-convert-ng enzyme (ACE) inhibitor
  - CPR, if appropriate, and how to activate the EMS if needed
  - Deep breathing and lung expansion
  - Wound care
- Instruct the patient to report the following to his or her provider:
  - Symptoms of infection
  - Palpitations, tachycardia, or irregular pulse
  - Change in the nature of chest pain, return of angina
  - Dizziness or increased fatigue
  - Sudden weight gain and increase in peripheral edema
  - Increase in shortness of breath or paroxysmal nocturnal dyspnea

Follow-Up Care

- Follow-up appointments with the cardiovascular surgeon and cardiologist are scheduled in the early post-hospital recovery phase.
- Provide information regarding follow-up phone calls to surgeons, cardiologist, or nurse.
- Make appropriate referrals to home care agency, cardiac rehabilitation, and community support groups.

VALVULAR REPAIR AND VALVULAR REPLACEMENT

Description

- Valvular repair is a surgical procedure to correct a stenotic or incompetent valve. Acquired valve disease most commonly affects the aortic and mitral valves, the two valves this section will focus on.
  - Commissurotomy is a procedure in which fused valve leaflets are split apart and then reconstructed.
  - Annuloplasty is the repair of the valve annulus, which is the junction of the valve leaflets with the muscular heart wall. Two different techniques are used.
    - The orifice of an incompetent valve is made smaller by remodeling, using a ring prosthesis attached to the valve leaflets and annulus.
    - The other technique involves tacking the valve leaflets to the atrium with sutures or taking tucks to tighten the annulus.
  - Chordoplasty is a procedure in which the elongated or ruptured chordae tendineae of the mitral valve are repaired.
- Valvular replacement is used when a dysfunctional valve is not suitable for repair. Two types of prosthetic valves are used, mechanical and biologic (tissue) valves.
  - Mechanical valves have excellent durability but are usually thrombogenic and require lifelong anticoagulation therapy. Types of mechanical valves include bileaflet, tilting disk, and caged-ball valves. Mechanical valves may be preferred over a biologic valve for patients with the following conditions:
    - Age younger than 65 years
    - History of atrial fibrillation
    - History of embolic cerebral vascular accident
    - Already on anticoagulant therapy
  - Biologic (tissue) valves are less thrombogenic and less durable than mechanical valves. Types of biologic valves include xenografts (porcine or bovine) and homografts or allografts (human valves). Biologic valves may be preferred over mechanical valves for patients with the following conditions:
    - Age older than 65 years
    - Unable or unwilling to take warfarin
      - Desire to become pregnant
      - Desire to maintain active, athletic lifestyle
    - History of bleeding

Procedure

Valvular heart surgery can be accomplished by standard median sternotomy, MIDCAB, or through port access using small incisions and endoscopic techniques. Valve surgery requires an arrested heart; therefore, CPB must be used:

- Types of surgery for valve disease:
  - Mitral stenosis (MS)
    - A stenotic mitral valve may be repaired by open chest commissurotomy and reconstruction.
    - The mitral valve is replaced when repair is not possible. Usually there is severe mitral regurgitation along with the stenosis caused by rheumatic heart disease.
    - Percutaneous balloon mitral valvuloplasty (PBMV) is an alternate, less invasive approach.
  - Mitral insufficiency or regurgitation (MR)
    - Mitral valve repair uses reconstructive techniques that may include direct suture of the valve cusps, repair of the valve annulus (annuloplasty) and remodeling with a rigid ring prosthesis, repair with a pericardial band, or repair of the ruptured or elongated chordae tendineae (chordoplasty).The most common mitral valve repair is surgical reconstruction of the posterior leaflet with ring placement.
    - With chronic MR, valve replacement should occur before the patient experiences irreversible left ventricular dysfunction.
  - Aortic stenosis (AS)
    - Aortic valve replacement is the only effective treatment for advanced AS and is recommended for patients with severe, symptomatic AS.
    - Percutaneous balloon aortic valvuloplasty (PBAV) may be used in symptomatic patients who are not candidates for surgery or as a temporary bridge to surgery.
  - Aortic insufficiency (AI)
    - Aortic valve replacement is the only effective treatment for acute and chronic AI.
      - Patients with acute AI because of infective endocarditis are treated with an appropriate course of intravenous antibiotics before valve replacement.
      - Patients with ascending aortic dissection or dilation contributing to AI require replacement of the ascending aorta. This occurs with Marfan syndrome.
      - With chronic AI, valve replacement should occur before left ventricular function deteriorates.

Indications

Acquired valvular disease of the aortic or mitral valve

Contraindications

Patients with high surgical risk as evaluated by cardiac surgeons

Complications
- Similar to those in patients undergoing CABG
- Specific complications related to prosthetic valves include:
  - Thromboembolism
  - Prosthetic valvular thrombosis
  - Bacterial endocarditis
  - Prosthesis malfunction, which has occurred with mechanical valves
  - Paravalvular leaks
  - Valve degeneration, which is a primary complication with tissue valves
  - Hemolytic anemia

Nursing Implications
- Pre- and postoperative care is the same as for the patient undergoing CABG.
- Assessment and appropriate intervention also should be taken for complications associated with prosthetic valves.
- Anticoagulation therapy may be started 48 hours after surgery.
  - Patients with mechanical valves require lifelong anticoagulation.
  - Patients with biologic valves, except homografts, may require anticoagulation for 6 to 12 weeks after surgery, after which time the patient is converted to aspirin therapy.
  - Clinical guidelines and protocols for postoperative anticoagulation differ among centers. The important point is that there is a designated person responsible for the monitoring of warfarin. This may be done through physicians or anticoagulation clinics.
- Postoperative atrial fibrillation has a higher occurrence in patients with valvular disorders but management postoperatively is the same.

Patient and Family Education
- Similar to the care of the CABG patient
- Medication regimen, including duration of anticoagulation therapy and the need for lab work with continuous follow-up of prothrombin time (PT) and international normalized ratio (INR)
- Teach the patient about the use of warfarin, side effects, and symptoms to report.
- Antibiotic Infective Endocarditis prophylaxis is prescribed before dental, invasive endoscopic, and surgical interventions.

Follow-Up Care
- Follow-up clinic appointments are similar to those for patients undergoing CABG.
- Anticoagulation guidelines differ among centers and according to valve type (mechanical versus biologic) and position (mitral versus aortic).
  - For patients with mechanical valves, INR is maintained between 2.5 and 3.5.
  - Laboratory testing may occur weekly until the effective warfarin dose is established, and then every 4 weeks unless dose changes require more frequent monitoring.
- The function of the valve can be evaluated by transthoracic echocardiogram or if needed, transesophageal echocardiography (TEE).

ARTERIAL BYPASS SURGERY

Description

Bypass grafts are performed to reroute blood flow around the peripheral stenosis or occlusion. The distal vessel must be at least 50% patent for the grafts to remain patent. Various locations along the arterial system can be reconstructed using either femoral artery bypass grafting or axillofemoral reconstruction. Bypass grafts may be either synthetic or autologous vein. Selection for surgery is based on careful history and physical and diagnostic assessments, including arteriography.

Procedure

- Lower abdominal aorta and iliac arteries are the most common areas of atherosclerotic disease. The most frequent operative procedure for aortoiliac occlusive disease is aortobifemoral bypass. Most surgeons place a bifurcated aortic graft using a transabdominal midline approach. Synthetic graft material includes expanded polytetrafluoroethylene (ePTFE, such as Gore-Tex®), and woven or knitted Dacron®. An aortoiliac endarterectomy, in which atheromatous plaque is removed, also can be performed. The surgeon identifies the area, clamps off the blood supply to the vessel, makes an incision into the artery, removes plaque, and sutures the vessel to restore vascular integrity.
- If the occlusion is below the inguinal ligament in the superficial femoral artery, the surgical procedure of choice is the femoral-to-popliteal graft. The grafts can be anastomosed into any of the three lower leg arteries, including the anterior tibial, posterior tibial, or peroneal artery. If the distal anastomosis is above the knee, prosthetic material may be used for the graft. If the distal anastomosis is below the knee, one of the patient's own veins (autologous) can be used.
  - In situ graft use the saphenous vein left in its anatomic position. A part of the proximal and distal vein is dissected and brought to the artery for anastomosis.
  - In reversed vein graft, the vein is harvested, removed from the extremity, reversed and tunneled back into the extremity at the site of the occlusion to form a bypass.
- Extra-anatomic bypass such as axillofemoral bypass, or femorofemoral bypass, are reserved for patients who have increased operative risk, such as patients with marginal cardiopulmonary status, or unable to tolerate abdominal surgery. In the axillofemoral bypass, the graft begins at the axillary artery and is tunneled subcutaneously along the lateral chest wall to the femoral artery.

Indications

- Severe unilateral or bilateral aortoiliac disease
- Distal aortic occlusion
- Critical limb ischemia with diffuse disease and long total occlusions

Contraindications

- Medically unstable
- Poor distal runoff

Complications
- Thrombosis and embolization
- Bleeding
- Arterial dissection
- Infection
- Restenosis
- Compartment syndrome
- Mesenteric ischemia or infarction
- Death

Nursing Implications
- Preoperative
  - Obtain baseline vital signs with careful documentation of the character of the peripheral pulses, particularly those that can be palpated and those that only can be assessed by Doppler.
  - Complete nursing history and physical assessment
  - Screen the patient for potential problems, including bleeding disorders and comorbid medical conditions.
  - Verify that informed consent is obtained and documented.
  - Antibiotic therapy is usually prescribed preoperatively.
  - Assess the patient and family's learning needs and the patient's functional level, coping mechanisms, and support systems.
- Postoperative
  - Hemodynamic stability and maintenance of adequate circulation through the arterial repair, as evidenced by normal tissue perfusion and skin integrity, is key.
    - Observe for signs and symptoms of hemorrhagic shock (e.g., increased pulse, decreased blood pressure [BP], pallor, cool clammy skin, decreasing level of consciousness).
    - Check hematocrit and hemoglobin levels.
    - Assess pedal pulses every hour for 24 hours, and compare the extremities.
      - Doppler evaluation of the vessels is usually done.
      - Measurement of ankle-brachial systolic pressure index may be ordered every 2 hours for 24 hours, and then routinely.
      - Color, temperature, capillary refill, sensory and motor functions are monitored hourly for 24 hours, then assessed every shift unless otherwise ordered.
    - Leg swelling is common after revascularization. Vascular boots are used for patients who had a loss of sensation before surgery or who are at risk for pressure ulcers. If edema worsens with the legs dependent, elastic wraps may be prescribed.
  - Assess for complications, including infection and compartment syndrome.
    - Compartment syndrome develops from swelling around the fascial compartments of the leg, which can compromise circulation in the limb. If severe and prolonged, the muscle cells become ischemic and eventually necrotic. The dead muscle cells release myoglobin, which can cause acute tubular necrosis from rhabdomyolysis.
      - Manifested by pain out of proportion to the surgery, a tense and swollen leg, and decreased sensation of the extremity.

        – Tissue pressure can be measured with a pressure monitoring system connected to a needle inserted into the peripheral tissue. The muscle should be at rest. Normal pressure is less than 20 mm Hg. Compartment syndrome is confirmed with pressures above 30 mm Hg. This should be treated as an emergency and a surgical fasciotomy is needed to relieve tissue pressure.

        – Urinalysis that is positive for hemoglobin but negative for red blood cells indicates myoglobin. The urine color changes to rusty brown.

    – Assess the patient's level of pain as to type, severity, duration, and location and provide comfort measures and medication.

    – Medication management may include:

- Anticoagulants, such as heparin or low molecular weight heparin (e.g., enoxaparin)
- Antiplatelet medication (e.g., clopidogrel) is recommended by some to preserve graft patency.
- Long-term use of anticoagulants such as warfarin may be prescribed for patients with poor outflow, complicated procedures, or a small-caliber graft.
- Aspirin is prescribed for most patients.
- Broad-spectrum antibiotics are continued postsurgically.

Patient and Family Education

- Discuss prescribed medications and give written instructions. Patients will be on long-term aspirin therapy and also may be on clopidogrel for 4 to 6 weeks or longer. If the patient has had problems with poor outflow or had a complicated procedure, warfarin is prescribed.
- Management of hypertension is critical, and discussion of antihypertensive medications, diet and weight management, and the importance of keeping a record of BP readings should be reviewed.
- Atherosclerosis risk factors should be assessed. Refer the patient to self-help clinics such as smoking cessation, weight management, and exercise programs.
- Foot care is an important aspect of care of the patient with peripheral vascular disease. Daily hygiene, inspection and lubrication of the skin, care of toenails, proper footwear, safety precautions, and activity are topics to be discussed.
- Review activity level and when the patient can anticipate return to normal activities or work.

Follow-Up Care

- Follow-up appointment with the vascular surgeon is made within one week of hospital discharge.
- Follow-up graft surveillance can be performed with duplex ultrasound.
- A foot care specialist (e.g., podiatrist) may be needed to address the issues of footwear and nail care.

ANEURYSM REPAIR

Description

Aneurysm resection and bypass grafting are the usual surgical repair procedures. An aneurysm is a localized sac or dilation that formed at a weak point of the vessel wall. The most common type of aneurysm is abdominal, and has been attributed to atherosclerotic changes in the aorta. Other areas include the thoracic aorta, subclavian artery, femoral artery, and popliteal artery. Surgical treatment of an aneurysm may be either an emergency surgery or an elective procedure.

Procedure

- Abdominal aortic aneurysm
  - The surgical technique involves an incision from the xiphoid process to the symphysis pubis. The aneurysm is exposed and aortic clamps are applied above and below the aneurysm. The aneurysm is opened and a polyester (Dacron®) graft is placed within the aneurysm. The aneurysm sac is then wrapped around the graft to protect it.
  - Elective aneurysm repair occurs when the benefits of the operation to prevent aneurysm rupture are greater than the risk of surgical complications.
  - Endovascular grafting is an alternative approach for treating infrarenal abdominal aortic aneurysm. This procedure involves the transluminal placement of a sutureless graft across the aneurysm. The procedure may be done under local or regional anesthesia. It cannot be used for a ruptured aneurysm.
- Ascending thoracic aneurysm
  - Repair of this type of aneurysm involves exposure of the aneurysm, clamp above the aneurysm, incision into the aneurysm, aortic valve replacement with aortic graft implant to repair the ascending aortic aneurysm. The aortic aneurysm is then trimmed and closed over the graft.

Indications

Abdominal aortic aneurysm or thoracic aneurysm as described above. In the event of a dissection, the procedure becomes emergent with increased mortality.

Contraindications

Medically unstable, although emergent surgery may be attempted.

Complications

- Postoperative bleeding
- Cardiac tamponade
- Myocardial infarction
- Pulmonary complications including atelectasis, pulmonary edema, or pulmonary emboli
- Renal impairment
- Gastrointestinal problems (e.g., abdominal distention, ileus, hepatic dysfunction, mesenteric ischemia)
- Hematoma or wound infection
- Distal ischemia or embolization, dissection or perforation of the aorta, graft thrombosis or infection

- Spinal cord ischemia resulting in paraplegia, rectal and urinary incontinence, or loss of pain and temperature sensation
- Death
- With endovascular repair, the surgical complications are not seen but you may find
  - Fracture of the graft placement clips
  - Retroperitoneal bleeding
  - Hematoma or bleeding from puncture site
  - Compartment syndrome

Nursing Implications

- Preoperative
  - Obtain baseline vital signs and ECG. Complete nursing history and physical assessment.
  - Screen the patient for potential problems, including bleeding disorder and comorbid medical conditions.
  - Verify that informed consent is obtained and documented.
  - Assess the patient and family's learning needs and the patient's functional level.
  - Assess for signs of impending rupture.
    - Abdominal aneurysm: severe back or abdominal pain, which may be persistent or intermittent.
      - Low back pain also may be present because of pressure of the aneurysm on the lumbar nerves.
    - Thoracic aneurysm: Intense chest, back, shoulder, or abdominal pain, often described as a "ripping pain."
    - Impending rupture of either thoracic or abdominal aneurysm may present with hypotension, symptoms of heart failure, and falling hematocrit.
  - BP management is critical preoperatively, and the systolic BP should be maintained at about 100 mm Hg to 120 mm Hg with antihypertensive agents.
    - Beta blockers, especially labetalol and ß blocker, are the drugs of choice because they reduce shear force on the aortic wall, as well as reducing HR and BP.
- Postoperative
  The following areas should be assessed. (See desirable parameters under CABG.)
  - Cardiac status
  - Respiratory status
  - Neurological status
  - Peripheral vascular status
  - Gastrointestinal status, particularly because ileus can occur as well as mesenteric ischemia, causing ischemic colitis
  - Pain status
  - Psychosocial status
  - Complications described above should be identified and measures instituted to reverse their progression.
- Post percutaneous infrarenal endovascular repair
  - Same postprocedure care as described under PCI
  - Assessment of peripheral perfusion
  - Assessment of puncture site
  - Maintain bed rest until puncture site is stable

Patient and Family Education
- Similar to the care of the patient undergoing CABG
- Provide verbal and written instructions to include activity, diet, and medication regimen.
- Assess the patient for atherosclerosis risk factors, including hyperlipidemia, smoking history, hypertension, diabetes, and obesity. Discuss resources for further interventions.

Follow-Up Care
- Follow-up appointment is usually made one week after surgery.
- Ultrasound or CT scanning is used to monitor graft patency.

CAROTID ENDARTERECTOMY

Description
Carotid endarterectomy (CEA) is a surgical procedure with the opening of the carotid artery to remove obstructing and embolizing plaque. After CABG, it is the second most common vascular surgery.

Procedure
- An incision is made on the anterior border of the sternocleidomastoid muscle, the vessel is clamped, and the plaque or atheroma is removed.
- Intraoperative electroencephalogram (EEG) and transcranial Doppler monitoring may be used to monitor cerebral blood flow.

Indications
- Severe carotid stenosis (more than 70% by duplex Doppler ultrasound) in symptomatic or asymptomatic patients
- Ulcerated or intermediate degrees of stenosis (more than 50% by duplex ultrasound) if they remain or become symptomatic despite use of antiplatelet therapy
- More than 50% stenosis (by duplex ultrasound) if it is in conjunction with contralateral internal carotid occlusion

Contraindications
- Thick, circular calcifications may increase operative risk
- Totally occluded arteries
- Patients with comorbid conditions, particularly cardiovascular disease, may have increased operative risk and may be better treated by PTA and stent.

Complications
- Thrombus formation and embolization
- Transient ischemic attack or stroke
- Cranial nerve injury
- Infection or hematoma of the surgical incision
- Intracerebral hemorrhage
- Restenosis
- Death

Nursing Implications

- Preoperative
  - Baseline vital signs, 12-lead ECG, complete nursing history and physical examination, and screen for comorbid conditions.
  - Assess and document baseline neurological status.
  - Assess patient and family learning needs.
- Postoperative
  - Neurological assessment is made every 1 to 2 hours, including level of consciousness, reflexes, motor strength, level of sensation, and pupil size and reaction to light.
  - Cranial nerve assessment for nerve damage is also important.
    - Facial nerve (VII)
    - Vagus nerve (X)
    - Spinal accessory (XI)
    - Hypoglossal (XII)
    - The most common cranial nerve damage causes vocal cord paralysis, difficulty in managing saliva, or tongue deviation.
  - Cardiopulmonary assessment, including HR and BP monitoring and lung status.
    - BP should be maintained within 20 mm Hg of the preoperative baseline.
    - Labile blood pressure is common.
    - Hypertension may precipitate cerebral hemorrhage, edema, or hemorrhage at the incision site.
    - Hypotension may cause cerebral ischemia and thrombosis.
  - Assess incision for evidence of excessive swelling or hematoma.
  - If neurologic deficits are identified, appropriate referral to speech, occupational, or physical therapy.

Patient and Family Education

- Discuss prescribed medications and give written instructions. Patients are instructed to take an aspirin daily, and may also be on clopidogrel for 4 to 6 weeks or longer.
- Management of hypertension is critical, and use of antihypertensive medications, diet and weight management, and the importance of keeping a record of BP readings should be reviewed.
- Review signs and symptoms to report to the provider.
  - Numbness or weakness of the face, arm, or leg, especially if one-sided
  - Trouble speaking or understanding speech
  - Sudden, severe headache
  - Visual disturbances
  - Difficulty walking
  - Confusion or memory loss
- Assess the patient for atherosclerosis risk factors such as smoking, diabetes, and hyperlipidemia and discuss resources for further intervention.
- Review activity level and when the patient can anticipate return to normal activities or work.

Follow-Up Care

- Follow-up appointment is usually made in the first week postoperatively.
- Follow-up Doppler studies are performed 3 months postoperatively to assess for artery patency, again at 6 months to a year, and then annually to detect restenosis on the operated side and disease on the other side.

PERIPHERAL THROMBOEMBOLECTOMY

Description
A balloon catheter technique is used to remove arterial emboli and restore peripheral circulation. Systemic arterial emboli may originate from a variety of sites, but 80% to 85% arise in the heart, usually because of atherosclerotic heart disease. The left ventricle in the setting of MI accounts for 60% to 65% of systemic emboli, which tend to travel to the lower extremities, with 75% to 79% lodging in the iliac, femoral, or popliteal arteries.

Procedure
- Aortic and iliac occlusions
  - The initial approach to an aortic occlusion is via bilateral vertical groin incisions. The superficial, common, and deep femoral arteries are isolated and looped with silastic tapes. The arteriotomy is made in the common femoral artery proximal to the bifurcation. The vessel is carefully palpated for location of the plaque.
  - The embolectomy catheter is passed through the affected artery and distal to the occlusion. The balloon is inflated with sterile saline solution and the thrombus is extracted as the catheter is extracted. Repeated passes are made to ensure all obstructing emboli are removed.
  - Heparinized solution is injected into the distal artery through an irrigating catheter.
  - A similar procedure is performed on the opposite leg after extraction of the clot from one side.
- Femoral and popliteal occlusions
  - The most current approach for occlusion at the level of the adductor tendon and popliteal areas is through an incision in the distal common femoral artery. This is a more satisfactory approach than making an incision over the site of the occlusion. The balloon technique is the same as described above.
- Adjunctive endovascular procedures such as balloon dilatation and atherectomy may be used if thromboembolectomy alone fails.
- Immediate anticoagulation and early operative embolectomy is the recommended treatment.

Indications
- Acute arterial occlusion with symptoms, including loss of sensation and proprioception of the affected limb, loss of motor function, and rigor.
- A surgeon may elect to proceed with embolectomy even in the presence of gangrene to achieve a lower level amputation.

Contraindications
- Advanced ischemia of 24 to 48 hours usually increases risk of poor outcome, and ischemia longer than 48 hours increases the risk of amputation.

Complications
- Thrombus formation
- Vessel vasospasm
- Hemorrhage
- Bleeding or hematoma formation along incision site
- Artery dissection
- Compartment syndrome

- In advanced ischemia with motor loss and rigor, significant complications and death can occur if not recognized or handled appropriately. Complications include:
  - Venous thrombosis and development of edema
  - Hyperkalemia and acidosis secondary to pooled blood in ischemic limbs, which may lead to hypotension and cardiac arrhythmia
  - Rhabdomyolysis and renal failure

Nursing Implications

- Preprocedure
  - Obtain baseline vital signs with careful documentation of the character of the peripheral pulses, particularly those that can be palpated and those that only can be assessed by Doppler. Keep the extremity level or slightly (15°) dependent.
  - Complete a nursing history and physical assessment.
  - Screen the patient for potential problems, including bleeding disorder and comorbid medical conditions.
  - Verify that informed consent is obtained and documented.
  - Administered heparin intravenously, as prescribed.
  - Assess the patient and family's learning needs and the patient's functional level, coping mechanisms, and support systems.
- Postprocedure
  - Similar to the care of patient undergoing peripheral bypass surgery, including:
    - Hemodynamic stability and maintaining adequate circulation through the arterial repair, as evidenced by normal tissue perfusion and skin integrity, is key, along with assessment of patient's pedal pulses (Doppler, ankle-brachial indices), leg swelling, and signs of hemorrhage.
  - Assess for complications, including infection and compartment syndrome.
  - Assess the patient's level of pain as to type, duration, and, location and provide comfort measures and appropriate medication.
  - Medication management also may include use of anticoagulants such as heparin or low molecular weight heparin (e.g., enoxaparin) postprocedure. Some recommend antiplatelet medication such as clopidogrel along with aspirin, while others recommend long-term use of anticoagulants.

Patient and Family Education

- Similar to the care of the patient undergoing peripheral bypass surgery, including diet, activity level, and management of hypertension. Other risk factors, including smoking and weight management, should be assessed, and appropriate referrals should be made. Tight glycemic control is recommended for patients with diabetes.
- Discuss prescribed medications and give written instructions. If the patient is taking warfarin, careful instructions are given including use, side effects, and need for monitoring of the PT and INR.
- Discussion with the vascular surgeon to explore further interventions that may be required.
  - Approximately 60% of patients sustaining an acute arterial occlusion require an additional operative procedure within 1 month of the original procedure.

Follow-Up Care

- Follow-up appointment is made within 1 week of discharge.
- Follow-up surveillance can be performed with duplex ultrasound.
- A foot care specialist (e.g., podiatrist) may be needed to address the issues of footwear and nail care.

OVERVIEW OF CARDIAC TRANSPLANTATION

Description

Cardiac transplantation is a surgical procedure for patients with end-stage heart disease.

Procedure

- An orthotopic heart transplant is the most common procedure. The recipient's heart is removed and the donor heart implanted with direct anastomosis to the aorta, pulmonary artery, and right and left atrial cuffs to include the vena cava and pulmonary veins.
  - The procedure involves a median sternotomy and the use of CPB.
  - The procedure denervates the heart so ischemia does not result in chest pain.
  - The procedure surgically interrupts the connection between the SA node of the recipient's heart and the SA node of the donor heart. Thus, the ECG may reveal 2 P waves, and the donor SA node drives the conduction of the heart.
  - Heart rate no longer responds to the autonomic nervous system and elevation in HR requires circulating catecholamines.
- The heterotopic heart transplant, in which the donor heart is placed parallel to the recipient's heart, is performed rarely. The right side of the patient's heart can continue to function, while the dysfunctional left ventricle is bypassed.
  - The United Network for Organ Sharing (UNOS) sets the guidelines for transplantation and rules for organ distribution, and maintains the list of patients waiting for transplantation. Local transplant programs work with UNOS to obtain the donor hearts.
  - Potential recipients are matched to donors based on blood type and body size (plus or minus 15%). Patients with the worst cardiac conditions are highest on the priority list.
  - Patients with a high panel of reactive antigens (PRA) also will have a longer wait for a suitable match.
  - Because patients may wait for months or even years for donor hearts, left ventricular assist devices may be implanted as either a bridge to transplant or in place of the transplant as destination therapy.
  - Once transplanted, the recipient is on life-long immunosuppressant therapy.

Indications

Selection criteria

- End-stage heart failure, New York Heart Association III or IV
- Maximum oxygen consumption less than 14 mL/kg/min or less than 50% of predicted maximum level
- Life expectancy of less than one year
- Nonsmoker, no drug or alcohol abuse
- Patient is psychologically stable and able to follow postoperative instructions and long-term medication use.

Contraindications

- Underlying conditions that would limit survival such as systemic infection; irreversible renal, pulmonary, or hepatic insufficiency; active peptic ulcer; or recent pulmonary emboli.
- History of cancer because the immunosuppressant drug regimen will increase risk of recurrence or new cancers.
- Age 65 years or older. However, a healthy older candidate may receive a donor heart than is older than what would normally be considered for transplant.

Nursing Implications

- Preoperative and perioperative care
  - Maximize heart failure treatment to keep the patient in optimal condition prior to transplant. The focus is on preventing infections, acute renal or liver failure, or irreversible right ventricular dysfunction.
  - Patients may be waiting at home for a long time so routine UNOS updates on status are needed. Also, the stress of waiting may take a toll on patients and family.
  - The care of the cardiac transplant patient is very complex, and the nurse works collaboratively with the multidisciplinary team. The care focuses on instituting immunosuppression while preventing infection.
- Postoperative and long-term care
  - Rejection, infection, and transplant coronary artery disease are the major long-term problems.
  - Other long-term problems resulting from the immunosuppressant therapies include:
    - infection
    - nephrotoxicity
    - hypertension
    - hyperlipidemia
    - transplant lymphoproliferative disease
    - malignancy
  - Isolation procedures are used postoperatively. Patients must wear masks for several months postoperatively and avoid working in the soil; eating raw, unpeeled vegetables or fruit; indoor plants; birds as pets; and cat litter boxes because these are sources for infection in someone who is immunosuppressed.
  - See postoperative CABG care for details of recovery.
  - Medication management includes immunosuppressive agents and antibiotic prophylaxis, and may include antihypertensive agents, diuretics, proton pump inhibitors or H2 blockers, and lipid-lowering drugs.
  - Right heart catheterizations with RV biopsy to detect rejection are done weekly, then at progressively longer intervals until it is annual. If rejection is detected, more aggressive immunosuppressant therapy is required.
  - Annual left heart catheterizations are done to examine the coronary arteries because patients will no longer experience chest pain with ischemia. A form of diffuse intimal disease occurs frequently after transplant and may be because of the immunosuppressant medications. Angioplasty can be performed on donor vessels with discrete lesions.
  - Cardiac rehabilitation exercise is recommended but patients should have a longer warmup to ensure increasing heart rate. Heart rate recovery after exercise takes longer.

Patient and Family Education

- Importance of rigorous medication regimen and side effects of the various medications
- Discuss the signs and symptoms of rejection and infectious complications and when to notify the healthcare team in order to intervene early.
- Cardiac rehabilitation provides a benefit of improving exercise tolerance and psychosocial support for the transplant participant and family members.

Follow-Up Care

- Follow-up visits are made with the multidisciplinary team, and the patient should adhere to these follow-up appointments. Follow-up visits may include laboratory surveillance and endomyocardial biopsies.
- Cardiac rehabilitation is recommended.

SUMMARY

This chapter provided an overview of care of the patient undergoing invasive cardiac procedures. These procedures include balloon angioplasty procedures for various arteries, stent placement in dilated areas of the arteries, pacemaker insertions, percutaneous valve procedures, and heart and vascular surgeries. The nurse plays a pivotal role in patient recovery from these varied approaches to treatment of cardiac and vascular disease. The next chapter covers the common pharmacologic approaches to care of these patients.

REFERENCES

Abdel-Latif, A., & Moliterna, D. J. (2009) Antiplatelet polypharmacy in primary percutaneous coronary intervention: Trying to understand when more is better. *Circulation, 119*, 3168–3170.

Adams, R. J., Albers, G., Alberts, M. J., Benavente, O., Furie, K., Goldstein, L. B., ... American Stroke Association. (2008). Update to the AHA/ASA recommendations for the prevention of stroke in patients with stroke and transient ischemic attack. *Stroke, 39*(5), 1647–1652.

Barkley, T. W., & Myers, C. M. (2008). *Practice guidelines for acute care nurse practitioners* (2nd ed.) St. Louis, MO: Elsevier Saunders.

Chen, K. Y., Rha, S. W., Podder, K. L., Jin, Z., Minami, Y., Wang, L., ... Korea Acute Myocardial Infarction Registry Investigators. (2009). Triple versus dial antiplatelet therapy in patients with acute ST segment elevation myocardial infarction undergoing primary percutaneous coronary intervention. *Circulation, 119*, 3207–3214.

Crawford, M. H. (2009). *Cardiology: Current diagnosis and treatment.* New York: McGraw Hill.

Efstratiadis, G., Pateinakis, P., Tambakoudis, G., Pantzaki, A., Economidou, D., & Memmos, D. (2008). Contrast media-induced nephropathy: Case report and review of the literature focusing on pathogenesis. *Hippokratia, 12*(2), 87–93.

Estes, N. A. M., Halperin, J. L., Calkins, H., Ezokowitz, M. D., Gitman, P., Go, A. S., ... Society of Thoracic Surgeons. (2008). ACC/AHA/Physician Consortium 2008 clinical performance measures for adults with nonvalvular atrial fibrillation or atrial flutter: A report of the American College of Cardiology/American Heart Association Task Force on Performance Measures and the Physician Consortium for Performance Improvement (Writing Committee to Develop Clinical Performance Measures for Atrial Fibrillation): developed in collaboration with the Heart Rhythm Society. *Circulation, 27*, 117(21), e350–408. Epub 2008 May 15.

Hill, K. M. (2009). Mitral valve repair: A new choice. *American Nurse Today, 4*(5), 8–10.

Hirsch, J., Guyatt, G., Albers, G. W., Harrington, R., & Schunemann, H. J. (2008). Antithrombotic and thrombolytic therapy: Executive summary. *Chest, 133*, 71S–109S.

Labus, D. (2008). *Cardiovascular care made incredibly easy.* Philadelphia: Springhouse.

McCaffrey, R., & Blum, C. (2009). Venothrombotic events: Evidence-based risk assessment, prophylaxis, diagnosis, and treatment. *Journal for Nurse Practitioners, 5*(5), 325–333.

Moser, D., & Reigel, B. (2008). *Cardiac nursing: A companion to Braunwald's heart disease.* St. Louis, MO: Elsevier Saunders.

Patel, M. R., Dehmer, G. J., Hirshfeld, J. W., Smith, P. K., & Spertus, J. A. (2009). ACCF/SCAI/STS/AATS/AHA/ASNC 2009 Appropriateness Criteria for Coronary Revascularization: A Report of the American College of Cardiology Foundation Appropriateness Criteria Task Force, Society for Cardiovascular Angiography and Interventions, Society of Thoracic Surgeons, American Association for Thoracic Surgery, American Heart Association, and the American Society of Nuclear Cardiology: Endorsed by the American Society of Echocardiography, the Heart Failure Society of America, and the Society of Cardiovascular Computed Tomography. *Circulation, 119*(9), 1330–1352.

Pearson, T. L. (2007). Correlation of ankle-brachial index values with carotid disease, coronary disease and cardiovascular risk. *Journal of Cardiovascular Nursing, 22*, 436–439.

Sandau, K. E., & Smith, M. (2009). Continuous ST segment monitoring: Protocol for practice. *Critical Care Nurse, 29*(4), 39–49.

Serruys, P. W., Morice, M. C., Kappetein, P., Colombo, A., Holmes, D. R., Mack, M. J., ... SYNTAX Investigators. (2009). Percutaneous coronary interventions versus coronary artery bypass grafting for severe coronary disease. *New England Journal of Medicine, 360*, 961–972.

Shoulders-Odom, B. (2008). Management of patients after percutaneous coronary interventions. *Critical Care Nurse, 28*(5), 26–43.

Soat, M. (2009). Aortic aneurysm: Causes, clues, and treatment options. *American Nurse Today, 4*(7), 7–9.

Stout, K. K., & Verrier, E. D. (2009). Acute valvular regurgitation. *Circulation, 119,* 3232–3241.

Swatzky, J. V., & Naimark, B. J. (2009). Coronary artery bypass graft surgery: Exploring a broader perspective of risks and outcomes. *Journal of Cardiovascular Nursing, 24,* 198–206.

Woods, S. L., Sivarajan Froelicher, E. S., Underhill Motzer, S., & Bridges, E. J. (2009). *Cardiac nursing* (6th ed.). Philadelphia: Lippincott.

Zipes, D. P., Libby, P., Bonow, R. O., & Braunwald, E. (2009). *Braunwald's heart disease: A textbook of cardiovascular medicine* (8th ed.). Philadelphia: Elsevier-Saunders.

15

Cardiovascular Pharmacology

The cardiovascular system consists of three anatomical components: the autonomic nervous system, the heart, and the vasculature. These three components interact in a complex manner to control blood flow to organs throughout the body. A clear understanding of the basic principles of cardiovascular physiology is needed to appreciate the complex mechanisms and pharmacological effects of many of the cardiovascular drugs. In this chapter, a hierarchy is used for the organization of cardiovascular drugs: groups, classes, and drugs. In this hierarchy, groups represent the major headings, classes represent categories of drugs within the groups, and drugs represent individual class members. For example, positive inotropic agents are a group, cardiac glycosides are a class of inotropic agent, and digoxin is a drug that is a cardiac glycoside. It is important to realize that some drugs may belong to two different groups (e.g., dobutamine is a sympathomimetic but it is also a positive inotropic agent). Another consideration is that many of the drug groups and classes are used for many forms of cardiovascular problems. See Table 15–1 for examples of the purpose for using several common cardiac drug groups.

ADRENERGIC GROUP

Classes within this group include sympathomimetics, alpha$_1$-selective adrenergic agonists, alpha$_2$-selective (centrally acting) adrenergic agonists, alpha-adrenergic antagonists, and beta-adrenergic antagonists.

Table 15–1. Uses of Common Classes of Cardiac Medications

	Hypertension	Coronary Artery Disease or Myocardial Infarction	Heart Failure	Dysrhythmias
Diuretics	Yes	No	Yes	No
Beta Blockers	Yes	Yes	Yes	Yes
Calcium Channel Blockers	Yes	Yes	No	Yes
ACE Inhibitors	Yes	Yes	Yes	No
ARB	Yes	Yes	Yes	No
Vasodilators	Yes	Yes	Yes	No

Sympathomimetics

- Drugs within class
  - Dobutamine (Dobutrex®)
  - Isoproterenol (Isuprel®)
  - Dopamine (Intropin®)
  - Epinephrine (Adrenalin®)
  - Norepinephrine (Levophed®)
  - Metaraminol (Aramine®)

Mechanisms of Action

- Sympathomimetic drugs mimic the effects of endogenous catecholamines and stimulate (to varying degrees) both alpha- and beta-adrenergic receptors.
- Epinephrine and norepinephrine are endogenous catecholamines that interact with both alpha and beta receptors.
- Metaraminol is a synthetic agent that is very similar to norepinephrine and has prominent, direct effects on alpha receptors. It is most often used under anesthesia. It has been used off-label in the treatment of priapism.
- Dopamine is another endogenous catecholamine that primarily interacts with dopamine receptors, in addition to alpha and beta receptors.
- Isoproterenol is a synthetic catecholamine with higher affinity for beta receptors.
- Dobutamine is another synthetic catecholamine with higher affinity for beta$_1$ receptors.

Pharmacological Effects

- Stimulation of alpha receptors causes vasoconstriction.
- Stimulation of cardiac beta$_1$ receptors increases the force and rate of cardiac contraction.
- Stimulation of dopamine receptors increases the force of cardiac contraction and dilates renal blood vessels.

Therapeutic Uses
- Hypotension and shock
    - Epinephrine and norepinephrine are used to treat shock or cardiac arrest.
    - Dopamine increases renal blood flow and does not cause the renal shutdown that has been associated with the other sympathomimetics.
    - Dobutamine is used in the treatment of severe, decompensated heart failure (HF) because it increases myocardial contractility without a marked increase in heart rate or oxygen demand.
    - Metaraminol is most often used for hypotension when undergoing anesthesia. It has been used off-label in the treatment of priapism.

Adverse Effects
- GI (gastrointestinal): nausea and vomiting
- CV (cardiovascular): tachycardia, dysrhythmia, hypertension, palpitations, and angina
- CNS (central nervous system): throbbing headache and cerebral hemorrhage

Contraindications
- Tachydysrhythmia and ventricular fibrillation
- Pheochromocytoma

Nursing Implications
- Use extreme caution in calculating and preparing doses of these drugs.
- Monitor patient response closely (monitor vital signs) and adjust dosage accordingly to ensure the most benefit with the least toxicity.
- Be careful to prevent extravasation because tissue sloughing can occur. Phentolamine or another adrenergic antagonist can be given to counter the vasoconstriction and prevent tissue damage by infiltration of the site with 5 mg to 10 mg dissolved in 10 mL to 15 mL saline.
- Administer via central line, if at all possible.

Alpha₁-Selective Adrenergic Agonists
- Drugs within class
    - Phenylephrine (Neo-Synephrine®)
    - Methoxamine (Vasoxyl®)
    - Midodrine (ProAmatine®)

Mechanisms of Action
- Stimulate alpha-adrenergic receptors in vascular smooth muscle

Pharmacological Effects
- Increase peripheral vascular resistance.
- Maintain or increase blood pressure (BP).

Therapeutic Uses
- Phenylephrine is the drug most commonly used in intensive care unit (ICU) settings.
- Midodrine may be useful in the treatment of some patients with persistent hypotension.

Adverse Effects
Extension of the therapeutic effects (e.g., increased BP, sweating).

Contraindications
- Hypertension
- Tachycardia
- Vasospasm
- Lactation

Nursing Implications
- Do not discontinue drug abruptly because sudden withdrawal can result in rebound hypertension, dysrhythmia, hypertensive encephalopathy, and death. Taper drug over 2 to 4 days.
- Do not discontinue prior to surgery; mark the patient's chart and monitor BP carefully during surgery. Sympathetic stimulation may alter the normal response to, and recovery from, anesthesia.
- Intravenous administration via central line only.

Alpha₂-Selective Adrenergic Agonists (Centrally Acting)
- Drugs within class
  - Clonidine (Catapres®)
  - Guanfacine (Tenex®)
  - Guanabenz (Wytensin®)
  - Methyldopa (Aldomet®)

Mechanisms of Action
- Activate alpha₂ receptors in the cardiovascular control centers of the central nervous system (CNS).
- Methyldopa is metabolized to alpha-methyl norepinephrine in the brain, and this compound is thought to activate central alpha₂ receptors in a manner similar to that of clonidine, guanfacine, and guanabenz.

Pharmacological Effects
Activation of alpha₂ receptors in the CNS suppresses the outflow of sympathetic nervous system activity from the brain, thus decreasing BP and heart rate.

Therapeutic Uses
- Alpha₂-selective adrenergic agonists are used primarily in the treatment of systemic hypertension.
- Methyldopa is the drug of choice in pregnant women who are hypertensive.

Adverse Effects
- CNS: depression, nightmares, sedation, drowsiness, fatigue, and headache
- CV: hypotension, HF, and bradycardia
- Other: dry mouth, sexual dysfunction, and decreased urinary output

Contraindications
- Severe coronary heart disease
- Vascular disease
- Chronic renal failure

Nursing Implications
- Withdrawal reactions may follow abrupt discontinuation of long-term therapy. This is primarily reflex tachycardia and hypertension (HTN).
- Clonidine is the most commonly used drug from this group.
  - It can be used in hypertensive urgencies or emergencies because of its rapid onset of action.
  - It is a useful third-line drug for people with resistant HTN but b.i.d. or t.i.d. dosing poses a problem for people who may miss doses. Significant reflex tachycardia and HTN, which develop as the drug level falls, can be prevented by use in conjunction with a beta blocker.
  - It is now available as a 3-day patch, which reduces the risk of rebound.

Alpha-Adrenergic Antagonists
- Drugs within class
  - Doxazosin (Cardura®)
  - Prazosin (Minipress®)
  - Terazosin (Hytrin®)
  - Phenoxybenzamine (Dibenzyline®)
  - Phentolamine (Regitine®)
  - Tolazoline (Priscoline®)

Mechanisms of Action
- Alpha-adrenergic receptor antagonists
  - Alpha$_1$ receptors are postsynaptic receptors that produce the effects of the sympathetic nervous system.
  - Alpha$_2$ receptors are presynaptic receptors that modulate norepinephrine release.
- Some of these drugs have markedly different affinities for alpha$_1$ and alpha$_2$ receptors.
  - Prazosin, terazosin, and doxazosin are more potent in blocking alpha$_1$ than alpha$_2$ receptors (and are termed alpha$_1$-selective).
  - Phenoxybenzamine and phentolamine have similar affinities for both of these receptor sites.

Pharmacological Effects
- Decrease vascular tone and produce vasodilation, which lowers blood pressure.
- Because alpha$_1$-selective antagonists do not block the presynaptic alpha$_2$ receptor sites, the reflex tachycardia that accompanies the reduction in blood pressure is less likely to occur.

Therapeutic Uses
- Hypertension, most often as a third-line drug with combination therapy
- Phenoxybenzamine and phentolamine are used in the treatment of pheochromocytoma.
- Phentolamine is also used to manage extravasation of tissue-toxic agents.
- Doxazosin, prazosin, and terazosin are commonly used for benign prostatic hypertrophy. In older men with uncontrolled hypertension, these drugs are ideal additional antihypertensives because they treat both conditions.

Adverse Effects

- CV: postural hypotension, dysrhythmia, edema, HF, and angina. Vasodilation from these agents can cause flushing, rhinitis, reddened eyes, nasal congestion, and priapism.
- CNS: dizziness, weakness, fatigue, drowsiness, and depression
- First-dose phenomenon: Marked postural hypotension and syncope are sometimes seen 30 to 90 minutes after a patient takes an initial dose. Therefore, a low dose is used to start therapy and it is commonly given at bedtime.

Contraindications

- Use cautiously in the presence of HF or renal failure, because drug effects could exacerbate these conditions. Caution also should be used with pregnancy and lactation.
- Use cautiously with other vasodilators (e.g., nitrates, hydralazine). Use with erectile dysfunction medications can cause profound hypotension.

Nursing Implications

- Monitor BP, pulse, rhythm, and cardiac output regularly to determine need to adjust dosage or discontinue drug if cardiovascular effects are severe.
- Observe the patient for any hypotensive effects for approximately 90 minutes following administration of first dose.
- Teach patient to take doxazosin, prazosin, and terazosin at bedtime and do not take sildenafil and similar erectile dysfunction drugs when on these medications.

Beta-Adrenergic Antagonists (Beta Blockers)

Drugs within class (see Table 15–2)

Mechanisms of Action

- Beta receptor antagonists occupy beta receptors and block receptor action.
  - Beta$_1$ receptors are found in the heart, where they stimulate myocardial contraction and increase heart rate.
  - Beta$_2$ receptors are found predominately in bronchioles (where they cause dilation), smooth muscle of blood vessels (where they cause dilation), and the uterus (where they cause relaxation).
  - Some of these drugs have markedly different affinities for beta$_1$ and beta$_2$ receptors, known as selectivity. However, at high doses most lose their selective affinity.
- Other mechanisms of action include partial agonist activity at beta receptors and local anesthetic action, which differ among the beta blockers.
- Table 15–2 summarizes the properties of various beta-adrenergic antagonists.

Pharmacological Effects

- Decrease heart rate and BP
- Reduce renin release in the kidneys
- Beta-receptor blockade has relatively little effect on the normal heart of a person at rest but has profound effects when sympathetic control of the heart is dominant, such as during exercise, stress, or from an underlying pathophysiology.

Table 15–2. Properties and Therapeutic Uses of Beta Receptor–Blocking Drugs

	Trade Name	Selectivity	Partial Agonist Activity	Therapeutic Uses
Acebutolol (A,C)	Sectral®	Beta$_1$	Yes	Hypertension, ventricular dysrhythmias
Atenolol	Tenormin®	Beta$_1$	No	Hypertension, chronic angina, status post MI
Betaxolol (A)	Kerlone®	Beta$_1$	No	Hypertension
Bisoprolol	Zebeta®	Beta$_1$	No	Hypertension
Carteolol	Cartrol®	None	Yes	Hypertension
Carvedilol (B)	Coreg®	None	No	Hypertension, HF
Esmolol	Brevibloc®	Beta$_1$	No	Supraventricular tachycardia
Labetalol (A,B)	Normodyne® Trandate®	None	Yes	Hypertension
Metoprolol (A)	Lopressor® Toprol®	Beta$_1$	No	Hypertension, angina, prevention of reinfarction after MI
Nadolol	Corgard®	None	No	Hypertension, angina
Penbutolol	Levatol®	None	Yes	Hypertension
Pindolol (A,C)	Visken®	None	Yes	Hypertension
Propranolol (A)	Inderal®	None	No	Hypertension, angina, idiopathic hypertrophic subaortic stenosis, dysrhythmias, pheochromocytoma
Sotalol	Betapace®	None	No	Ventricular dysrhythmias
Timolol	Blocadren®	None	No	Hypertension, prevention of reinfarction after MI

(A) Beta blockers with local anesthetic action. (B) Carvedilol and labetalol also provide alpha$_1$-adrenergic receptor blockade. (C) Beta blockers with intrinsic sympathomimetic activity (ISA).

Therapeutic Uses
- Several beta blockers have the property of intrinsic sympathomimetic activity (ISA) because they are antagonists with a partial agonist effect (e.g., pindolol, acebutolol). ISA mitigates the degree of HR and BP reduction, making it more tolerable for the person who exercises or a person prone to hypoglycemia. It also reduces the metabolic effect of beta blockers.
- Therapeutic cardiac uses include hypertension, angina, post myocardial infarction (MI), tachydysrhythmias, and heart failure. Additional uses include migraine headache prophylaxis, benign tremor, panic disorder, stage fright, glaucoma, esophageal varices, perioperative prophylaxis for noncardiac surgery, and thyroid toxicosis.

Adverse Effects
- CV: bradycardia, heart block, HF, hypotension, and peripheral vascular insufficiency
- Pulmonary (with nonselective beta blockers): difficulty breathing, coughing, and bronchospasm
- CNS: fatigue, dizziness, depression, paresthesia, sleep disturbances, memory loss, and disorientation
- Metabolic: decreased glycogenolysis and glucagon secretion, which can exacerbate fasting hypoglycemia.
- Other: nausea, vomiting, diarrhea, colitis, decreased libido, sexual dysfunction, masking of signs of hypoglycemia, slowed recovery from hypoglycemia, and decreased exercise tolerance

Contraindications
- CV: bradycardia or heart block; use with caution in HF (e.g., metoprolol); avoid starting or increasing dose during episodes of fluid overload. Wait until the patient is euvolemic.
- Pulmonary: bronchospasm, chronic obstructive pulmonary disease, or acute asthma
- Nonselective beta blockers should be used with great caution in people with diabetes and frequent hypoglycemic reactions.
- Traditionally, beta blockers were contraindicated for the cocaine user because of unopposed alpha stimulation. Recent studies have reported safety when using beta blockers in the acute setting of cocaine-induced chest pain.

Nursing Implications
- Do not withdraw these drugs abruptly after chronic therapy; taper gradually over 2 weeks because long-term use of these drugs can sensitize the myocardium to catecholamines and severe reactions can occur.
- Give the oral form of these drugs with food to improve absorption.
- If beta blockers are used in people with HF, be aware that HF symptoms may worsen initially. Dosage may need to be adjusted if the person experiences weight gain, significant bradycardia, or dizziness.
- Selectivity may be lost with high doses of beta1 selective antagonists.

INOTROPIC AGENTS

Classes within this group include cardiac glycosides, phosphodiesterase inhibitors, and sympathomimetics (dopamine and dobutamine) discussed at the beginning of this chapter.

Cardiac Glycosides
- Drugs within class
  - Digitalis
  - Digitoxin (Crystodigin®)
  - Digoxin (Lanoxin®)

Mechanisms of Action
Cardiac glycosides act by inhibiting the enzyme Na+/K+ adenosine triphosphatase ([ATPase] "the sodium pump"), which is responsible for maintaining the resting membrane potential of nerve and muscle cells.

Pharmacological Effects
- Inhibition of the sodium pump increases sodium and calcium influx during the cardiac action potential. Thus, the cardiac glycosides allow more calcium to enter myocardial cells during depolarization, resulting in the following effects:
  - Increased force of contraction of the heart (positive inotropic effect), increased cardiac output, and increased renal perfusion
  - Decreased heart rate (negative chronotropic effect) caused by decreased rate of repolarization (increased duration of the "plateau phase" of the cardiac action potential) and from indirect stimulation of the vagal nerve
  - Decreased conduction velocity through the atrioventricular (AV) node
  - ECG can show the "dig effect," which is slurring of the ST segment in all leads. This does not indicate toxicity and may be seen after just one dose.

Therapeutic Uses
- Treatment of HF
- Treatment of atrial flutter, atrial fibrillation, and paroxysmal atrial tachycardia (PAT)

Adverse Effects
- CV: Cardiac effects are the most dangerous and include premature ventricular contractions (PVC), dysrhythmia, and bradycardia.
- GI: Nausea, vomiting, and anorexia are caused by central stimulation of the chemoreceptor trigger zone (CTZ), an area of the brainstem responsible for producing nausea and vomiting.
- CNS: Neurologic effects include the presence of yellow-green halos in the visual field, headaches, fatigue, confusion, and depression.
- Toxicity and drug interactions
  - Factors influencing toxicity
    - Electrolyte imbalances (decreased potassium levels potentiate toxicity because potassium competes with cardiac glycosides for binding to Na+/K+ ATPase)
    - Renal (digoxin) and hepatic (digitoxin) insufficiency
  - Treatment of digitalis-related toxicity
    - Decontamination (emesis)
    - Continuous monitoring of plasma potassium levels
    - Administration of antidysrhythmics such as phenytoin (Dilantin®) or lidocaine if necessary
    - Administration of digitalis antibodies (digoxin immune Fab [Digibind®])
  - Pharmacokinetic drug interactions
    - Examples of drugs that decrease the effect of digoxin are antacids, cholestyramine, neomycin, and sulfasalazine.
    - Examples of drugs that increase the effect of digoxin are albuterol, amiodarone, captopril, cyclosporine, diltiazem, erythromycin, nifedipine, omeprazole, tetracycline, and thyroxine.

Contraindications
- Ventricular tachycardia or fibrillation
- Heart block
- Idiopathic hypertrophic subaortic stenosis
- Acute MI
- Wolff-Parkinson-White (WPW) syndrome

Nursing Implications
- Digoxin is the drug within this class most often used to treat HF.
  - Rapid onset of action
  - Available for parenteral and oral use
- Digitoxin is only available in the oral form and has a slow onset of action and a long duration, making it less useful than digoxin in managing acute HF. Digitoxin is metabolized by the liver and can reach toxic levels in patients with diminished liver function.
- Cardiac glycosides have a very narrow margin of safety (that is, the therapeutic dose is very close to the toxic dose), so extreme care must be taken when using these drugs. Periodic blood levels should be determined to assure appropriate dosing.

Phosphodiesterase Inhibitors
- Drugs within class
  - Amrinone (Inocor®)
  - Milrinone (Primacor®)

Mechanisms of Action
- Inhibit phosphodiesterase, the enzyme responsible for the inactivation of the second messengers cAMP and cGMP. These second messengers mediate calcium levels within the cell.
- By blocking phosphodiesterase metabolism, these agents increase calcium levels within the myocardial cell.

Pharmacological Effects
- Increased intracellular calcium causes a stronger contraction, thus increasing cardiac output with little or no effect on heart rate or blood pressure.
- Although the acute effects are beneficial in some patients, the toxicity of these agents prevents their long-term use.

Therapeutic Uses
Treatment of decompensated HF in patients who do not respond to conventional HF therapy (digoxin, diuretics, and vasodilators)

Adverse Effects
- CV: dysrhythmia
- GI: nausea and vomiting (high incidence), liver enzyme changes
- Heme: thrombocytopenia (TCP), bone marrow toxicity

Contraindications
- Aortic or pulmonary valvular disease
- Acute MI
- Ventricular dysrhythmia

Nursing Implications
- Use caution with older adults because they are more likely to develop adverse effects.
- Life support equipment should be available in case of severe reaction to drug or development of ventricular dysrhythmia.
- Assure accurate dosing because these drugs are given intravenously (IV) only.
- May be used as continuous IV therapy at home for the end-stage heart failure patient or someone awaiting transplant. Patients should know that these drugs treat symptoms but increase the risk of dysrhythmic death.

ANTIDYSRHYTHMICS

Classes and drugs within this group are listed in Table 15–3.

Mechanisms of Action
- Class I antidysrhythmic drugs block sodium channels to varying degrees.
- Class II drugs are beta-adrenergic receptor antagonists.
- Class III drugs block potassium efflux during repolarization.
- Class IV agents are calcium channel blockers.
- Digitalis and related compounds slow conduction velocity (discussed with cardiac glycosides).
- Adenosine is an endogenous nucleoside that activates adenosine receptors. The mechanism of action of adenosine involves enhanced potassium conductance and inhibition of camp-induced calcium influx.

Pharmacological Effects
- Class IA antidysrhythmic drugs have moderate potency for activated sodium channel blockade and prolonging repolarization, thus lengthening the refractory period between action potentials.
  - Class IA drugs have little effect on sinoatrial (SA) node automaticity, while most other antidysrhythmics reduce SA node automaticity. (Automaticity occurs when one or more regions of the heart are beating asynchronously with the rest of the heart.)
    - Class IB agents block both activated and inactivated sodium channels and shorten action potential duration.
    - Class IC agents are the most potent sodium channel blockers and have limited effects on repolarization.
    - Class II agents decrease heart rate and SA automaticity.
    - Class III agents block potassium channels, thus prolonging repolarization and slowing the conduction rate of the heart.
    - Class IV agents are calcium channel antagonists, causing a depression of depolarization and prolongation of repolarization, which acts to slow automaticity and conduction.
    - Adenosine can produce a bradycardia that is resistant to atropine, and it depresses SA automaticity, conduction velocity, and AV nodal conduction.
  - Administration of adenosine could be considered the pharmacological "shocking" of the heart.

Table 15–3. Antidysrhythmic Drug Classification and Major Therapeutic Uses

Class	Drugs	Therapeutic Uses
IA	Quinidine (Cardioquin®, etc.)	Atrial dysrhythmias, ventricular tachycardia
	Procainamide (Pronestyl®)	Atrial dysrhythmias, WPW, life-threatening ventricular dysrhythmias
	Moricizine (Ethmozine®)	Life-threatening ventricular dysrhythmias
	Disopyramide (Norpace®)	Life-threatening ventricular dysrhythmias
IB	Lidocaine (Xylocaine®)	Life-threatening ventricular dysrhythmias, WPW
	Tocainamide* (Tonocard®)	Life-threatening ventricular dysrhythmias
	Mexiletine* (Mexitil®)	Life-threatening ventricular dysrhythmias
	Phenytoin (Dilantin®)	Digitalis-induced dysrhythmias
IC	Flecainamide (Tambocor®)	Ventricular dysrhythmias, prevention of PAT
	Propafenone (Rythmol®)	Ventricular dysrhythmias, prevention of PAT
II	Propranolol (Inderal®)	Atrial dysrhythmias, sinus tachycardia, AV reentry, WPW
	Acebutolol (Sectral®)	Premature ventricular contractions
	Esmolol (Brevibloc®)	Short-term or intraoperative management of supraventricular tachycardia
III	Bretylium (Bretylol®)	Ventricular tachycardia and as last resort for ventricular fibrillation
	Amiodarone (Cordarone®)	Life-threatening ventricular dysrhythmias
	Ibutilide (Corvert®)	Atrial fibrillation or flutter
	Sotalol† (Betapace®)	Ventricular tachycardia, life-threatening ventricular dysrhythmias
	Dofetilide (Tikosyn®)	Cardioversion of atrial fibrillation and flutter
IV	Verapamil (Calan, Isoptin®)	Atrial tachycardia, atrial flutter
	Diltiazem (Cardizem, etc. ®)	Atrial tachycardia, atrial flutter
Others	Digoxin (Lanoxin®)	Atrial fibrillation, atrial flutter, PAT
	Adenosine (Adenocard®)	PAT, ventricular tachycardia

Note. WPW = Wolff-Parkinson-White syndrome, PAT = paroxysmal atrial tachycardia.
*Mexiletine and tocainide are analogs of lidocaine with structures that have been modified to reduce first-pass hepatic metabolism (associated with lidocaine) to make chronic oral therapy effective.
†Sotalol is a nonselective beta blocker, but acts as a Class III antidysrhythmic that prolongs the action potential.

Therapeutic Uses

See Table 15–3.

Adverse Effects

- CV: All antidysrhythmic agents include the development of new dysrhythmia ("prodysrhythmia"), heart block, hypotension, vasodilation, and the potential for cardiac arrest.
- Some of the more notable, noncardiovascular side effects of individual antidysrhythmic agents are listed below.
    - Quinidine: nausea and vomiting are common; quinidine syncope, hypersensitivity, hemolytic anemia, anticholinergic effects, "cinchonism" (tinnitus, headache, blurred vision)
    - Procainamide: hypersensitivity, systemic lupus-like syndrome (arthralgia and arthritis)
    - Moricizine: orthostatic dizziness, euphoria, perioral numbness
    - Lidocaine: agitation, disorientation, paraesthesia, tremor, lightheadedness, slurred speech, seizures
    - Tocainamide: bone marrow suppression
    - Propranolol: bronchospasm; see beta-adrenergic receptor antagonists
    - Amiodarone: photosensitivity, ophthalmic deposits, skin color changes, pulmonary infiltrates, liver infiltrates, thyroid dysfunction. Amiodarone may have effects for many months after discontinuation because of its extremely long half-life.
    - Verapamil: constipation, lassitude, nervousness, peripheral edema
    - Adenosine: shortness of breath, flushing, headache, nausea, paresthesia

Contraindications

- Contraindicated with allergy, bradycardia, sick sinus syndrome, AV block, shock, hypotension, and respiratory depression
- Use with caution in patients with HF. Only amiodarone and sotalol are advised for use in HF.

Nursing Implications

- Continually monitor cardiac rhythm when initiating therapy or changing dose to detect potentially serious adverse effects and to evaluate drug effectiveness.
- Arrange for periodic monitoring of cardiac rhythm when the patient is on long-term therapy to evaluate the effects on cardiac status.
- Maintain life support equipment on standby to treat adverse reactions that might occur.
- Give parenteral forms only if the oral form is not feasible; convert to an oral form as soon as possible to decrease potential for adverse effects.
- Consult the prescriber to reduce the dosage in patients with renal or hepatic insufficiency.

VASODILATORS

The three main classes of drugs used in the treatment of angina are beta blockers, calcium channel blockers, and direct-acting vasodilators (nitrates and nitrites). Because beta blockers and calcium channel blockers are discussed elsewhere within this chapter, the emphasis of this section will be on the direct-acting vasodilators used in the treatment of angina, as well as vasodilators used in the treatment of hypertension and afterload reduction. Classes within the vasodilator group are anti-anginal vasodilators (nitrates and nitrites) and antihypertensive vasodilators.

Anti-Anginal Vasodilators (Nitrates and Nitrites)
- Drugs within class
  - Amyl nitrite (Aspirols®, Vaporole®)
  - Isosorbide dinitrate (Isordil®, Sorbitrate®)
  - Isosorbide mononitrate (Imdur®, Ismo®, Monoket®)
  - Nitroglycerin (Nitrobid®, Nitrostat®, Nitrong®, Nitro-Dur®, Nitrol®, Nitrogard®)

Mechanisms of Action
- Nitrates and nitrites directly relax all types of vascular smooth muscle (from large arteries to large veins) by releasing nitric oxide, a potent vasodilator.

Pharmacological Effects
- Vasodilators increase coronary blood flow by relaxing coronary blood vessels, leading to an increase in the supply of oxygen to myocardial cells.
  - Because coronary heart disease causes stiffening and decreased responsiveness in coronary arteries, nitrates probably have little effect on increasing blood flow through these vessels.
  - Nitrates do, however, increase blood flow through healthy coronary arteries.
- Vasodilators decrease cardiac oxygen demand and workload by decreasing venous return (preload) and peripheral resistance (afterload).
- Vasodilators relax all types of smooth muscle, but have practically no direct effect on cardiac or skeletal muscle.

Therapeutic Uses
- Nitroglycerin is the most commonly used anti-anginal agent and is useful in treating all types of angina.
- Isosorbide is used for prophylaxis of angina and is not used for acute attacks.
- Amyl nitrate is used as an inhalant in the treatment of acute attacks, with an onset of action of about 30 seconds.
- In addition, the utility of nitrates and nitrites to relieve pulmonary congestion and to increase cardiac output in HF is well-established.

Adverse Effects
- CV: hypotension, rebound tachycardia, bradycardia, flushing, and sweating
- CNS: throbbing headache, and dizziness
- Other: nausea, vomiting, incontinence, and contact dermatitis

Contraindications
- Head trauma
- Cerebral hemorrhage
- Pregnancy and lactation

Nursing Implications
- Bioavailability of the traditional oral nitrates is very low. The sublingual route, which avoids the first-pass effect, is therefore preferred for achieving a therapeutic blood level rapidly.
- Sublingual or buccal preparations produce a fizzing or burning sensation, which indicates potency.
- Ensure that translingual spray is used under the tongue and not inhaled.
- With continuous exposure to nitrates, smooth muscle may develop complete tolerance (tachyphylaxis), and patients may become more tolerant when long-acting preparations (oral, transdermal) or continuous intravenous infusions are used for more than a few hours without interruption.
  - Transdermal nitrates should be discontinued during the night (or at another nitrate-free interval of approximately 12 hours) to prevent tolerance development.
  - Increasing the dose of nitrates also can overcome tolerance.
  - Transdermal nitrates should be applied in areas with good perfusion. However, if it is prescribed for peripheral vascular disease, it may be applied for a more local effect in areas of poor perfusion or with vasospastic disorders (e.g., Raynaud's phenomenon).

Antihypertensive Vasodilators
- Drugs within class
  - Diazoxide (Hyperstat®)
  - Minoxidil (Loniten®)
  - Fenoldopam (Corlopam®)
  - Nitroprusside (Nipride®)
  - Hydralazine (Apresoline®)
  - Tolazoline (Priscoline®)

Mechanisms of Action
- These agents act directly on vascular smooth muscle.
- All vasodilators used in hypertension produce direct relaxation of the arterioles. Nitroprusside also relaxes the veins.

Pharmacological Effects
- Decreased arteriolar resistance and decreased arterial blood pressure elicit compensatory responses, mediated by baroreceptors and the sympathetic nervous system, as well as the renin-angiotensin-aldosterone system.
  - These compensatory responses oppose the antihypertensive effect of vasodilators. Because sympathetic reflexes are intact, antihypertensive vasodilator therapy usually does not cause orthostatic hypotension or sexual dysfunction.
- Vasodilators work best in combination with other antihypertensive drugs that oppose the compensatory cardiovascular responses.

Therapeutic Uses
- Hypertension
- Hypertensive crisis (nitroprusside, diazoxide, fenoldopam)
- Pulmonary hypertension in the newborn (tolazoline)
- Hydralazine often is combined with isosorbide dinitrate to provide a balanced vasodilatation reducing preload and afterload in heart failure or hypertension.

Adverse Effects
- CV: sweating, flushing, edema, dizziness, hypotension, and reflex tachycardia
- CNS: throbbing headache
- Other
    - Systemic lupus-like syndrome (hydralazine)
    - Hypertrichosis (increased hair growth; minoxidil)
    - Nitroprusside can increase thiocyanate levels, and therefore should be used with caution in patients with renal failure.

Contraindications
- Pregnancy and lactation
- Use with caution with peripheral vascular disease, coronary heart disease (CHD), HF, or tachycardia

Nursing Implications
- Monitor BP closely during administration to evaluate for effectiveness and to ensure quick response if BP falls rapidly or too much.
- Monitor carefully in any situation that might lead to reduced fluid volume (e.g., excessive sweating, vomiting, diarrhea, dehydration).

Natriuretic Peptide
- There is only one drug in this class: nesiritide (Natrecor®). It is a recombinant drug derived from *E. coli.*

Mechanisms of Action
Increases cGMP, resulting in smooth muscle relaxation and vasodilation of arteries and veins

Pharmacological Effects
- Vasodilation results in lowering of preload and reduced pulmonary artery occlusive pressure.
    - The drug is administered as a continuous intravenous infusion.
    - The effect is quickly obtained and the half-life is 18 minutes.

Therapeutic Uses
Reduces the dyspnea associated with heart failure exacerbations.

Adverse Effects
- Caution should be taken with this drug because hypotension may occur, but it is generally not as frequent or severe as what might occur with other intravenous vasodilators.

Contraindications
- Hypotension
- Cardiogenic shock
- Hypersensitivity

Nursing Implications
- This drug is generally used in the ICU but it has been given in the step-down unit (SDU).
- In the past, this drug was used for outpatient infusion and safety is established.
- Dyspnea, blood pressure perfusion, and output should be monitored.

CALCIUM CHANNEL BLOCKERS (CCB)

Drugs Within Class
See Table 15–4.

Mechanism of Action
- These agents act by antagonizing L-type calcium channels in both smooth and cardiac muscle. There are three different classes of calcium channel blockers.
  - Diphenylalkylamines: Verapamil is the only drug available in the United States in this class. It has significant effects on cardiac and vascular smooth muscle.
  - Benzodiazepines: Diltiazem is the only drug available in the United States in this class. It also affects cardiac and vascular smooth muscles with less negative inotropic effect.
  - Dihydropyridine: Nifedipine was the first generation but more second-generation drugs in this class are now available. These drugs have greater affinity for vascular calcium channels than for cardiac cells and thus are used for hypertension treatment.

Pharmacological Effects
- Marked reduction in transmembrane calcium current
  - Long-lasting relaxation in smooth muscle
  - Reduced contractility, decreased SA pacemaker rate, and decreased AV conduction velocity in heart.

Therapeutic Uses, Adverse Effects, and Contraindications
See Table 15–4.

Table 15–4. Therapeutic Uses and Special Considerations of Calcium Channel–Blocking Drugs

	Trade Name	Therapeutic Uses	Adverse Effects and Contraindications
Amlodipine	Norvasc®	Prinzmetal angina, chronic angina, hypertension, HF	Headache, dysrhythmias, edema, bleeding gums
Bepridil	Vascor®	Chronic, stable angina	Serious dysrhythmia, agranulocytosis, dizziness, nausea
Diltiazem	Cardizem®	Prinzmetal angina, chronic angina, exercise flushing, bradycardia-associated angina, hypertension, Raynaud's phenomenon, atrial tachycardia, atrial flutter	Serious dysrhythmia, dizziness
Felodipine	Plendil®	Hypertension, Raynaud's phenomenon, HF	Dizziness, headache
Isradipine	DynaCirc®	Hypertension	Headache, fatigue
Nicardipine	Cardene®	Chronic, stable angina; hypertension	Dysrhythmia, severe GI upset, edema, headache, constipation
Nifedipine	Adalat® Procardia®	Prinzmetal angina, chronic angina, hypertension	Dysrhythmia, tachycardia, GI upset, edema, dizziness, flushing, constipation
Nimodipine	Nimotop®	Subarachnoid hemorrhage	Headache, diarrhea
Nisoldipine	Sular®	Hypertension	Dysrhythmia, GI upset, edema, dizziness, flushing, constipation
Verapamil	Calan® Isoptin®	Prinzmetal angina, chronic angina, unstable preinfarction angina, hypertension, atrial tachycardia, atrial flutter	Hypotension, myocardial depression, constipation, edema; do not use with any heart block; has strong negative inotropic effects

Nursing Implications
- Monitor blood pressure very carefully if the patient is also on nitrates or beta blockers because there is increased risk of hypotensive episodes.
- Provide comfort measures to help the patient tolerate drug effects, including small, frequent meals, and access to bathroom facilities if GI upset is severe. Institute preventive dietary measures to reduce constipation.
- Monitor for edema resulting from vasodilation.
- Monitor for AV block if taking verapamil.

DRUGS INFLUENCING THE RENIN-ANGIOTENSIN-ALDOSTERONE SYSTEM

Classes within this group: angiotensin converting enzyme (ACE) inhibitors; angiotensin II antagonists, and a new renin inhibitor. Also, beta blockers, which were discussed previously, will inhibit the release of renin from the kidney by blocking beta1 receptors in that organ. Spironolactone and eplerenone block aldosterone and these drugs are discussed in the section on diuretics.

ACE Inhibitors (ACE-I)
- Drugs within class
  - Benazepril (Lotensin®)
  - Moexipril (Univasc®)
  - Captopril (Capoten®)
  - Perindopril (Aceon®)
  - Enalapril (Vasotec®)
  - Quinipril (Accupril®)
  - Fosinopril (Monopril®)
  - Ramipril (Altace®)
  - Lisinopril (Prinivil®, Zestril®)
  - Trandolapril (Mavik®)

Mechanisms of Action
These drugs inhibit the converting enzyme that hydrolyzes angiotensin I to angiotensin II and that inactivates bradykinin, a potent vasodilator.

Pharmacological Effects
- Inhibits the renin-angiotensin system
  - Blocks the formation of angiotensin II, a potent vasoconstrictor
  - Blocks the release of aldosterone from the adrenal glands, thus decreasing sodium and water reabsorption in the kidneys
- Stimulates the kallikrein-kinin system
  - By inhibiting ACE, increases bradykinin
  - Bradykinin is a vasodilator
- Cumulative effect of ACE inhibition is a decrease in BP

Therapeutic Uses
- Primary therapeutic use is in the treatment of hypertension.
- Particularly useful in treating patients with diabetic nephropathy because ACE inhibitors diminish proteinuria and stabilize renal function (even in the absence of lowering of blood pressure).
  - These benefits probably result from improved intrarenal hemodynamics, with decreased glomerular efferent arteriolar resistance and a resulting reduction of intraglomerular capillary pressure.
- Extremely useful in the treatment of HF and after MI.
  - ACE inhibitors result in better preservation of left ventricular function in the years following MI by reducing postinfarction remodeling.

Adverse Effects
- Hypotension
- Glomerular damage, acute renal failure, hyperkalemia
- Dry cough (resulting from increased bradykinin and substance P
  - Dry cough is sometimes accompanied by wheezing but is usually only a nuisance, not a problem.
- Agranulocytosis
- GI upset, skin rash, or other hypersensitivities
- Pay particular attention to the possibility of angioedema development, which can occur either early after starting the drug or many years later.
  - Angioedema begins with swelling of the dermis and subcutaneous tissue of the face and tongue, and can progress to airway blockage over minutes to hours. It is a medical emergency.
  - If angioedema occurs, the patient should never be on any ACE inhibitors again and some recommend avoiding any angiotensin receptor blockers (ARBs) or a renin inhibitor.

Contraindications
Second and third trimesters of pregnancy, because of the risk of fetal hypotension, anuria, and renal failure, sometimes associated with fetal malformations or death

Nursing Implications
- All of the ACE inhibitors except fosinopril and moexipril are eliminated primarily by the kidneys; doses of renally excreted ACE-I should be reduced in patients with renal insufficiency.
- Monitor the patient carefully in any situation that might lead to decreased fluid volume (e.g., excessive sweating, vomiting, diarrhea, dehydration) to detect and treat excessive hypotension that may occur.
- Potassium and renal function should be monitored periodically.
- Teach patients the signs of angioedema and that it requires prompt attention by calling EMS.

Angiotensin II Receptor Antagonists (ARBs)
- Drugs within class
  - Candesartan (Atacand®)
  - Losartan (Cozaar®)
  - Eprosartan (Teveten®)
  - Telmisartan (Micardis®)
  - Irbesartan (Avapro®)
  - Valsartan (Diovan®)

Mechanisms of Action
- Block angiotensin II receptors (specifically blocking a subtype of angiotensin II receptor known as AT1)
- No effect on bradykinin metabolism and therefore more selective than ACE inhibitors

Pharmacological Effects
- By blocking AT1 receptors in blood vessels and in the adrenal cortex, angiotensin II antagonists block the pressor and aldosterone-releasing effects of angiotensin II, resulting in decreased blood pressure caused by a decrease in both peripheral resistance and blood volume.
- Because the angiotensin II antagonists do not alter the levels of bradykinin, patients may escape the cough and other related side effects of ACE inhibition.

Therapeutic Uses
- Hypertension
- In place of an ACE-I if a patient with HF is not able to tolerate an ACE-I

Adverse Effects
- GI upset, dry mouth, tooth pain
- Headaches, dizziness
- Some cough
- Dry skin, alopecia
- Angioedema can occur, but it is has a lower incidence than found with ACE-I.

Contraindications
- Second and third trimesters of pregnancy because of associated fetal malformations or death

Nursing Implications
- Administer with food to decrease GI distress if necessary.
- Monitor the patient carefully in any situation that might lead to decreased fluid volume (e.g., excessive sweating, vomiting, diarrhea, dehydration) to detect and treat excessive hypotension.
- Potassium and renal function should be monitored periodically.
- Teach patients the signs of angioedema and that it requires prompt attention by calling EMS.

Selective Renin Inhibitor
There is only one drug in this category: aliskiren (Tekturna®).

Mechanisms of Action
- Blocks renin receptors
- Reduces plasma renin level

Pharmacological Effects
- Reduces catecholamines
- Lowers blood pressure

Therapeutic Uses
- Hypertension
- It can be combined with other antihypertensives including ACE-I and ARBs.

Adverse Effects
- Diarrhea
- Cough
- Angioedema has been noted but the incidence is less than with other drugs in this category.
- Hyperkalemia is more common when combined with another drug from this group.

Contraindications
- Pregnancy
- Renal insufficiency

Nursing Implications
- Encourage fiber in the diet. Administer with food to decrease GI distress if necessary.
- Potassium and renal function should be monitored periodically.
- Teach patients the signs of angioedema and that it requires prompt attention by calling EMS.

Aldosterone Antagonists

Spironolactone and eplerenone are two drugs that block aldosterone and are classified as potassium-sparing diuretics. They are discussed in the next section. Both drugs are useful in the management of heart failure.

DIURETICS

See Table 15–5 for classes and drugs within this group.

Mechanisms of Action
- Diuretics prevent cells lining the tubules of the nephron from reabsorbing sodium ions from the glomerular filtrate.
  - As a result, sodium and other ions (and therefore water) are lost in the urine instead of being reabsorbed into the blood.
- Each class of diuretic drugs works at a slightly different site in the nephron, and therefore produces effects by a slightly different mechanism.
- The specific mechanisms of each of the diuretic classes are listed below.
  - Thiazide diuretics inhibit sodium and chloride reabsorption in the distal convoluted tubule of the nephron. The resulting loss of sodium, chloride, and potassium causes an increase in urine output. Sodium loss also decreases the glomerular filtration rate. These agents are associated with a moderate potassium loss.
  - Loop diuretics inhibit sodium and chloride reabsorption from the thick ascending limb of the loop of Henle. The resulting loss of sodium, chloride, and potassium causes an increase in urine output. These agents are powerful and associated with a high potassium loss.

Table 15–5. Diuretic Drug Classification and Major Therapeutic Uses

Class	Drugs	Therapeutic Uses
Thiazide Diuretics	Bendroflumethiazide (Naturetin®) Benzthiazide (Exna®) Chlorothiazide (Diuril®) Chlorthalidone (Hygroton®) Hydrochlorothiazide (Hydrodiuril®, etc.) Hydroflumethiazide (Diucardin®) Indapamide (Lozol®) Methyclothiazide (Enduron®) Metolazone (Mykrox®) Polythiazide (Renese®) Quinethazone (Hydromox®) Trichlormethiazide (Diurese®)	HF, hypertension, edema
Loop Diuretics	Bumetanide (Bumex®) Ethacrynic Acid (Edecrin®) Furosemide (Lasix®) Torsemide (Demadex®)	HF; pulmonary edema; hypertension; edema from HF, renal, or liver disease
Potassium-Sparing Diuretics	Amiloride (Midamor®) Spironolactone (Aldactone®) Triamterine (Dyrenium®)	Hypertension; edema from HF, renal, or liver disease; replacement diuretic if patient develops hypokalemia
Osmotic Diuretics	Glycerin (Osmoglyn®) Mannitol (Osmitrol®)	Intracranial pressure, brain edema

- Potassium-sparing diuretics increase sodium excretion and decrease potassium secretion from the distal convoluted tubule. These agents are associated with less potassium loss compared to the thiazide and loop diuretics.
- Osmotic diuretics inhibit sodium and water reabsorption from the proximal convoluted tubule and descending limb of the loop of Henle.
- Carbonic anhydrase inhibitors are rarely used as diuretics. They are, however, useful in treating glaucoma and in preventing altitude sickness. The only drug in this category is acetazolamide (Diamox®). It is not included in the table because it has little use as a cardiovascular medication.

Pharmacological Effects

The net result of diuresis is a decrease in intravascular volume, resulting in decreased BP and decreased workload of the heart (from decreased stroke volume and cardiac output).

Therapeutic Uses

See Table 15–5.

Adverse Effects
- The most common adverse effects are imbalances in electrolytes and fluids, hypotension, oliguria, anuria, and dizziness.
- Specific adverse effects of each of the diuretic classes are listed below.
  - Thiazide diuretics: hypokalemia, hyponatremia, hypocalcemia, hyperglycemia, hyperuricemia, GI distress
  - Loop diuretics: hypokalemia; hyponatremia; hypocalcemia; dehydration with elevation of creatinine; hyperglycemia; hyperuricemia; and ototoxicity resulting in hearing loss, GI distress, and tolerance
  - Potassium-sparing diuretics: hyperkalemia, some hyponatremia, glucose intolerance in patients with diabetes, gynecomastia, GI distress
  - Osmotic diuretics: dehydration, electrolyte imbalance

Contraindications
Thiazides and loop diuretics should be used with caution with renal disease, hypokalemia, dysrhythmia, glucose intolerance, and gout.

Nursing Implications
- Use of the potassium-sparing diuretic triamterene may cause the urine to turn blue.
- Administer these agents early in the day so increased urination will not interfere with sleep. Loop diuretics often are administered in divided doses about 5 to 6 hours apart.
- Monitor the dose carefully and reduce the dosage of one or both drugs if administered with an antihypertensive drug.
- Patients can develop tolerance to loop diuretics over time. Furosemide has the lowest bioavailability.
- Braking can occur with loop diuretics, meaning that as higher doses are needed, the rennin-angiotensin-aldosterone response is enhanced in an attempt to hold more fluid.
- Provide a potassium-rich or potassium-poor diet as appropriate for the administered drug to maintain electrolyte balance. Electrolyte and renal function should be monitored periodically.

ANTICOAGULANT, ANTITHROMBOTIC (ANTIPLATELET), AND THROMBOLYTIC (FIBRINOLYTIC) DRUGS

Classes within this group are anticoagulants, antithrombotics, and thrombolytic (fibrinolytic) drugs. Anticoagulant and antithrombotic drugs play an important role in the prevention of thrombus during an acute event or chronic use in high-risk people. Thrombolytics are used in an acute situation to lyse a clot.

Anticoagulants
- Drugs within class
  - Antithrombin III (Thrombate III®)
  - Heparin (Liquaemin®)
  - Lepirudin (Refludan®)
  - Warfarin (Coumadin®)
  - Danaparoid (Orgaran®)

- Low molecular weight (LMW) heparins: ardeparin (Normiflo®), dalteparin (Fragmin®), enoxaparin (Lovenox®), tinzaparin (Innohep®)
- Argatroban (Acova®)
- Bivalirudin (Angiomax®)

Mechanisms of Action
- Antithrombin III is a naturally occurring clotting inhibitor.
- Heparin is a naturally occurring protein that inhibits the conversion of prothrombin to thrombin, thus blocking the conversion of fibrinogen to fibrin, the final step in clot formation.
- Lepirudin is a recombinant hirudin (leech polypeptide) that directly inhibits thrombin formation.
- LMW heparins inhibit thrombus and clot formation by blocking factors Xa and IIa.
- Warfarin acts by interfering with the formation of vitamin K–dependent clotting factors in the liver.
- Bivalirudin is a synthetic, reversible, direct thrombin inhibitor given intravenously.

Pharmacological Effects
The eventual effect of all anticoagulants is a depletion of clotting factors (or inhibition of their formation or activity) and a prolongation of clotting times.

Therapeutic Uses
- Antithrombin III is used in patients with hereditary antithrombin III deficiency who are undergoing surgery or obstetric procedures that might put them at risk for thromboembolism.
- Heparin is indicated for acute treatment and prevention of venous thrombosis and pulmonary embolism; treatment of atrial fibrillation with embolization; prevention of clotting in blood samples and dialysis and venous tubing; and diagnosis and treatment of disseminated intravascular coagulation (DIC), as well as an adjunct in the treatment of MI and stroke.
- Lepirudin and argatroban are used for anticoagulation in patients with heparin-induced thrombocytopenia (HIT).
- Bivalirudin also protects against HIT and is growing in popularity as an intravenous anticoagulant during percutaneous coronary intervention (PCI).
- LMW heparins are used for the prophylaxis or treatment of deep venous thrombosis and pulmonary emboli.
- Warfarin is used to treat patients with atrial fibrillation, artificial heart valves, or valvular damage that makes them susceptible to thrombus or embolus formation.

Adverse Effects
- Bleeding, hemorrhage
- Nausea, GI upset
- Thrombocyotopenia (TCP), hepatic dysfunction

Contraindications

- Conditions that could be compromised by increased bleeding tendencies; these include hemorrhagic disorders, recent trauma, spinal puncture, GI ulcers, recent surgery, intrauterine device placement, tuberculosis, the presence of indwelling catheters, and threatened abortion.
- Warfarin is contraindicated in pregnancy (if an anticoagulant must be used, use heparin only).
- Use with caution in HF, thyrotoxicosis, diarrhea (which could alter the normal clotting process by loss of vitamin K from the intestines), and fever (which could activate plasminogen).

Nursing Implications

- Warfarin's onset of action is about 3 days, and its effects last for about 5 days.
  - Because of this time delay, warfarin is not the drug of choice for acute situations, but is convenient and useful for prolonged effects.
  - A heparin bridge is needed until warfarin reaches therapeutic levels.
  - A bolus dose of warfarin is never recommended.
  - Two genetic factors can be used to predict patient response to warfarin and dosage needed to reach a therapeutic level. These tests are now available in labs that do genetic testing. While not widely done at this time, the Food and Drug Administration suggests that it be used and growth will increase as more testing sites and more rapid reporting of results is available.
    - CYP2C9 produces the enzymes responsible for metabolism of warfarin. People with polymorphisms in alleles 2 and 3 of CYP2C9 required much lower doses of warfarin to reach therapeutic level. These people have a higher risk of supratherapuetic International Normalized Ratio (INR) and higher risk of bleeding.
    - Vitamin K epoxide reductase complex 1 (VKROC) genetic mutation affects the metabolism of vitamin K, the antidote for warfarin. If the level of vitamin K in the blood is changed, it can alter the amount of warfarin needed.
  - Teach patients the importance of following the recommended schedule for INR monitoring with warfarin (at least monthly but more often with dose changes). Also, teach patients about dietary concerns related to vitamin K intake, which should remain stable.
  - Warfarin has documented drug–drug interactions with a vast number of drugs. It is wise practice never to add or remove a drug from the drug regimen of a patient receiving warfarin without careful patient monitoring and possible adjustment of the warfarin dosage to prevent serious adverse effects.
- Heparin is injected IV or subcutaneously (SC) and has an almost immediate onset of action.
- Maintain availability of antidotes to anticoagulants in case of overdose.
  - Protamine sulfate for heparin
  - Vitamin K for warfarin

Antithrombotic (Antiplatelet) Drugs

Drugs within class (see Table 15–6).

Table 15-6. Mechanism of Action and Therapeutic Uses of Antithrombotic and Antiplatelet Drugs

	Trade Name	Mechanism of Action	Therapeutic Uses
Abciximab	ReoPro®	Glycoprotein IIb/IIIa inhibitor; blocks platelet aggregation	Used to treat ischemia in high-risk patients; adjunct to percutaneous coronary intervention (PCI)
Aspirin Ibuprofen Sulfinpyrazone	Easpirin®, etc. Motrin®, etc. Anturane®	Cyclooxygenase inhibitor; inhibits formation of thromboxanes; blocks platelet aggregation	Reduction of risk of recurrent TIAs in males (aspirin only); reduction of risk of death or MI in patients with history of MI or unstable angina (aspirin only); reduction of emboli in rheumatic valve disease, atrial fibrillation
Clopidogrel	Plavix®	ADP receptor blockade; blocks ADP from binding to platelets; blocks platelet aggregation	Treatment of patients with high risk for ischemic events (history of MI, peripheral artery disease, stroke)
Dipyridamole	Persantine®	Phosphodiesterase inhibitor; increases cAMP, which potentiates prostacyclin (platelet aggregation inhibitor)	With warfarin to prevent thromboembolism; with aspirin to enhance life span of platelets in patients with thrombotic disease
Eptifibatide	Integrilin®	Glycoprotein IIb/IIIa inhibitor; blocks platelet aggregation	Treatment of acute coronary syndrome; prevention of cardiac ischemic complications; often used with heparin
Prasugrel	Effient®	Inhibits platelet activation and aggregation by irreversibly binding to P2Y12 class of ADP receptors on platelets	Acute coronary syndrome with stent placement
Ticlopidine	Ticlid®	ADP receptor blockade; blocks ADP from binding to platelets; blocks platelet aggregation	Prevention of thrombotic stroke, especially in patients intolerant of aspirin or ibuprofen
Tirofiban	Aggrastat®	Glycoprotein IIb/IIIa inhibitor; blocks platelet aggregation	With heparin to treat acute coronary syndrome; prevention of cardiac ischemic complications

Mechanisms of Action
- See Table 15–6.
  - The glycoprotein IIb/IIIa inhibitors block the receptors on the activated platelet strands of fibrin, prohibiting fibrinogen from attaching to the receptors and thus blocking the mesh formation of the fibrin clot. These drugs are used intravenously during acute interventions to prevent a clot.
  - Cyclooxygenase inhibitors (aspirin) are irreversible and prevent platelet activation. Because platelets have a life span of 7 to 10 days, it takes that long to rid the body of the effect.
  - Thienopyridines are oral agents that irreversibly prohibit the binding of adenosine diphosphate (ADP) to the glycoprotein IIb/IIIa receptor on the platelets, preventing platelets from binding with fibrinogen.

Pharmacological Effects
The end result of the various actions of all antithrombotic drugs is the inhibition of platelet aggregation.

Therapeutic Uses
See Table 15–6.

Adverse Effects
- Bleeding and hemorrhage. Some of the more notable, noncardiovascular side effects of some of the individual antithrombotic agents are listed below.
  - Aspirin, clopidogrel, prasugrel: GI ulceration
  - Dipyridamole: may worsen angina, dizziness, headache, syncope, GI upset, rash
  - Eptifibatide, tirofiban: headache, dizziness, thrombocytopenia purpura (TCP)
  - Ticlopidine: neutropenia, rash, nausea, diarrhea, and TCP
  - Abciximab: TCP

Contraindications
- Caution should be used in the following conditions:
  - Presence of any known bleeding disorder because of the risk of excessive blood loss
  - Recent surgery
  - Closed head injuries

Nursing Implications
- Provide comfort measures and analgesia for headache to relieve pain and improve compliance.
- Suggest safety measures, including the use of an electric razor and avoidance of contact sports.
- When chronic oral therapy is prescribed, teach patients that continued therapy is needed.

Thrombolytic (Fibrinolytic) Drugs

- Drugs within class
  - Alteplase (t-PA, Activase®)
  - Streptokinase (Streptase®)
  - Anistreplase (Eminase®)
  - Urokinase (Abbokinase®)
  - Reteplase (Retavase®)
  - TNK t-PA (TNKase®, Tenecteplase®)

Mechanisms of Action

- Streptokinase, urokinase, and anistreplase activate the conversion of plasminogen to plasmin and inhibit the formation of fibrin.
- Alteplase, tenecteplase, and reteplase are recombinant forms of tissue plasminogen activator (t-PA) and activate the conversion of fibrin-bound plasminogen to plasmin.

Pharmacological Effects

The production of plasmin causes the digestion of fibrin. The result is the degradation of fibrin clots to open up blood vessels and restore blood flow to the dependent tissue.

Therapeutic Uses

- Lysis of thrombi in ischemic, but not necrotic, coronary arteries after infarction, acute MI, pulmonary embolism, deep venous thrombosis, occluded AV cannulas in dialysis patients, and peripheral artery thrombosis
- Lysis of thrombi in a cerebral vascular accident (CVA), after ensuring that there is no intracerebral bleeding

Adverse Effects

- Bleeding, bruising, anaphylaxis, hematoma
- Aminocaproic acid (Amicar®) is a fibrinolytic inhibitor that can be administered to antagonize the action of the thrombolytic drugs.

Contraindications

- These drugs should not be used with any conditions that could be compromised by dissolution of clots, including:
  - Recent surgery
  - Hemorrhage
  - Cerebrovascular accident within the past 2 months
  - Aneurysm
  - Obstetric delivery
  - Organ biopsy
  - Serious GI bleeding
  - Major trauma
  - Hypertension

Nursing Implications

- Evaluate the patient regularly for any sign of blood loss.
- Initiate treatment within 6 hours of the onset of symptoms of acute MI to achieve optimum therapeutic effectiveness.
- Initiate treatment within 3 hours of symptoms in a CVA.

ANTIHYPERLIPIDEMICS

Classes within group: resins (bile acid sequestrants), statins (HMG-CoA reductase inhibitors), cholesterol absorption inhibitors, niacin, fibric acid derivatives

Resins (Bile Acid Sequestrants)
- Drugs within class
    - Cholestyramine (Questran®)
    - Colestipol (Colestid®)
    - Colesevelam (WelChol®)

Mechanisms of Action
These agents act as bile acid sequestrants by forming an insoluble complex with bile salts that is excreted in the feces. The resulting low level of bile acids feeding back to the hepatic circulation stimulates the production of more bile acids. The body compensates by increasing liver low-density lipoprotein (LDL) receptors, removing LDL from the circulation, and oxidizing the cholesterol from LDL to form bile acids.

Pharmacological Effects
- Decrease LDL lipoprotein (15% to 30%)
- Increase HDL lipoprotein (3% to 5%)
- No effect on triglyceride

Therapeutic Uses
- Single-drug therapy should be evaluated before drug combinations are used.
- Second line in the treatment of hypercholesterolemia and hyperlipidemia; primarily used in those unable to take statins.
    - Provided that diet therapy has failed, these agents are used if LDL is above 160 mg/dL, or if LDL is above 130 mg/dL with the presence of two or more risk factors (e.g., obesity, poor diet, smoking, HDL below 40 mg/dL).
    - The LDL goal for people with coronary heart disease (CHD) or CHD equivalents and for people at highest risk for CHD is below 100 mg/dL.
    - Resins can be given to children 11 through 17 years of age.

Adverse Effects
- GI irritation, bloating, constipation
- Malabsorption of vitamins A, D, and K

Contraindications
- Hypertriglyceridemia, biliary obstruction, abnormal intestinal function
- Pregnancy and lactation (to avoid malabsorption of important vitamins)

Nursing Implications
- Do not administer powder in dry form; the drug must be mixed with fluids to be effective.
- Tablets must not be cut, chewed, or crushed. Tablets are designed to break down in the GI tract, and if the tablet is crushed the active ingredients will be ineffective.

Statins (3-Hydroxy–3-Methylglutaryl-Coenzyme-A [HMG-CoA] Reductase Inhibitors)

- Drugs within class
  - Atorvastatin (Lipitor®)
  - Pravastatin (Pravachol®)
  - Fluvastatin (Lescol®)
  - Simvastatin (Zocor®)
  - Lovastatin (Mevacor®)
  - Rosuvastatin (Crestor®)

Mechanisms of Action

- Competitive inhibition of HMG-CoA reductase
- HMG-CoA reductase catalyzes an early, rate-limiting step in cholesterol biosynthesis
- Depletion of intracellular cholesterol from the previous steps leads to an increase in the number of LDL receptors in an effort to bring more LDL to the cells. The increased number of receptors further decreases the serum level of LDL.
- Other therapeutic benefits include plaque stabilization, improvement of coronary endothelial function, inhibition of platelet function, and anti-inflammatory activity.

Pharmacological Effects

- The statins are the best-tolerated and most effective agents for treating dyslipidemia.
- Decrease LDL (18% to 55%)
- Increase HDL (5% to 15%)
- Higher doses of the more potent statins (atorvastatin, rosuvastatin) can also reduce triglyceride (7% to 30%).
- Generally, doubling a dose of a statin will result in another 7% to 9% reduction in LDL.

Therapeutic Uses

- Single-drug therapy should be evaluated before drug combinations are used. When statins are combined with a cholesterol absorption inhibitor, the reduction of LDL can be 23% to 25%.
- Treatment of hypertriglyceridemia, hypercholesterolemia, and hyperlipidemia
  - Provided that diet therapy has failed, these agents are used if LDL is above 160 mg/dL, or if LDL is above 130 mg/dL with the presence of two or more risk factors (e.g., obesity, poor diet, smoking, HDL below 40 mg/dL).
  - The LDL goal for people with CHD or CHD equivalents and for people at highest risk for CHD is below 100 mg/dL or below 70 mg/dL in those with the highest risk.

Adverse Effects

- Statins can cause liver dysfunction and increase liver transaminases. Therefore, a liver function test to measure alanine aminotransferase (ALT) is recommended at baseline and 3 to 6 months after initiation of therapy. If the ALT values are normal, it is not necessary to repeat the ALT test more than every 6 to 12 months. If ALT is greater than three to six times the upper limit of normal, the drug should be stopped.
- Statins can cause myopathy and rhabdomyolysis, both associated with myalgia and fatigue. These side effects can be severe, and prompted the removal of cerivastatin (Baycol®) from the market after the drug had been linked to rhabdomyolysis, particularly when used with gemfibrozil.
- These agents also can cause cataracts, hypersensitivities, and renal failure.

Contraindications
- Liver disease
- Pregnancy

Nursing Implications
- Administer the drug at bedtime for some of the statins (simvastatin, fluvastatin, lovastatin) because the highest rates of cholesterol synthesis occur between midnight and 5 a.m., and these drugs have a better effect at night.
- Arrange for periodic ophthalmic exams to monitor for cataract development.
- Monitor liver function tests prior to and periodically during therapy.
- Ensure that patients adhere to a cholesterol-lowering diet and an exercise plan in conjunction with the drug therapy. Patients should continue to limit their fat intake and to exercise routinely after drug therapy is initiated.
- Instruct patients to report muscle or joint pain.

Cholesterol Absorption Inhibitor
- There is only one drug in this category: ezetimibe (Zetia®). Ezetimibe is also available in combination with simvastatin (Vytorin®).

Mechanisms of Action
Inhibition of cholesterol absorption at the brushy border of the small intestine.

Pharmacological Effects
- Lowering of LDL by 17%
- Lowering of triglycerides by 6%
- Elevation of HDL by 1% to 2%
- When added to a statin, the additional lowering of LDL is 23%.

Therapeutic Uses
- Minimal effectiveness as a single-drug approach but may be useful if the person is intolerant of a statin.
- Synergistic effect with a statin can allow for better LDL goal attainment while reducing the risk of myopathy from higher doses of statins.
- Long-term studies have not demonstrated the benefit of reduced cardiac events.

Adverse Effects
Primarily GI distress

Contraindications
- Active liver disease
- Gallstones

Nursing Implications
- Ensure that patients adhere to a low-cholesterol diet and an exercise plan in conjunction with the drug therapy. Patients should continue to limit their fat intake and to exercise routinely after drug therapy is initiated.
  - Try different timing of drug administration to reduce GI distress.

Niacin
- Drugs within class
  - Niacin (nicotinic acid, Nicobid®, Niaspan®)

Mechanisms of Action
- Inhibits lipolysis of triglycerides in adipose tissue, which reduces the transport of free fatty acids to the liver and decreases hepatic triglyceride synthesis.
- Decreased triglyceride synthesis reduces very low density lipoprotein (VLDL) production by the liver, which results in reduced LDL levels.

Pharmacological Effects
- Best agent available for increasing HDL (increase of 15% to 35%)
- Lowers triglyceride (decrease of 20% to 50%)
- Lowers LDL (decrease of 5% to 25%)

Therapeutic Uses
- Single-drug therapy should be evaluated before drug combinations are used.
- Treatment of hypertriglyceridemia, hypercholesterolemia, and hyperlipidemia
  - Provided that diet therapy has failed, these agents are used if LDL is above 160 mg/dL, or if LDL is above 130 mg/dL with the presence of two or more risk factors.
  - The LDL goal for people with CHD or CHD equivalents and those at highest risk for CHD is below 100 mg/dL.

Adverse Effects
- Niacin can cause cutaneous flushing, pruritus or dry skin, hyperpigmentation, GI distress, liver dysfunction (transaminase activity should be monitored), abnormal glucose tolerance, and hyperuricemia. Flushing and dyspepsia are two of the most common adverse effects, limiting patient compliance with this drug.
  - Starting niacin at a low dose and increasing very gradually reduces the flushing.
  - Drugs designed to provide the niacin benefits but inhibit flushing are in developmental testing.

Contraindications
- Gout
- Pregnancy

Nursing Implications
- Oral nicotinamide (source of niacin in many vitamin supplements) does not affect lipid levels.
- The dose of niacin for antihyperlipidemic therapy is high: 1 to 2 grams per day or more.
- Flushing is worse when therapy is initiated or the dosage is increased, but after 1 or 2 weeks of a stable dose, most patients no longer flush.
- Taking an aspirin (30 minutes prior to taking niacin) alleviates the flushing in many patients.
- Flushing is more likely to occur when niacin is consumed with hot beverages or alcohol.
- Taking the niacin at bedtime may be helpful and improve tolerance of the drug.

Fibric Acid Derivatives

- Drugs within class
  - Clofibrate (Atromid-S®)
  - Fenofibrate (TriCor®)
  - Gemfibrozil (Lopid®)

Mechanisms of Action
Unclear

Pharmacological Effects
- Decrease VLDL synthesis, with subsequent decrease in LDL (decrease 5% to 20%)
- Reduce triglycerides (20% to 50%) by stimulating lipoprotein lipase activity
- Increase HDL levels (10% to 20%)

Therapeutic Uses
- Single-drug therapy should be evaluated before drug combinations are used.
- Treatment of hypertriglyceridemia, hypercholesterolemia, and hyperlipidemia
  - Provided that diet therapy has failed, these agents are used if LDL is above 160 mg/dL, or if LDL is above 130 mg/dL with the presence of two or more risk factors.
  - The LDL goal for people with CHD or CHD equivalents and those at highest risk for CHD is below 100 mg/dL.
  - Fibric acid derivatives are the drugs of choice for type III hyperlipidemia and hypertriglyceridemia.

Adverse Effects
- GI distress, rash, alopecia, fatigue, headache, impotence, and anemia
- A myositis flu-like syndrome also can occur.

Contraindications
Renal or liver failure

Nursing Implications
- Fibric acid derivatives have potential antiplatelet effects, so potential drug interactions need to be addressed.
- Gemfibrozil should not be combined, or used with extreme caution, with statins because of increased risk of rhabdomyolysis.

OTHER APPROACHES TO HYPERLIPIDEMIA

- Hormone replacement therapy as a treatment for hyperlipidemia or for cardioprotection is no longer recommended. Several large studies found no benefit and the Women's Health Initiative found a higher risk of thrombotic events occurring early in the therapy.
- Omega-6 fatty acids found in oily fish have been found to raise HLD and lower LDL. Supplements are available over the counter but vary in the strength of the active ingredients. These can be used in conjunction with other drugs.
- Plant stanols and sterols are dietary products that interfere with the intestinal uptake of cholesterol. Daily intake of 2 to 3 grams can reduce LDL by 6% to 15%.
- Exercise can increase HDL and lower LDL.
- Dietary intake of unblanched almonds (75 g per day) or walnuts can decrease LDL by 14% and raise HDL by 4%. Cranberry juice, pomegranate juice, and black teas have shown lipid improvements near that of almonds.

REFERENCES

Abdel-Latif, A., & Moliterna, D. J. (2009). Antiplatelet polypharmacy in primary percutaneous coronary intervention: Trying to understand when more is better. *Circulation, 119,* 3168–3170.

Adams, R. J., Albers, G., Alberts, M. J., Benavente, O., Furie, K., Goldstein, L. B., ... American Stroke Association. (2008). Update to the AHA/ASA recommendations for the prevention of stroke in patients with stroke and transient ischemic attack. *Stroke, 39*(5), 1647–1652.

Ayala, C., & Spellberg, B. (2007). *Pharmacology for the boards and wards* (2nd ed.). Philadelphia: Lippincott Williams & Wilkins.

Barkley, T. W., & Myers, C. M. (2008). *Practice guidelines for acute care nurse practitioners* (2nd ed.) St. Louis, MO: Elsevier Saunders.

Chen, K. Y., Rha, S. W., Podder, K. L., Jin, Z., Minami, Y., Wang, L., ... Korea Acute Myocardial Infarction Registry Investigators. (2009). Triple versus dial antiplatelet therapy in patients with acute ST segment elevation myocardial infarction undergoing primary percutaneous coronary intervention. *Circulation, 119,* 3207–3214.

Cole, T. A. (2009). Evidence for ACE inhibitor use in LV systolic dysfunction and heart failure. *American Journal for Nurse Practitioners, 13*(6), 21–31.

Crawford, M. H. (2009). *Cardiology: Current diagnosis and treatment.* New York: McGraw Hill.

DiPiro, J. T., Talbert, R.L., Yee, G. C., Matzke, G. R., Wells, B. G., & Posey, L. M. (2009). *Pharmacotherapy: A pathophysiologic approach* (7th ed.). Stamford, CT: Appleton Lange.

Edmunds, M. W., & Mayhew, M. S. (2009). *Pharmacology for primary care providers* (3rd ed.). Philadelphia: Elsevier Mosby.

Garavalia, L., Garavalia, B., Spertus, J. A., & Decker, C. (2009). Exploring patients' reasons for discontinuance of heart medications. *Journal of Cardiovascular Nursing, 24,* 371–379.

Golan, D., Tashijian, A. H., Armstrong, E., & Armstrong, A. (2008). *Principles of pharmacology: The pathophysiologic basis of drug therapy* (2nd ed.). Philadelphia: Lippincott Williams & Wilkins.

Gutierrez, K. (2008). *Pharmacotherapeutics: Clinical reasoning in primary care* (2nd ed.). St. Louis, MO: Saunders.

Hardman, J. G., & Limbird, L. E. (2009). *Goodman and Gilman's the pharmacological basis of therapeutics* (12th ed.). New York: McGraw-Hill.

Harvey, R. A., Champe, P. C., Finkel, R., Cubeddu, L. X., & Clark, M. A. (2009). *Lippincott's illustrated reviews: Pharmacology* (4th ed.). Philadelphia: Lippincott Williams & Wilkins.

Hirsch, J., Guyatt, G., Albers, G. W., Harrington, R., & Schunemann, H. J. (2008). Antithrombotic and thrombolytic therapy: Executive summary. *Chest, 133,* 71S–109S.

Holcomb, S. S. (2009). Common herb drug interactions: What you should know. *The Nurse Practitioner, 34*(5), 21–29.

Howe, L. A. (2009). Pharmacogenomics and management of cardiovascular disease. *The Nurse Practitioner, 34*(8), 28–35.

Katzung, B. G. (2007). *Basic and clinical pharmacology* (10th ed.). New York: McGraw-Hill.

Lindenauer, P. K., Pekow, P., Wang, K., Maidi, D. K., Gutierrez, B., & Benjamin, E. M. (2005). *New England Journal of Medicine, 353,* 349–361.

Moser, D., & Reigel, B. (2008). *Cardiac nursing: A companion to Braunwald's heart disease.* St. Louis, MO: Elsevier-Saunders.

Prudente, L. A. (2008). Quelling atrial chaos: Current approaches to managing atrial fibrillation. *American Nurse Today, 3*(8), 21–25.

Russell, J. A., Walley, K. R., Singer, J., Gordon, A. C., Herbert, P. C., Cooper, J., ... VASST Investigators. (2008). Vasopressin versus norepinephrine infusion in patients with septic shock. *New England Journal of Medicine, 358,* 877–887.

Woods, S. L., Sivarajan Froelicher, E. .S., Underhill Motzer, S., & Bridges, E. J. (2009). *Cardiac nursing* (6th ed.). Philadelphia: Lippincott.

Wynne, A. L., Woo, T. M., & Millard, M. (2007). *Pharmacotherapeutics for nurse practitioner prescribers* (2nd ed.). Philadelphia: F. A. Davis.

Zagaria, M. A. (2009). Renal dosing: Understanding glomerular filtration rate and estimating creatinine clearance. *American Journal of Nurse Practitioners, 13*(7), 32–35.

Zipes, D. P., Libby, P., Bonow, R. O., & Braunwald, E. (2009). *Braunwald's heart disease: A textbook of cardiovascular medicine* (8th ed.). Philadelphia: Elsevier-Saunders.

16

Special Situations

This chapter addresses some of the special situations encountered in cardiac and vascular nursing practice. It provides a brief overview of cardiac and vascular emergency conditions that often are treated in the emergency department or intensive care unit. Individual differences of race, ethnicity, and culture that influence cardiac and vascular nursing practice are described. Comorbid and concomitant conditions are discussed and the chapter concludes with a section on adults with congenital cardiac defects.

EMERGENCY CONDITIONS

Cardiac Arrest

Description
Sudden cessation of cardiac function that may be reversible if appropriate actions are taken but will lead to death if no intervention is initiated.

Etiology
- Ventricular fibrillation
- Bradydysrhythmia
- Asystole
- Sustained ventricular tachycardia

- Pulseless electrical activity
- Ventricular rupture
- Cardiac tamponade
- Acute disruption of blood flow

Risk Factors
- Coronary heart disease (CHD)
- Myocardial infarction (MI)
- Cardiac dysrhythmia
- Multiple conditions, including pericardial effusion, cardiac surgery, pulmonary embolism, and acute respiratory failure, may be risk factors for cardiac arrest.

Assessment
- History
  - Symptoms of chest pain, dyspnea, fatigue, and palpitations preceding arrest
  - Increased cardiac electrical ectopic activity, such as tachycardia and ventricular ectopy, prior to ventricular fibrillation
  - Symptoms of conditions associated with cardiac arrest before the event
- Physical findings
  - Loss of effective cardiac function
  - Loss of effective circulation (pulseless)
  - Loss of consciousness
- Diagnostic tests
  - Electrocardiography (ECG) to identify cardiac rhythm if present.

Management
- Nonpharmacologic
  - Assess that the collapse is because of cardiac arrest
  - Once confirmed, start basic life support (BLS) and activate the emergency medical system (EMS).
- Pharmacologic
  - Initiate advanced cardiac life support (ACLS) protocol based on the cause of the cardiac arrest or type of dysrhythmia

Outcomes and Follow-Up
- Predictors of outcomes
  - Prehospital care and admission to the hospital alive
    - Increased survival with the initiation of bystander cardiopulmonary resuscitation (CPR)
    - Increased survival with immediate defibrillation
- Predictors of in-hospital mortality
  - Before arrest: presence of hypotension, pneumonia, renal failure, cancer, or home-bound lifestyle
  - During arrest: duration of arrest longer than 15 minutes, intubation, hypotension, pneumonia, or home-bound lifestyle
  - After resuscitation: coma, need for vasopressors, or arrest duration of longer than 15 minutes

- Post cardiac arrest care
  - Acute MI: conventional treatment
  - Chronic CHD
    - Diagnostic testing: cardiac catheterization, angiography, stress testing, or imaging
    - Ischemic therapy: medical or surgical management
    - Electrophysiology evaluation: surgery, devices, medications
  - Nonischemic heart disease
    - Diagnostic testing: cardiac catheterization, angiography, stress testing, imaging, and electrophysiology evaluation (surgery, devices, medications), if indicated
    - Medical or surgical treatment
  - Nonstructural arrhythmogenic factors
    - Discontinue prodysrhythmic medications, correct electrolyte imbalance, and initiate treatment for hypoxemia
- Protocols for induced hypothermia post cardiac arrest have demonstrated improved outcomes if initiated as soon as stabilized post-arrest.
  - Protocols are initiated in the emergency department or intensive care unit (ICU). Unconscious adult patients with spontaneous circulation after out-of-hospital cardiac arrest should be cooled to 32° C to 34° C for 12 to 24 hours when the initial rhythm was ventricular fibrillation (VF).
  - Such cooling also may be beneficial for other rhythms or in-hospital cardiac arrest.

ACUTE HEART FAILURE AND PULMONARY EDEMA

Description
Acute heart failure (HF) and pulmonary edema is a complex syndrome that is characterized by an abnormality of cardiac function that results in the heart's inability to pump blood to the tissues at the rate required to meet metabolic needs. Decreased cardiac output, inadequate tissue perfusion, and acute pulmonary congestion characterize the syndrome. Pulmonary edema is caused by increased fluid in the interstitial compartment and alveoli because of elevated pulmonary capillary pressures.

Etiology
- Left ventricular systolic and diastolic dysfunction may lead to biventricular failure.
- Aortic or mitral valve dysfunction, including rupture of the papillary muscle
- Congenital arteriovenous fistulas
- Acute cardiac events associated with elevated left atrial and pulmonary capillary pressures, such as rupture of the ventricular septum

Risk Factors
- Exacerbation of cardiac condition associated with acute HF
- Inadequate treatment, lack of compliance, uncontrolled hypertension (HTN), dysrhythmia, MI, and administration of cardiac depressant medications

Assessment

- History
  - HTN, MI, aortic or mitral valvular dysfunction, rheumatic heart disease, dysrhythmia, cardiomyopathy, congenital arteriovenous fistula, and cardiotoxic drugs
  - Symptoms of left-sided HF: dyspnea on exertion, paroxysmal nocturnal dyspnea, orthopnea, nocturia, activity intolerance, and fatigue
  - Symptoms of right-sided HF: weight gain, anorexia, nausea, early satiety, and abdominal pain
- Physical findings
  - Left-sided HF: crackles, wheezes, S3, S4, and tachycardia
  - Right-sided HF: increased jugular venous pressure (JVP), increased central venous pressure (CVP), hepatojugular reflux, dependent edema, and hepatomegaly
- Diagnostic tests
  - Chest x-ray to detect ventricular hypertrophy, pleural effusion, and pulmonary edema
  - ECG to identify areas of infarction or ischemia, ventricular hypertrophy, and dysrhythmia
  - Echocardiogram to evaluate ventricular function, ejection fraction (EF), valvular function, and wall motion abnormalities
  - Coronary angiography to evaluate ventricular filling pressures, EF, and coronary artery stenosis
  - Arterial blood gases (ABG) to determine acid–base imbalance and hypoxemia
  - Laboratory tests to detect electrolyte imbalance, renal insufficiency, and other causes of HF including anemia, and thyroid dysfunction

Management

- Invasive management
  - Cardiac surgery to repair or replace impaired valves
  - Intra-aortic balloon pump (IABP) or left ventricular assist device (VAD) to decrease workload of the left ventricle
  - Continuous arteriovenous hemofiltration, continuous venovenous hemofiltration, or ultrafiltration to decrease fluid overload
  - Pacemaker or implanted cardioverter defibrillator for patients with symptomatic dysrhythmia or conduction defects
- Pharmacologic management
  - Morphine to decrease anxiety, decrease systemic vascular resistance (afterload), and increase venous capacitance (decrease preload)
  - Vasodilators to decrease afterload
    - Nesiritide (Natrecor®) intravenous infusion for arterial and venous dilation offers rapid effect, reducing preload as seen with a decrease in pulmonary artery occlusive pressure.
    - Nitrates intravenously (nitroglycerine or nitroprusside) or transdermally may be used.
  - Diuretics to remove excess fluid in the vascular compartment (decrease preload)
  - Cardiac glycosides for cardiac rate control and to enhance contractility

– Inotropes to enhance myocardial contractility
– Antidysrhythmics for treatment of dysrhythmia; beta-adrenergic blockers and calcium channel blockers may be contraindicated
– Vasopressor support to treat severe hypotension

Cardiogenic Shock

Description
Cardiogenic shock is the failure of the heart as pump to meet the metabolic demands of the body.

Etiology
• MI
• Congenital cardiac defects
• Valvular dysfunction
• Dysrhythmia
• Cardiomyopathy
• Cardiac trauma or rupture of the ventricular septum

Risk Factors
A major risk factor for cardiogenic shock is MI. Cardiogenic shock usually occurs as a result of damage to the left ventricle that impairs the pumping and ejection of blood.

Assessment
• History
  – History of MI, congenital cardiac defects, valvular dysfunction, cardiomyopathy, or cardiac trauma
  – Typical or atypical symptoms associated with MI and other conditions causing HF
  – Symptoms of left-sided HF: dyspnea on exertion, paroxysmal nocturnal dyspnea, orthopnea, nocturia, activity intolerance, and fatigue
  – Symptoms of right-sided HF: weight gain, anorexia, nausea, early satiety, and abdominal pain
• Physical findings
  – Left-sided HF: crackles, wheezes, S3, S4, tachycardia, and hypotension
  – Right-sided HF: elevated JVP, increased CVP, hepatojugular reflux, dependent edema, and hepatomegaly
  – Cardiac dysrhythmia
  – Impaired tissue perfusion: mottled or cyanotic extremities; cool, clammy skin; gastric hypomotility; oliguria; or change in level of consciousness
• Diagnostic tests
  – ECG to identify MI, myocardial ischemia, or dysrhythmia
  – Chest x-ray to detect cardiomegaly and pulmonary edema
  – Echocardiogram to evaluate ventricular function, EF, and valvular function
  – Laboratory tests to detect electrolyte imbalance, renal or liver impairment, anemia, and shock state (such as lactic acid level and ABG)

Management
- Invasive management
  - Intubation and mechanical ventilation to improve oxygen supply to the myocardium
  - Pulmonary artery catheter to monitor hemodynamic parameters (cardiac output, cardiac index, systemic vascular resistance, pulmonary artery and pulmonary capillary wedge pressure) at baseline and effect of treatment. CVP is elevated in right and biventricular failure.
  - IABP or left VAD to decrease ventricular workload. VAD may be temporary, bridge to transplant, or destination therapy.
  - Cardiac surgery to repair the cause of cardiogenic shock or emergent heart transplant
- Pharmacologic management
  - Inotropes to enhance myocardial contractility
  - Vasodilators to decrease afterload
  - Antidysrhythmics for treatment of dysrhythmia; beta-adrenergic blockers and calcium channel blockers may be contraindicated.
  - Vasopressors to treat severe hypotension

Cardiac Tamponade

Description
Cardiac tamponade is compression of the heart caused by accumulation of fluid in the pericardial space. Cardiac compression by pericardial fluid causes increased intracardiac pressures, decreased diastolic filling, and reduced cardiac output.

Etiology
Pericarditis, cancer, uremia, MI, diagnostic cardiac procedures, cardiac trauma, bacterial infection, cardiomyopathy, and cardiac surgery

Risk Factors
- Diseases or illnesses that cause excessive accumulation of pericardial fluid
- Diagnostic procedures that result in movement of fluid into the pericardial space

Assessment
- History
  - Acute or chronic pericarditis, cardiac disease, renal failure, infection, injury to the heart, or systemic diseases
- Physical findings
  - Hypotension
  - Tachycardia
  - Diminished heart sounds
  - Pericardial friction rub
  - Pulsus paradoxus
  - Tachypnea

- Diagnostic tests
  - Chest x-ray to identify enlarged cardiac silhouette
  - ECG to detect electrical alternans of the QRS complex
  - Echocardiogram to diagnose the presence of pericardial effusion
  - Angiography

Management
- Invasive management
  - Pericardiocentesis (percutaneously with a needle or catheter), pericardiotomy, or surgical pericardiectomy to remove pericardial fluid

Aortic Dissection

Description
Aortic dissection usually starts with either a tear in the intima, or a medial hemorrhage that ruptures the integrity of the aortic wall. Blood penetrates into the aortic wall, separates the layers, and creates a false lumen.

Etiology
- Medial degeneration is the most common cause
- Trauma

Risk Factors
- Hereditary connective tissue diseases such as Marfan and Ehlers-Danlos syndromes
- HTN
- Increasing age; peak incidence is the sixth and seventh decades
- Gender; affects men twice as frequently as women

Assessment
- History
  - In acute dissection, the pain often has a sudden onset. If the chest pain is located anteriorly, the site of dissection is often the ascending aorta. Other associated symptoms for this site may be neck, throat, or jaw pain. If the pain is located in the interscapular region, the area of involvement is usually the descending thoracic aorta. Pain in the back, abdomen, or lower extremities frequently is indicative of a dissection of the descending aorta.
- Physical findings
  - HTN or hypotension
  - Pulse deficits
  - With proximal aortic dissection, decrescendo diastolic murmur of aortic regurgitation
  - With involvement of the innominate or left common carotid arteries, changes in level of consciousness
  - Paraparesis or paraplegia may occur as a result of changes in spinal cord perfusion.
- Diagnostic tests
  - Aortography to identify the presence and extent of aortic dissection
  - CT scan or MRI study to detect extent of aortic dissection
  - Transthoracic or transesophageal echocardiography to identify aortic dissection

Management
- Invasive management
  - Aortic aneurysm repair is indicated for acute proximal dissection and those distal aortic dissections that are complicated by continued pain, rupture, expansion, saccular aneurysm, Marfan syndrome, and ischemia of organs or lower extremities.
- Medical management
  - For those patients with uncomplicated distal aortic dissection, particularly the elderly, medical therapy is associated with similar outcomes as surgical repair.
  - Medical management is also recommended for those patients with stable arch dissection or uncomplicated distal dissection.
  - Patients experiencing acute aortic dissection should be admitted to the hospital for monitoring of their hemodynamic status and emergent surgical intervention.
    - Acute reduction of arterial pressure may be accomplished with intravenous medications such as beta-adrenergic blockers, calcium channel blockers, ACE inhibitors, or nitrates.
    - Unstable patients or those requiring short-acting intravenous medications should be admitted to an intensive care unit or operating suite.

Acute Arterial Occlusion

Description
Acute arterial occlusion occurs when a thrombus or embolism obstructs an artery, producing significant tissue ischemia. Prompt recognition and treatment are critical to avoid loss of limb or death.

Etiology
- Embolism from atrial fibrillation, recent MI, valvular heart disease, or ventricular aneurysm
- Thrombosis because of atherosclerosis, aneurysms, hypercoagulable diseases (see Table 16–1 for a list of etiologies), and vascular grafts
- Iatrogenic emboli (e.g., catheter tips, dislodged atherosclerotic debris)

Table 16–1. Causes of Hypercoagulable States

Acquired	Congenital
Cancer	Antithrombin III deficiency
Inflammatory disorders	Factor V Leiden
Postoperative state	Protein C deficiency
Estrogens, pregnancy	Protein S deficiency
Lupus anticoagulant	Dysfibrinogenemia
Heparin-induced thrombocytopenia	Abnormal plasminogen
Paroxysmal nocturnal hemoglobinuria	Activated protein C resistance

Risk Factors

Presence of diseases or conditions that can cause either embolism or thrombosis

- Assessment
  - History
    - History of prior peripheral vascular disease, aortic aneurysm, or other conditions associated with embolism or thrombosis
    - Sudden onset of symptoms such as pain, coolness, and paresthesia distal to the arterial occlusion
  - Physical findings
    - Absence of peripheral pulses—may be acute loss of pulse distal to occlusion
    - Pallor
    - Poikilothermia (inability to determine hot or cold with touch)
    - Paralysis
  - Diagnostic tests
    - Arterial Doppler studies
    - Arteriography before embolectomy
    - Echocardiogram may be indicated to evaluate cardiac source

Management

- Invasive management
  - Balloon embolectomy
  - Arterial bypass procedure
  - Fasciotomy may be required after revascularization is achieved
- Pharmacologic management
  - Fibrinolytic therapy
  - Emergent heparinization to prevent propagation of the clot

RACE, ETHNIC, GENDER, AND CULTURAL CONSIDERATIONS

Race and Ethnicity

Heart disease is the leading and stroke the third highest cause of death for people in the United States. Despite the gains achieved with the programs associated with Healthy People 2000 and 2010, health disparities for specific racial and ethnic groups remain. The overall number of cardiovascular deaths has decreased but there are disparities related to race and ethnicity. Blacks have the highest rates of CHD deaths, HF hospitalizations, and stroke. They also have the highest rate of death from HTN of any racial or ethnic group. Statistics related to cardiac and vascular disease morbidity and mortality rates for specific racial and ethnic groups are as follows.

- According to the Centers for Disease Control and Prevention, in 2007 the overall heart disease crude death rates per 100,000 population for the five largest U.S. racial and ethnic groups were
  - Hispanics, 69.2
  - Asians and Pacific Islanders, 73
  - Native Americans, 82.5
  - Blacks, 189.8
  - Whites, 235.5

- Among Native Americans ages 65 through 74, the rates (per 1,000 population) of new and recurrent heart attacks are 25.1 for men and 9.1 for women.
- Heart disease prevalence data from the CDC in 2007
  - White males, 8.8%
  - White females, 6.6%
  - Black males, 9.6%
  - Black females, 9.0%
  - Hispanic males, 5.4%
  - Hispanic females, 6.3%

Gender

Women experience major cardiovascular events approximately 10 years later than men. The difference between men and women decreases with advancing age.

- Because of the older age at onset of CHD and the presence of comorbid conditions, women are more likely than men to die in the first few weeks after MI.
- Black females and White males have the highest rate of CHD deaths of any racial or ethnic groups.
- Women may experience atypical symptoms during an acute coronary syndrome. It may be more diffuse, and chest pain may be less severe.
- Recent public education from the American Heart Association (Red Dress Campaign) efforts have been successful in warning women of their risk of cardiovascular disease. Studies show that women now realize that heart disease is responsible for more women's deaths than breast cancer.

Cultural Considerations

- Cultural phenomena that vary among racial and ethnic groups may affect their receptivity to care delivered by healthcare providers.
  - Environmental control is the ability of people to control nature. Cultural groups that believe they have mastery over nature or the environment may accept medications or invasive procedures. Cultural groups that believe they do not have control over nature or the environment may not accept medications and procedure and may seek alternative treatments such as folk medicine.
  - Biologic variation is the genetic susceptibility of people to illness.
    - Racial and ethnic variations in the incidence of cardiac and vascular diseases and the presence of risk factors (described previously) may have a genetic component.
    - Most cardiovascular diseases are the result of multiple genetic foci that are triggered by some environmental or intrinsic factor that results in the appearance of the disease.
    - There are genetic differences in the way many medications are metabolized and that may play a role in why some drugs are more effective in certain groups than others.
      - If a drug is metabolized faster, it wears off quickly and higher doses are needed.
      - If metabolism is slower, the person has a greater risk of developing toxic reactions to the drug.
  - Social organization is the family unit and the role of family members. There are cultural differences in the composition (nuclear or extended) of families and the values placed on the respective roles. Some cultural groups have extended family units with multiple members involved in decision-making. Other cultural groups are matriarchal in their decision-making processes.

- Communication is the verbal and nonverbal behaviors that are used in personal interactions. Acceptable forms of expression for people are often culturally based. Some cultures are formal while others are informal in their conversations with healthcare providers.
- Personal space refers to the boundaries or acceptable distances between people that affects their personal comfort. Some cultural groups are comfortable with close contact with healthcare providers while others are not. Space or closeness is an important concern for nurses caring for cardiac and vascular patients because many procedures cross these boundaries and may result in personal discomfort.
- Time orientation is a culture's view of the past, present, and future. Some cultures are future-oriented while others have strong beliefs in practices of their ancestors.
- Nursing care that is culturally competent is knowledgeable and sensitive to the patient's cultural needs. Care of people from different cultures should be based on the following principles:
  - Care is designed for the specific patient.
  - Care is based on the patient's cultural norms and values.
  - Care incorporates interventions that facilitate the patient's decision-making about his or her care.
  - Care is sensitive to the patient's cultural uniqueness.

COMORBID OR CONCOMITANT CONDITIONS

Cardiopulmonary Disease
Cardiopulmonary diseases and their related risk factors contribute to an increased incidence of cardiac and vascular health problems. Smoking is linked to CHD and chronic obstructive pulmonary diseases (COPD). Pulmonary health problems such as COPD may result in secondary pulmonary HTN and cardiac disorders such as cor pulmonale, a form of right ventricular failure. The presence of cardiopulmonary diseases among patients experiencing cardiac or vascular health problems can complicate recovery and increase mortality.

Diabetes
Diabetes mellitus is a major risk factor for the development of cardiovascular diseases including CHD, stroke, and arterial occlusive diseases. The rate of newly diagnosed cases of non–insulin-dependent diabetes mellitus in the United States is climbing at an alarming rate in adults and children. Diabetes is a leading associated cause of mortality for men and women in this country. Approximately two-thirds of people with diabetes will die of cardiovascular disease. People with diabetes who have intensive or tight control of their blood glucose have lower incidence of diabetic complications including retinopathy, microalbuminuria, and neuropathy as well as lower low-density lipoprotein and total cholesterol levels than people with less intensive control. Cardiovascular mortality is less when hemoglobin A1C levels are low. Diabetes mellitus complicates the recovery of people from cardiovascular events. Hyperglycemia increases risk of postoperative wound infections in people having surgical procedures such as coronary artery bypass surgery. For these reasons and the statistics from the Framingham Heart Study, diabetes is considered an equivalent of cardiovascular disease when setting goals for risk reduction.

Renovascular Disease

Renovascular diseases contribute to an increased incidence of cardiac and vascular problems. The development of end-stage renal disease has been linked to HTN. End-stage renal disease (ESRD) and its sequel, chronic renal failure, has been associated with the development of HF, hypertrophic cardiomyopathy, and accelerated coronary atherosclerosis. The perioperative care of cardiac and vascular patients with renovascular disease presents many challenges because of complications associated with the disease including HTN, electrolyte imbalance, and fluid management issues. Many drugs used in the treatment of cardiovascular disease need to be dosed in a reduced amount based on estimated creatinine clearance or glomerular filtration rate.

Cerebrovascular Disease

Cerebrovascular diseases can be risk factors for the development of cardiac diseases, and abnormalities of the heart also can cause acute cerebrovascular injury. Patients may have carotid artery occlusive disease and coexisting CHD because the risk factors are similar. Increased incidences of dysrhythmia, MI, and cardiopulmonary arrest have been associated with acute cerebrovascular injury. The presence of CHD adversely affects survival of patients with cerebrovascular accident (CVA). Stroke is the third leading cause of death and most CVAs are because of atherosclerosis. Patients undergoing cardiac or vascular surgical procedures may have an increased incidence of acute cerebral injury because of embolization from the aorta or carotid arteries, respectively.

Congenital Heart Disease

Many persons with congenital heart disease who in the past would have died during childhood are now living to adulthood. Some people will not have a congenital problem identified until adulthood. It is important to mention a few conditions that are included in the test content outline for the certification examination.

- Adult survivors of congenital heart disease
  - A possible outcome is right side heart failure because of pulmonary hypertension. You may see signs of peripheral congestion, fluid overload, and dyspnea.
  - Be sure to understand the original and corrected flow of blood through the heart.
  - These patients may have special needs when undergoing a cardiac catheterization or other noninvasive cardiac diagnostic tests.
  - If the cardiac condition worsens, another surgical correction may be needed or a heart transplant may be the only option.
- Marfan syndrome is a connective tissue disorder and is associated with a tall, gangly appearance (like Abraham Lincoln). People with this disorder have a higher incidence of aortic root dilation and other disorders and may require a aortic valve and aortic grafting.
- Atrial septal defects can be acquired (post MI or trauma) or congenital. In some cases, this may be a very small opening that is not hemodynamically significant. This opening does provide a site for emboli to travel from the right atrium to the left atrium. If that happens, the embolus can travel to the brain, causing a CVA, or to the periphery, causing an arterial occlusion. The foramen ovale is a connection needed for fetal circulation that is located in the atrial septum. At times it does not close and this patent foramen ovale (PFO) can be the

cause of a number of embolic strokes. It should be suspected in persons unlikely to otherwise suffer a CVA.

- PFO can be detected on an echocardiogram bubble study. The patient is positioned on his or her side during the echocardiogram, a safe gas is injected intravenously, and if the PFO exists, the bubbles will pass through the septal opening.
- Chronic anticoagulation is no longer routinely recommended for an asymptomatic PFO.
- Warfarin is recommended for the person who has had symptomatic emboli.
- The PFO can be closed with a transeptal patch placed during a right heart catheterization. The patch is deployed across the septum and eventually endothelializes so that only short-term warfarin is needed. (See Figure 16–1.)

Figure 16-1. Transseptal Patch Used for ASD and PFO Closure

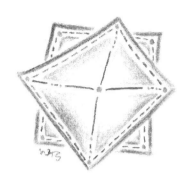

One side of the umbrella device is on either side of the atrium.

SPECIFIC NURSING INTERVENTIONS

General Measures

- Activity progression including bed rest, out of bed to the chair or commode, or ambulation is based on the patient's diagnosis and activity tolerance.
- Vital signs are monitored to detect any changes in the patient's condition. The frequency of vital signs depends on the patient's acuity.
- Neurovascular checks are used to assess the temperature, color, capillary refill, sensation, movement, and pulses of the upper and lower extremities. The frequency of neurovascular checks is determined by the presence of vascular disease or procedures that may cause changes in the peripheral circulation.
- Intravenous access is indicated for acutely ill patients with cardiac and vascular diseases and those at risk for complications.
- Oxygen is used for patients with ischemic symptoms or respiratory distress. Pulse oximetry or ABGs are used to monitor the effectiveness of oxygen therapy.
- Intake and output are monitored to determine the patient's fluid status. The frequency of intake and output is based on the patient's diagnosis and acuity.
- Daily weights are used to measure the patient's overall volume status and may be used as an indicator for diuretic or fluid therapies.

Specific Interventions

- A cardiac monitor may be used to continuously assess the electrical activity of the heart. It is used to identify cardiac dysrhythmia and ischemia in high-risk patients and those with acute health problems.
- ECG is a graphic recording of the electrical impulses generated during the cardiac cycle. This procedure provides information on the electrical activity of specific segments of the heart. The ECG may be used to measure electrical impulses, identify cardiac dysrhythmia, and diagnose MI.
- Unna boots are used in the management of venous ulcers. The plaster boot is a dressing composed of gauze moistened with specific medications. The boot is changed at specific time intervals (every 1 to 2 weeks) depending upon the amount of ulcer drainage. A boot should not be used and is discontinued if signs of infection are present.
- Compression stockings promote venous return and are also used to decrease leg swelling and prevent ulceration. Patients are measured for these stockings to ensure proper fit. The pressure at the ankle should be at least 30 mm Hg to 40 mm Hg and should decrease proximally.

SUMMARY

This chapter provided an overview of special conditions that the cardiovascular nurse must recognize and manage. Gender, racial, and ethnic influences are also described. Common comorbidities and congenital conditions were included to provide an overview of additional clinical concerns that the cardiac nurse must know.

REFERENCES

Adams, R. J., Albers, G., Alberts, M. J., Benavente, O., Furie, K., Goldstein, L. B., ... American Stroke Association. (2008). Update to the AHA/ASA recommendations for the prevention of stroke in patients with stroke and transient ischemic attack. *Stroke, 39*(5), 1647–1652.

American Heart Association. (2009). *2009 heart and stroke statistical update*. Dallas: Author.

Barkley, T. W., & Myers, C. M. (2008). *Practice guidelines for acute care nurse practitioners* (2nd ed.) St. Louis, MO: Elsevier Saunders.

Buchanan, L., & Likness, S. (2008). Evidence based practice to assist women in hospital settings to quit smoking and reduce cardiovascular disease risk. *Journal of Cardiovascular Nursing, 23*(5), 397–406.

Crawford, M. H. (2009). *Cardiology: Current diagnosis and treatment*. New York: McGraw Hill.

Garavalia, L., Garavalia, B., Spertus, J. A., & Decker, C. (2009). Exploring patients' reasons for discontinuance of heart medications. *Journal of Cardiovascular Nursing, 24*, 371–379.

Kozik, T. M. (2007). Induced hypothermia for patients with cardiac arrest: Role of a clinical nurse specialist. *Critical Care Nurse, 27*, 36–42.

Kozik, T. M., & Wung, S. F. (2009). Cardiac arrest from acquired long QT syndrome: A case report. *Heart and Lung, 38*, 238–342.

Moser, D., & Reigel, B. (2008). *Cardiac nursing: A companion to Braunwald's heart disease*. St. Louis, MO: Elsevier Saunders.

Russell, J. A., Walley, K. R., Singer, J., Gordon, A. C., Herbert, P. C., Cooper, J., ... VASST Investigators. (2008). Vasopressin versus norepinephrine infusion in patients with septic shock. *New England Journal of Medicine, 358*, 877–887.

Woods, S. L., Sivarajan-Froelicher, E. S.. Motzer, S., & Bridges, E. J. (2010). *Cardiac nursing* (6th ed.). Philadelphia: Lippincott.

Zagaria, M. A. (2009). Renal dosing: Understanding glomerular filtration rate and estimating creatinine clearance. *American Journal of Nurse Practitioners, 13*(7), 32–35.

Zipes, D. P., Libby, P., Bonow, R. O., & Braunwald, E. (2009). *Braunwald's heart disease: A textbook of cardiovascular medicine* (8th ed.). Philadelphia: Elsevier-Saunders.

INTERNET RESOURCES

American Heart Association: http://americanheart.org/
Centers for Disease Control and Prevention: http://www.cdc.gov/
Framingham Heart Study: (http://www.framinghamheartstudy.org/
National Health and Nutrition Examination Survey (NHANES): http://www.cdc.gov/nchs/nhanes/
National Institutes of Health: http://www.nhlbi.nih.gov/guidelines/cholesterol/index.htm
Women's Health Initiative: http://www.whiscience.org/

17

Psychosocial Aspects

Cardiovascular health problems not only affect the physiological status of patients but can also have a major impact on their coping and adaptation. The psychosocial aspects of illness can result in adaptive and maladaptive responses that can influence a person's interpersonal relationships, vocation, sexuality, and spirituality. Nurses can encourage patients to use positive coping mechanisms as they adapt to their cardiovascular health problems.

COPING AND ADAPTATION

Coping is the continuously changing cognitive and behavioral actions used by a person to manage the external and internal demands that are appraised as challenging or exceeding personal resources. Coping is a dynamic process between the person and the environment.

Functions of Coping
- Reduce tension and maintain equilibrium
- Facilitate independence and freedom
- Enhance personal decision-making
- Manage reactions to stressors
- Facilitate meeting social environmental demands
- Avoid negative self-evaluation
- Maintain a stable psychological, social, and physiological state

Coping Styles
- A person's way of coping may change according to specific situational variables.
- A flexible coping style is more adaptive to different events and stressors than one that is rigid.
- Coping styles involve a continuum of behaviors, from approaching the situation to avoidance.

Adaptive Responses
- Lifestyle modification: The patient changes certain aspects of his or her lifestyle to meet the demands of the illness. For the patient with newly diagnosed cardiac or vascular disease, lifestyle modification may mean starting an exercise routine, losing weight, and following a low-fat diet. The patient learns to avoid those activities that may exacerbate the disease.
- Enhancing knowledge and self-care strategies: The patient increases his or her understanding about the disease and its treatment. The patient copes by being aware of his or her symptoms and, based on his or her assessment of the symptom, either alters self-care activities or seeks help from healthcare providers.
- Maintaining a positive self-concept: The patient integrates the illness and treatment into the sense of self to maintain feelings of normalcy. The patient engages in activities to enhance self-esteem and adapts to an altered body image.
- Adjusting to changes in social relationships: The patient's illness and decreased energy alter his or her participation in social activities. Other people in social relationships may choose to limit contact with the patient either because of their discomfort with the situation or because of the need for respite. The patient must adapt to decreasing contacts and inquiries from other people and modifies his or her support systems.
- Grieving over losses: The patient grieves over the losses associated with illness such as functional ability, energy, body image, roles, sexuality, and social relationships. The patient works to maintain self-concept by adapting to these losses.
- Dealing with role changes: The patient adapts to changes in personal, social, and professional roles. Adaptation means either relinquishing or modifying previous roles and responsibilities. The person assumes the new role of patient also.
- Adjusting to physical discomfort: The patient attempts to cope with the discomfort associated with the illness and its treatment. The patient seeks ways to alleviate or decrease the discomfort through pharmacological and nonpharmacological interventions.
- Maintaining a sense of control: The patient has multiple intrusions into his or her personal space and privacy because of the illness. The patient attempts to maintain privacy and preserve personal dignity. Maintaining control involves making decisions about treatments and the subsequent timing of this care.
- Maintaining hope: The patient embraces a positive attitude that he or she will recover from the illness with the use of new therapies. The patient adjusts to deteriorating physical health and declining treatment options by having hope and attempts to avoid feelings of despair about the illness.
- Confronting impending death: The patient realizes that his or her life will be short. The patient has comfort in his or her personal accomplishments and relationships. Confronting death involves the anticipation and acceptance of the prognosis.

Maladaptive Responses

The person who is unable to cope with his or her illness is at risk for developing maladaptive responses. Maladaptive responses include anxiety, anger, depression, denial, dependence, and noncompliance. While these responses are labeled as maladaptive, that is individually determined and time-sensitive. A "maladaptive response" may be appropriate as a person is regaining resources to respond in a more productive manner.

- Anxiety is a response to an actual or perceived threat. It is characterized by feelings of apprehension, tension, and uneasiness. Anxiety may result from a fear of the illness and its associated diagnostic and therapeutic procedures. It also can occur because of fear of disfigurement and death. Mild anxiety has been associated with enhanced learning performance. Severe symptoms of acute anxiety, such as panic, include agitation and feeling out of control.
- Anger is a reaction associated with feelings of extreme displeasure, hostility, or rage. The stimulus for this emotion may be an actual or perceived threat to the person's self-concept. Anger occurs as a result of the person's perceived vulnerability because of the illness and the loss of independence and roles.
- Depression is a state associated with the loss of roles, functional status, and changes in self-concept. Symptoms associated with depression include feeling sad, guilty, anxious, apathetic, or confused. The person may experience disturbances in sleep and appetite and may have somatic complaints also. Severe or major depression can impair the ability to function at work and in social situations. The person with major depression often has feelings of hopelessness, worthlessness, and fearfulness and may be at risk for committing suicide.
- Denial is a defense mechanism that involves avoiding emotional conflict or anxiety by refusing to acknowledge thoughts, feelings, or facts that are intolerable. A person may deny the presence of an illness or the need for prescribed therapy.
- Dependence is a condition in which the person is overly dependent on others to meet his or her physical and emotional needs. This response may be precipitated also by a significant other's response to the illness.
- Noncompliance is a reaction to the limitations imposed by the illness and its related treatment. The person refuses to comply with the management of the condition. The response may be a rebellion against the feelings of vulnerability, temporary respite from the prescribed therapies, or a depressive withdrawal from the stress.
- Treatment of depression and anxiety
  - Nonpharmacological interventions
    - Cognitive behavioral therapy
    - Psychotherapy
    - Electroconvulsive therapy for selected depressive disorders
    - Light therapy for seasonal affective disorder
  - Pharmacological therapy
    - Selective serotonin reuptake inhibitors (SSRIs) such as fluoxetine, sertraline, paroxetine, and fluvoxamine are the first line of treatment for most anxiety disorders. They also are the medications of choice for depressive disorders.
    - Tricyclic antidepressants including imipramine, nortriptyline, desipramine, amitriptyline, and doxepin are useful in the treatment of generalized anxiety disorders and panic disorder. They are also used in the treatment of depressive disorders.
      - Tricyclics are extremely dangerous when taken in overdose quantities.
      - May cause cardiovascular adverse effects such as orthostatic hypotension, conduction defects, and dysrhythmia

- Benzodiazepines such as diazepam, lorazepam, and oxazepam are effective in the treatment of generalized anxiety. Alprazolam and clonazepam usually are used for panic disorder.
- Monoamine oxidase inhibitors (MAOIs) are used to treat atypical depression and treatment-resistant patients. MAOIs include phenelzine, tranylcypromine, L-deprenyl, and moclobemide.
- Atypical antidepressants include bupropion, mirtazapine, nefazodone, and trazodone.
  - Bupropion (Zyban®, Wellbutrin®) has the additional benefit of increasing success with smoking cessation.
  - Bupropion may cause vivid nightmares and lowers the threshold for seizures.

Nursing Diagnoses Related to Coping and Adaptation

- Ineffective coping is the inability to form a valid appraisal of the stressors, inadequate choices of practiced responses, inability to use available resources, or any combination of these.
- Defensive coping is the repeated projection of falsely positive self-evaluation based on a self-protective pattern that defends against underlying perceived threats to positive self-regard.
- Compromised family coping occurs when the usually supportive primary person provides insufficient, ineffective, or compromised support, comfort, assistance, or encouragement to manage adaptive tasks.
- Ineffective denial is the conscious or unconscious attempt to disavow knowledge or meaning of an event to reduce anxiety, but leading to the detriment of health.

Nursing Interventions to Enhance Coping and Adaptation

- Assess the patient's psychosocial responses to the illness and its treatment.
- Identify whether these responses are adaptive or maladaptive.
- Determine if there is a physiological cause of the maladaptive response.
- Plan a personalized psychosocial nursing care plan with the patient and family.
- Establish a therapeutic relationship with the patient and family.
- Promote the use of adaptive coping mechanisms by the patient and family.
- Provide educational materials to enhance knowledge about the disease and prescribed therapies.
- Encourage patient and family participation in support groups composed of people with similar illnesses.
- Consult with the patient's physician or advanced practice nurse about referral for psychiatric evaluation for maladaptive responses. Some patients may benefit from psychotherapy, psychopharmacology, or both.
- Evaluate the effectiveness of the psychosocial nursing care plan for the patient and family and revise as necessary.

QUALITY OF LIFE

The World Health Organization defined quality of life as "a broad-ranging concept affected in a complex way by the person's physical health, psychological state, level of independence, social relationships, and relationships to salient features of the environment." A person's perception of his or her quality of life, either positive or negative, can have broad implications for the ability to cope with cardiovascular disease and treatment. Some divide quality of life into global and health-related. Many reliable and valid tools and questionnaires have been developed to measure both forms of quality of life.

Influencing Factors

Factors influencing a person's perception of his or her quality of life include health, functional status, symptoms, and life satisfaction. The acuity or chronic nature of the illness afflicting the person affects these factors.

- Health is the state of physical, mental, and social well-being and not merely the absence of disease. Health exists on a continuum, with health and illness being on opposite ends.
- Functional status is the person's ability to perform his or her roles and related activities. The activities that may be affected by cardiovascular disease include physical, psychological, and social interactions.
- Symptoms are the person's responses to his or her physical, emotional, or cognitive states. These responses may be manifested as adaptive or maladaptive coping mechanisms.
- Life satisfaction is the fulfillment or contentment that a person feels from different facets of life including family, health, sexuality, spirituality, friendships, job, education, housing, standard of living, and finances.

Support Systems

- The spouse, family members, and significant others have an important role in the support of people with cardiovascular health problems. People who have a high level of social integration or social links to family and friends have better outcomes after acute myocardial infarction. As a result of their positive support systems, these people often have a perceived higher quality of life. The care by the spouse or significant other may come at a physiological or psychological cost to the caregiver. For some caregivers, the burden of caring may result in physical exhaustion and negative emotional responses. These factors can have a negative effect on the perceived quality of life of the caregivers.
- Community resources such as support groups, counseling services, and health care agencies can assist patients, their families, and significant others in their psychosocial adjustment to illness. Healthcare providers can help to improve the quality of life for patients and their family members. In some areas, respite care is also available to provide caregivers temporary relief from care-giving responsibilities.

Work

Vocational issues are related to quality of life for people with cardiovascular diseases. For many people, self-concept is linked to the roles in their lives including their occupations. Depending upon the type of work that the person does, there may be changes in some or all of his or her responsibilities, especially for those with physically demanding positions. Changes in work responsibilities and routines can cause stress and lowered self-esteem. These factors can have an effect on a person's perceived quality of life and psychosocial responses to the illness. The time that a person can return to work, along with any work limitations, should be discussed with his or her healthcare provider.

Sexuality

Sexuality is a concern for many cardiovascular patients. It is a subject that is not easily discussed in the therapeutic relationship. Some patients and their significant others may fear that sexual activity will result in angina or death. There are guidelines related to sexual activity after cardiovascular illnesses. For example, the American Heart Association recommends that patients having an uncomplicated myocardial infarction may resume sexual intercourse in 7 to 10 days. Some medications used to treat people with cardiovascular conditions, such as angiotensin converting enzyme inhibitors, beta adrenergic blockers, and calcium channel blockers, may have a negative effect on libido. Sexual dysfunction can cause feelings of anxiety, anger, or depression for the patient and partner. Patients with sexual dysfunction should be referred to their healthcare providers for evaluation.

Spirituality

Spirituality and religion give value to people's beliefs and behaviors. People may be spiritual but may not endorse a religion. Religious involvement has been associated with a lower incidence of cardiovascular disease and mortality. Additionally, people who have religious involvement and spirituality have a lower incidence of depression and anxiety related to physical illness. These factors have also been linked to higher levels of perceived quality of life for people with cardiovascular and other illnesses.

Stress Management

Stress management techniques are strategies that can be used to enhance a person's ability to cope with stressors. Conditions that may activate the stress response may be physical, emotional, cognitive, social, economic, or spiritual. Stressors may be events that have actually occurred or may be perceived as threats that are not reality-based. The body's response to the actual or perceived threat results in physiologic and psychological responses.

General Adaptation Syndrome

The general adaptation syndrome, identified by Hans Selye, depicts the stages associated with the body's response to a stressor.
- Alarm Stage is the initial response to the stressor. The central nervous system is stimulated and physiologic defense mechanisms are activated. This process often is called the fight-or-flight syndrome.
- Stage of Resistance or Adaptation is the process whereby the person continues the fight or flight response.
- Stage of Exhaustion is the point in which the continued stress precipitates the disruption of the compensatory mechanisms, leading to the onset of stress-related dysfunction such as disease or illness.

Physiologic and Psychologic Responses

- Physiologic responses to stress include the interactions among the sympathetic nervous system, anterior and posterior pituitary gland, and adrenal gland.
  - Sympathetic stimulation causes the release of norepinephrine, resulting in increased blood pressure, pupil dilation, skeletal muscle vasodilation, bronchodilation, and decreased gastric secretion.

- – Adrenal medulla activation stimulates epinephrine secretion, causing increased cardiac output, bronchodilation, increased glycogenolysis, increased gluconeogenesis, increased glucagon, increased free fatty acids, increased serum cholesterol, and decreased insulin.
  - – Anterior pituitary stimulation causes the release of adrenocorticotropic hormone (ACTH), growth hormone, and prolactin. ACTH acts on the adrenal cortex to secrete aldosterone and cortisol, resulting in increased sodium and water retention, increased blood glucose from gluconeogenesis, increased amino acids from protein catabolism, increase polymorphonucleocytes, decreased monocytes and macrophages, decreased lymphocytes, and decreased eosinophils.
  - – Posterior pituitary activation causes the release of vasopressin or antidiuretic hormone, thereby stimulating increased water retention.
- Psychologic responses to stress such as cardiovascular illness may result in the use of adaptive and maladaptive coping mechanisms.

Identification of Personal Traits and Responses
- Self-concept plays an important role in a person's response to actual or perceived stressors. People with high self-esteem use more adaptive coping responses while people with lower self-esteem are more vulnerable to psychological stressors and may respond with feelings of anger, denial, or depression. Negative self-concept has been proposed to have a significant role in the eventual onset of disease in vulnerable people.
- The "Type A Personality" was originally identified by Friedman and Rosenman. Personality traits of people with this syndrome include the need to accomplish tasks in the shortest amount of time, aggressive behavior that borders on hostility, highly motivated, very competitive, achievement-oriented, labile temper, and involvement in multiple tasks at the same time. People with this profile have been associated with a higher incidence of coronary heart disease. It has been proposed that these people have a heightened sympathetic responsiveness to stressors, which may be the key factor in pathological process leading to their increased cardiovascular risk.

Stress Management Techniques
- Autogenics is a technique used to promote deep relaxation. It involves the repeating of verbal phases and concentrating on sensations and actions in certain parts of the body. The rituals are focused on exercises that involve muscular relaxation, vascular dilation, regulation of the heart, regulation of breathing, regulation of visceral organs, and regulation of thoughts.
- Cognitive restructuring involves using the mind to alter the stress response. Negative feelings can trigger physiological aspects of the stress response. This technique requires the patient to identify maladaptive negative thoughts to stressors and to counter them with adaptive positive thoughts.
- Imagery is another method for stress reduction. The person creates a mental image of a place that is relaxing. Imagery is especially effective when combined with physical relaxation techniques such as diaphragmatic breathing exercises.
- Progressive muscle relaxation reduces stress by interfering with the autonomic arousal of the sympathetic nervous system by decreasing muscle tension. This technique involves tension–relaxation exercises of each of the major muscle groups of the body. It is used to decrease the impact of the physiological responses to stress and to enable the person to learn adaptive responses to stimuli.

- Meditation is a process that produces deep physiological relaxation. It involves limiting stimuli from conscious awareness, repeating verbal phrases or mantra, and concentrating on a focal point to relax the body.
- Aerobic exercise reduces anxiety and stress along with having a positive effect on subjective mood states. The exercise prescription usually involves repetitive movement of large muscle groups. The goal of aerobic exercise is to elevate the heart rate to a specified level. There are often positive cardiovascular benefits from aerobic exercise.

Self-Monitoring Techniques

Instructions for the person learning self-monitoring techniques include:

- Change your lifestyle by eating a well-balanced diet, engaging in regular exercise, getting adequate sleep, enjoying leisure activities, and using stress management techniques.
- Modify stressful situations by managing time and finances, being assertive, engaging in problem-solving, and possibly changing work situations or relationships.
- Change thinking by being positive, seeing problems as new opportunities, decreasing negative thoughts, and having a sense of humor.
- Modify reactions to stressors by being aware of your feelings. Learn to control these reactions with positive adaptive behaviors.

SUMMARY

This chapter provided an overview of the varied psychological and social factors that affect the well-being and quality of life of patients with cardiovascular disorders. Important points to consider are that there are many ways to cope in a situation. Some of the negative coping responses may be helpful in the short term as the person gathers the resources to manage over time. Depression and anxiety should be treated with medications to gain the best outcomes. Nursing interventions play a major role in helping the patient adjust to a life with a chronic disorder.

REFERENCES

Allman, E., Berry, D., & Nasir, L. (2009). Depression and coping in heart failure patients: A review of the literature. *Journal of Cardiovascular Nursing, 24*(2), 106–117.

Anderson, K. L. (1999). Conceptualization and measurement of quality of life as an outcome variable for health care intervention and research. *Journal of Advanced Nursing, 29*(2), 298–306.

Azzopardi, S., & Lee, G. (2009). Health-related quality of life 2 years after coronary artery bypass graft surgery. *Journal of Cardiovascular Nursing, 24*(3), 232–240.

Baas, L. S. (2004). Self care resources and activity as predictors of quality of life in persons after myocardial infarction. *Dimensions of Critical Care Nursing, 23*(3), 131–138.

Baas, L. S., Beery, T. A., Allen, G. A., Wizer, M., & Wagoner, L. E. (2004). An exploratory study of body awareness in persons with heart failure or transplant. *Journal of Cardiovascular Nursing, 19*(1), 32–40.

Beery, T., Baas, L. S., & Henthorn, C. (2007). Self reported adjustment to implanted cardiac devices. *Journal of Cardiovascular Nursing, 22*(6), 516–524.

Beery, T., Baas, L. S., Mathews, H., Burrough, J., & Henthorn, R. (2005). Development of the implanted devices adjustment scale. *Dimensions of Critical Care Nursing, 24*(5), 242–248.

Benson, H. (2001). *The relaxation response.* New York: Quill/Harper Collins.

Dennison, C. R., & Hughes, S. Progress in prevention: Imperative to improve care transitions for cardiovascular patients. *Journal of Cardiovascular Nursing, 24*(3), 249–251.

Dossey, B. M., Keegan, L., & Guzzetta, C. (2005). *Holistic nursing: A handbook for practice* (4th ed.). Boston: Jones & Bartlett.

Erickson, H. C. (2006). *Modeling and role-modeling: A view from the client's world.* Cedar Park, TX: Unicorn Press.

Erickson, H. C., Tomlin, E., & Swain, M. A. (1988). *Modeling and role-modeling: A theory and paradigm for nursing.* Lexington, SC: Pine Press of Lexington.

Fowler, C., Kirschner, M., Van Kuiken, D., & Baas, L. S. (2007). Promoting self-care through symptom management: A theory-based approach for nurse practitioners. *Journal of the American Association of Nurse Practitioners, 19*, 221–227.

Lazarus, R. S., & Folkman, S. (1984). *Stress, appraisal and coping.* New York: Springer.

Lee, C. S., Tkacs, N. C., & Riegel, B. (2009). The influence of heart failure self-care on health outcomes: Hypothetical cardioprotective mechanisms. *Journal of Cardiovascular Nursing, 24*(3), 179–187.

Selye, H. (1956). *The stress of life.* New York: McGraw-Hill.

Smith, M. J., & Liehr, P. R. (2008). *Middle range theory for nursing* (2nd ed.). New York: Springer.

Vollman, M. W., LaMontagne, L. L., & Hepworth, J. T. (2007). Coping and depressive symptoms in adults living with heart failure. *Journal of Cardiovascular Nursing, 22*(2), 125–130.

World Health Organization. (1947). *Constitution of the World Health Organization: Chronicle of the World Health Organization.* Geneva: Author.

Review Questions

1. On her application for a nursing license, a nurse indicates that she received a baccalaureate degree in nursing from a state university; however, she actually received an associate's degree from the university and has completed all but one course required for the baccalaureate. This nurse's actions are an example of:
   A. Fraud
   B. Miscarriage of justice
   C. Intentional tort
   D. Invasion of privacy

2. When a person begins to explore ways to quit smoking, he or she is in which stage of the transtheoretical model of behavior change?
   A. Contemplation
   B. Preparation
   C. Action
   D. Termination

3. A case management model that focuses on employee health and wellness and return to work is:
   A. Long-term health care
   B. Occupational health
   C. Managed care
   D. Private

4. A researcher wants to determine the relationship between perceived self-efficacy and attendance at a cardiac rehabilitation program. Which research design helps to best answer this question?
    A. Descriptive
    B. Correlational
    C. Phenomenological
    D. Controlled clinical trial

5. The measurement scale in which data are rank-ordered with equal distance between classes is:
    A. Nominal
    B. Ordinal
    C. Interval
    D. Categorical

6. Which strategy is most effective when teaching a patient to fill his or her weekly medication box?
    A. Lecture with discussion
    B. Role-playing with feedback
    C. Demonstration with return demonstration
    D. Instructional manual or booklet with illustrations

7. Which type of prevention is described as an intervention used to alter the susceptibility of individuals to illness?
    A. Primary
    B. Secondary
    C. Tertiary
    D. Quaternary

8. What has been the major role of professional and national healthcare organizations in promoting the health of the country?
    A. Rely on federal initiatives such as Healthy People 2010
    B. Assist local governments to develop regulations for their constituents
    C. Develop community education programs focused on the public and healthcare providers
    D. Work with academic institutions to research common health problems

9. The most desirable fasting lipid profile for a man with known coronary artery disease is:
    A. Total cholesterol 210, HDL 35, LDL 96, triglycerides 126
    B. Total cholesterol 223, HDL 38, LDL 116, triglycerides 163
    C. Total cholesterol 183, HDL 48, LDL 68, triglycerides 135
    D. Total cholesterol 146, HDL 44, LDL 110, triglycerides 178

10. While conducting a cardiovascular disease (CVD) risk assessment, the nurse discovers that a female patient has a waist circumference of 42 inches, a fasting glucose level of 124 mg/dL, and blood pressure (BP) of 144/92 mm Hg. From this information the nurse concludes that the patient has:
    A. Obesity
    B. Hypertension
    C. Metabolic syndrome
    D. Hyperlipidemia

11. The diagnosis of hypertension is based on:
    A. One BP reading of 140/90 mm Hg or higher
    B. At least three BP readings with an average of 140/90 mm Hg or higher
    C. Average BP reading of 140/90 mm Hg or higher on three different occasions
    D. Positional decrease in BP of 10 mm Hg or more

12. What is the first intervention for dyslipidemia in individuals with low to medium risk?
    A. Increase physical activity
    B. Decrease intake of dietary saturated fat and cholesterol
    C. Control blood glucose
    D. Increase soluble fiber

13. Water moves from an area of lesser sodium concentration to an area of greater sodium concentration by:
    A. Filtration
    B. Diffusion
    C. Osmosis
    D. Facilitated diffusion

14. The usual sequence of cardiovascular examination techniques is:
    A. Inspection, palpation, percussion, and auscultation
    B. Palpation, auscultation, inspection and percussion
    C. Auscultation, inspection, percussion, and palpation
    D. Inspection, auscultation, palpation and percussion

15. Which noninvasive diagnostic test will provide clinically useful information regarding the structure and movement of heart valves and the left ventricle?
    A. Echocardiogram
    B. Left heart catheterization
    C. Thallium study
    D. CT with calcium score

16. Which risk factor is considered unmodifiable?
    A. Family history
    B. Hypertension
    C. Obesity
    D. Diabetes mellitus

17. On auscultation, the sound of mitral stenosis is a:
    A. Holosystolic murmur at the apex *Mitral reg*
    B. Decrescendo, diastolic murmur at the base
    C. Systolic ejection crescendo–decrescendo murmur at the base *Aortic sten*
    D. Holodiastolic murmur at the apex *Aortic reg.*

18. The most life-threatening adverse effect of taking a statin (HMG coenzyme A reductase inhibitor) is:
    A. Angioedema
    B. Renal failure
    C. Myalgia
    D. Rhabdomyolysis

19. Which long-term therapy is considered for patients with heart failure when medical therapy fails and surgical revascularization is not appropriate?
    A. Coronary artery bypass graft (CABG) surgery
    B. Temporary left ventricular assist device
    C. Cardiac transplantation
    D. Implantable cardiac defibrillator

20. Primary pulmonary hypertension is caused by:
    A. An unknown etiology
    B. Cardiac dysfunction
    C. Lung parenchymal disease
    D. Pulmonary vascular obstruction

21. A 66-year-old man is hospitalized with a diagnosis of acute myocardial infarction. Four hours after his admission, his left arm has a purplish rubor and diminished pulses. His vital signs are: temperature 97.2° F (36.2° C); heart rate 166 bpm and irregular; respiration 24 bpm; and BP 82/50 mm Hg. The most likely cause of this patient's left arm symptoms is:
    A. Embolism from atrial fibrillation
    B. Thrombosis from venous catheters
    C. Intimal damage from chronic repetitive work
    D. Thromboembolism from trauma

22. What does the cardiac/vascular nurse include in the teaching for a patient scheduled for a percutaneous transluminal coronary angioplasty (PTCA)?
    A. The procedure is done in the operating room under general anesthesia
    B. After the procedure, angina will be completely gone
    C. There are no complications associated with the procedure when it is done at this facility
    D. A special catheter will be inserted through the femoral or brachial artery

23. Which nursing intervention has highest priority when a home healthcare nurse visits a patient after discharge following surgical repair of an abdominal aneurysm?
    A. Assess understanding of the activity prescription
    B. Monitor and control blood pressure and circulation
    C. Assess wound healing and reapply a sterile dressing
    D. Instruct the patient and his spouse about a low-fat, high-carbohydrate diet

24. Lisinopril (Prinivil®) is which type of medication?
    A. Calcium channel blocker
    B. Vasodilator
    C. Angiotensin II antagonist
    D. ACE inhibitor

25. A syndrome that results in the profound failure of the heart as a pump to meet the metabolic demands of the body is:
    A. Myocardial infarction
    B. Cardiogenic shock
    C. Unstable angina pectoris
    D. Acute coronary syndrome

26. Which intervention can be used in the treatment of draining venous stasis ulcers?
    A. Neurovascular monitoring
    B. Compression stockings
    C. Unna boots
    D. Elastic stockings

27. A 26-year-old woman has cardiomyopathy that was diagnosed 2 years ago after a viral illness. She has been informed that the only treatment option for her is a heart transplant. Lately, she has been feeling sad and has experienced symptoms of insomnia and anorexia. This patient's feelings are indicative of:
    A. Depression
    B. Anxiety
    C. Anger
    D. Dependence

28. Some people limit their contacts with someone who is ill because of their discomfort with the disease. A person's adaptive response to such changes in his or her support systems is:
    A. Adjusting to changes in social relationships
    B. Grieving over losses
    C. Maintaining a positive self-concept
    D. Dealing with role changes

29. The major factor associated with the increased survival of people experiencing cardiac arrest outside of the hospital is:
    A. Initiation of cardiopulmonary resuscitation and use of automatic advisory defibrillators by bystanders
    B. Activation of resources for emergency care (e.g., calling 911) by family members
    C. Accurate assessment by healthcare personnel that the collapse is a cardiac arrest
    D. Initiation of advanced cardiac life support (ACLS) protocols once the person arrives in the emergency room

30. Which diuretic agent has been associated with hearing loss, especially when administered intravenously?
    A. Spironolactone (Aldactone®)
    B. Furosemide (Lasix®)
    C. Chlorothiazide (Diuril®)
    D. Mannitol (Osmitrol®)

31. When caring for a patient with a temporary transvenous pacemaker, the cardiac/vascular nurse:
    A. Keeps the patient in a semi-Fowler position
    B. Encourages active range of motion at the insertion site to prevent frozen shoulder
    C. Maintains an electrically safe environment
    D. Prepares the patient for eventual placement of a permanent device

32. Which statement best describes intermittent claudication?
    A. Cramping pain of the lower extremity that is aggravated by increased activity
    B. Rest pain that is decreased by putting the lower extremity in a dependent position
    C. Cramping pain of the lower extremity that is precipitated by activity and is relieved by rest
    D. Activity pain of the lower extremity that is not affected by position or rest

33. Use of a transcutaneous pacemaker is indicated for which dysrhythmia?
    A. Atrial flutter with a 2:1 conduction
    B. Ventricular tachycardia
    C. Second-degree AVB type II with an atrial rate of 80 and a 2:1 conduction
    D. First-degree AVB with sinus rhythm

34. The most common cause of diastolic heart failure is:
    A. Coronary ischemia or infarction
    B. Hypertension
    C. Valvular dysfunction
    D. Anemia

35. A 65-year-old man comes to the clinic with a chief complaint of retrosternal chest pain that radiates to his back. The pain decreases when he leans forward in a sitting position and increases when he lies down. The patient had coronary artery bypass graft (CABG) surgery 2 weeks ago. Based on his symptoms and past surgical history, the cardiac/vascular nurse suspects:
    A. Rheumatic fever
    B. Endocarditis
    C. Pericarditis
    D. Angina pectoris

36. Which is the appropriate medication to treat substernal chest pain that radiates to the left arm in a patient on a coronary telemetry unit?
    A. Maalox®
    B. Ranitidine (Zantac®)
    C. Nitroglycerin (Nitrostat®)
    D. Metoprolol (Lopressor®)

37. Which lipid profile presents the lowest risk for cardiac and vascular disease in a healthy person?
    A. Total cholesterol 190 mg/dL; LDL cholesterol 100 mg/dL; HDL cholesterol 45 mg/dL
    B. Total cholesterol 190 mg/dL; LDL cholesterol 90 mg/dL; HDL cholesterol 45 mg/dL
    C. Total cholesterol 200 mg/dL; LDL cholesterol 90 mg/dL; HDL cholesterol 65 mg/dL
    D. Total cholesterol 200 mg/dL; LDL cholesterol 100 mg/dL; HDL cholesterol 65 mg/dL

38. Which disorder is characterized by arterial spasm?
    A. Abdominal aortic aneurysm
    B. Takayasu's disease
    C. Temporal arteritis
    D. Raynaud's phenomenon

39. After an acute myocardial infarction, the nurse teaches the patient about usual discharge medications, which include:
    A. Lisinopril, metoprolol, atorvastatin, aspirin
    B. Amiodarone, warfarin, vitamin B
    C. Carvedilol, furosemide, nifedipine
    D. There are no routine medications; it is patient-dependent

40. The goal of treatment for hypertension is to reduce:
    A. Symptoms
    B. Risk of cardiac and vascular disease
    C. Systolic BP to less than 110 mm Hg
    D. Diastolic BP to less than 70 mm Hg

41. Which statement about peripheral vascular disease (PVD) is true?
    A. PVD is an independent predictor for increased risk of cardiac death.
    B. If symptomatic, PVD carries a 30% risk of death within 10 years.
    C. PVD is more likely to develop in patients with hypertension than with diabetes.
    D. Symptomatic PVD carries a two- to fivefold increased risk of fatal or nonfatal CV events.

42. Diabetes mellitus is identified as a clinical cardiovascular disease equivalent because:
    A. People with diabetes have a poor prognosis after a myocardial infarction.
    B. Age-adjusted rates for CHD are two to three times higher in people with diabetes.
    C. Diabetes is associated with an accelerated atheromatous process.
    D. By age 70, CHD is the leading cause of death in men with diabetes.

43. Which person is the best description of Stage A heart failure?
    A. Person with symptomatic shortness of breath associated with aortic valve stenosis
    B. Person with end-stage heart failure undergoing transfer to hospice care
    C. Person with Stage I hypertension that is controlled with a calcium channel blocker
    D. Person after an acute myocardial infarction

44. Learning the signs and symptoms of peripheral vascular disease is an example of which domain of learning?
    A. Affective
    B. Cognitive
    C. Psychomotor
    D. Sensory–preparatory

45. Three hours after a scheduled percutaneous coronary intervention, Mr. Bailey complains of an increase in back pain and a feeling like he has to void but is unable to do so. His blood pressure has dropped to 104/70 mm Hg and heart rate is now 110 and regular. He has a +1 dorsalis pedis pulse bilaterally equal and no bleeding or hematoma at the puncture site. You call the physician to see the patient. What do you suspect is happening?
    A. Renal failure from contrast material
    B. A thrombus at the arterial puncture site
    C. Retroperitoneal bleed
    D. New onset atrial fibrillation

46. The major population trend that will have the largest effect on the future of case management is:
    A. Aging of the population
    B. Early discharges from hospitals
    C. Diversity of the population
    D. Acuity of patients

47. The nurse encourages a patient with intermittent claudication to begin walking a few blocks and gradually increase the distance. Which theoretical process supports this intervention?
    A. Negligence
    B. Vicarious learning
    C. Mastery
    D. Theory of reasoned action

48. A 74-year-old man with vascular dementia is admitted to the hospital from the nursing home with dehydration. He has difficulty swallowing liquids and has been restricted to thickened liquids. He does not have any advance directives and his wife believes a feeding tube is in his best interest. This situation poses an ethical dilemma based on which principles?
    A. Justice versus autonomy
    B. Beneficence versus autonomy
    C. Beneficence versus nonmaleficence
    D. This does not represent an ethical dilemma

49. Beta blockers are effective drugs used for many reasonsm including coronary artery disease, hypertension, heart failure, and dysrhythmias. Which of the following is a potential adverse effect of beta blockers?
    A. Increases myocardial oxygen demand
    B. Masks symptoms of hypoglycemia
    C. Increases renin release, worsening renal function
    D. Causes bronchodilation in asthma

50. Patients with a valve replacement who are scheduled for dental procedures need which type of medication prophylactically?
    A. Anti-inflammatory agents to prevent gingival swelling
    B. Aspirin to prevent clot formation
    C. Antibiotics to prevent endocarditis
    D. Analgesics to prevent pain management

B

Answers to the Review Questions

1. **Correct Answer: A.** Claiming an academic degree not yet earned is providing false or misleading information to a legal body, which constitutes fraud. The Board of Nursing has the right and duty to deny a license to persons who provide false information.

2. **Correct Answer: B.** Exploring ways to quit smoking is the preparation stage of behavior change.

3. **Correct Answer: B.** Occupational health is the model that focuses on the health and wellness of employees and their return to work. The long-term care model targets people with extended care needs. The managed care model manages access to services and advocates cost-effective care for its subscribers. The private model coordinates services for individuals or other groups as a subcontractor.

4. **Correct Answer: B.** The research question asks about the relationship between two concepts, perceived self-efficacy and attendance at a cardiac rehabilitation program. There is a relatively mature body of knowledge about both perceived self-efficacy and cardiac rehabilitation. Therefore, a correlational design is appropriate.

5. **Correct Answer: C.** A rank-ordered measurement scale in which data are rank-ordered with equal distance between classes meets the criteria for interval-level data: numbers are mutually exclusive and exhaustive, they are ordered, and there is an equal interval between data points. The interval level measurement scale does not include absolute zero.

6. **Correct Answer: C.** Demonstration with return demonstration is the most effective strategy for teaching psychomotor skills. Information, discussion, cuing, and feedback may all be used with this strategy to enhance learning and build skill, but are less effective than demonstration.

7. **Correct Answer: A.** Primary prevention is an intervention used to alter the susceptibility of individuals to illness. Secondary prevention involves strategies aimed at the early identification and treatment of disease. Tertiary prevention is focused on preserving or restoring function in people with health problems.

8. **Correct Answer: C.** The greatest contribution of professional healthcare organizations has been the development of community education programs to educate the public and healthcare providers about risk factors and health problems affecting individuals in this country.

9. **Correct Answer: C.** ATP III treatment goals for patients with CHD or CHD equivalent are total cholesterol below 200 mg/dL, HDL above 40 mg/dL, LDL below 70 mg/dL, and triglycerides below 150 mg/dL.

10. **Correct Answer: C.** Metabolic syndrome is defined clinically as the presence of at least three of the following factors: abdominal obesity (waist circumference > 35 inches in women; > 40 inches in men), triglycerides 150 mg/dL or higher, low HDL cholesterol (< 50 mg/dL in women; < 40 mg/dL in men), elevated blood pressure (130/85 mm Hg or higher), and a fasting blood glucose 110 mg/dL or higher.

11. **Correct Answer: C.** The diagnosis of hypertension is based on the average of two or more BP readings taken at each of two or more visits after an initial screening.

12. **Correct Answer: B.** The first intervention for most individuals with dyslipidemia is to reduce the intake of dietary saturated fat and cholesterol.

13. **Correct Answer: C.** Water moves from an area of lesser sodium concentration to an area of greater sodium concentration by osmosis.

14. **Correct Answer: A.** The usual sequence of cardiovascular examination technique is inspection, palpation, percussion, and auscultation. This sequence is different for the abdominal examination in which auscultation precedes palpation and percussion.

15. **Correct Answer: A.** Of these studies, the echocardiogram provides a dynamic picture of the heart that provides a view of valve structures opening and closing as well as muscle contraction.

16. **Correct Answer: A.** Family history is unmodifiable. The effects of other risk factors such as hypertension, obesity, and diabetes mellitus may be modified with lifestyle changes such as diet, exercise, and weight reduction.

17. **Correct Answer: B.** Mitral regurgitation has a holosystolic (pansystolic) murmur heard at the apex. The sound from aortic stenosis is a systolic ejection murmur while aortic regurgitation produces a holodiastolic murmur.

18. **Correct Answer: D.** Rhabdomyolysis is the most life-threatening adverse effect of taking statins, which are metabolized in the liver and more likely to be associated with liver damage. Angioedema is associated with the use of an ACE-I. Myalgia is associated with statin use, but only becomes a problem if there is massive breakdown of muscle tissue associated with rhabdomyolysis. If this occurs, renal failure ensues.

19. **Correct Answer: C.** Cardiac transplantation is used when medical management of heart failure is no longer effective and revascularization surgery is not considered an option. Coronary artery bypass graft surgery is contraindicated in this situation. Left ventricular assist devices are not approved for long-term management of heart failure. Implantable cardiac defibrillators are used for the management of problems such as ventricular fibrillation.

20. **Correct Answer: A.** There are several risk factors associated with the development of primary pulmonary hypertension, but the actual cause has not been determined.

21. **Correct Answer: A.** This patient's rubor and diminished pulses are from arterial ischemia and the most likely cause, based on his diagnosis of myocardial infarction and vital signs, is atrial fibrillation.

22. **Correct Answer: D.** A special catheter will be inserted through a peripheral artery. PTCA is done in the cardiac catheterization laboratory under conscious sedation. Complications of the procedure include coronary restenosis (reoccurrence of angina), abrupt closure of the coronary artery, myocardial infarction, bleeding or hematoma at the vascular access site, arterial embolization, pseudoaneurysm, retroperitoneal bleeding, and death.

23. **Correct Answer: B.** Hypertension is the major risk factor for aneurysm formation and must be controlled for life.

24. **Correct Answer: D.** Lisinopril is an angiotensin-converting enzyme (ACE) inhibitor used in the treatment of heart failure and hypertension. All generic (chemical) names of ACE inhibitors end in "-pril."

25. **Correct Answer: B.** Cardiogenic shock results in the profound failure of the heart as a pump to meet the metabolic demands of the body. The other health problems may result in the development of cardiogenic shock but are actually caused by inadequate blood flow to the myocardium.

26. **Correct Answer: C.** The Unna boot is a gauze dressing with specific medications that is used to treat this health problem.

27. **Correct Answer: A.** The patient's feelings of sadness and symptoms of insomnia and anorexia indicate depression. Anxiety is characterized by feelings of apprehension, tension, and uneasiness. Anger is associated with feelings of extreme displeasure and hostility. Dependence is a regressive reaction that causes the person who is ill to rely on others for their physical and emotional needs.

28. **Correct Answer: A.** The individual who is ill must adjust to changes in their social relationships. Other individuals impose some of the limitations. The individual who is ill may limit their interactions with others because of discomfort and fatigues associated with the disease.

29. **Correct Answer: A.** The start of CPR immediately after cardiac arrest as part of prehospital care is associated with increased survival.

30. **Correct Answer: B.** The loop diuretics are associated with ototoxicity and hearing loss; therefore, furosemide (Lasix®) is a diuretic agent associated with this adverse effect.

31. **Correct Answer: C.** A pacing wire goes directly from the skin (insertion site) to the heart; even small electrical currents can cause cardiac dysrhythmia or arrest. Therefore, the nurse must maintain an electrically safe environment.

32. **Correct Answer: C.** Intermittent claudication is cramping pain of the lower extremity that is precipitated by activity and is relieved by rest. It is a manifestation of lower arterial occlusive disease.

33. **Correct Answer: C.** Second-degree AVB type II and complete heart block are considered high degrees of heart block. The rate that results from these blocks often is not fast enough to support adequate cardiac output. Medications such as atropine are ineffective. Transcutaneous pacemakers can be used effectively to increase the heart rate until the blood pressure stabilizes.

34. **Correct Answer: B.** Hypertension is highly associated with the development of diastolic heart failure, which is more often found in older women.

35. **Correct Answer: C.** Retrosternal chest pain that radiates to the back, decreases when the patient leans forward in a sitting position, and increases when the patient lies down are the classic symptoms of acute pericarditis. A risk factor for this health problem is invasive procedures such as cardiac surgery.

36. **Correct Answer: C.** Nitroglycerin is the appropriate medication to treat substernal chest pain that radiates to the left arm in a patient on a coronary telemetry unit. The patient is probably experiencing angina pectoris and needs to be treated with a vasodilator.

37. **Correct Answer: C.** Although total cholesterol below 200 mg/dL is desirable, in this case the total cholesterol is explained, in part, by the high level of protective HDL cholesterol. LDL cholesterol is below 100 mg/dL, which is optimal.

38. **Correct Answer: D.** Raynaud's phenomenon is caused by arterial spasm in the arteries that supply blood to the skin, limiting blood circulation to affected areas (most commonly the fingers and toes).

39. **Correct Answer: A.** After MI, an ACE-I and beta blocker are routinely ordered to prevent the remodeling of the left ventricle that could result in heart failure. These drugs also block aspects of the renin-angiotensin-aldosterone system. A statin and aspirin (ASA) are used for anti-inflammatory effect. Statins produce a favorable lipid profile while ASA reduces the risk of platelet adhesiveness. These drugs are part of evidence-based practice recommended unless there is a contraindication for their use.

40. **Correct Answer: B.** The goal of treatment for hypertension is to reduce the risk of cardiac and vascular disease. Hypertension is symptomless unless target organ damage or very high levels of BP are present. The desired BP level for average-risk individuals with hypertension is less than 140/90 mm Hg.

41. **Correct Answer: A.** If symptomatic, PVD carries a 30% risk of death within 5 years, not 10. PVD is more likely to develop in patients with diabetes rather than hypertension due to the tendency of diabetes toward smaller distal vessels. If asymptomatic, patients with PVD have a two- to fivefold increased risk of CV events.

42. **Correct Answer: C.** Although people with diabetes have a higher mortality rate than those without diabetes after an MI, it is the accelerated pathology of atherosclerosis that places diabetes in the category of a CHD equivalent. Age-adjusted rates for CHD are two to three times higher only for men with diabetes; for women with diabetes, the rates are three to seven times higher. By age 40, the leading cause of death is CHD in both men and women with diabetes.

43. **Correct Answer: C.** A person with Stage A heart failure is the person with no symptoms of heart failure and no indication of LV dysfunction. However, this is the person at risk of developing HF eventually. People with hypertension are also Stage A heart failure because of the high (50%) risk of developing the disorder.

44. **Correct Answer: B.** Cognitive learning deals with the intellectual or knowledge area and involves acquiring facts, reaching conclusions, or making decisions.

45. **Correct Answer: C.** This patient is beginning to have the signs and symptoms associated with bleeding. BP is falling and the heart rate is becoming more rapid. With a retroperitoneal bleed, the person often experiences more severe back pain or abdominal pressure due to the blood entering the retroperitoneal space and applying additional pressure. This is an emergent situation.

46. **Correct Answer: A.** Even though all of these factors will have an effect on case management and the delivery of healthcare services, the aging of the population will have the greatest impact because of the increasing numbers of older adults requiring care.

47. **Correct Answer: C.** Mastery is a source of efficacy information. It provides the patient with positive reinforcement through achievement.

48. **Correct Answer: D.** An ethical dilemma requires a choice between courses of action that involve fundamental concepts of right and wrong. Because there is no advance directive, the surrogate decision-maker (the wife) is legally and ethically bound to make the decision she believes to be in the best interest of the patient.

49. **Correct Answer: B.** Because beta blockers can decrease the heart rate and blood pressure, the person with diabetes experiencing a hypoglycemic response will not have the tachycardia or other signs of sympathetic stimulation associated with the drop in blood glucose.

50. **Correct Answer: C.** Patients with valve replacement are at risk for endocarditis and need to receive antibiotic prophylaxis.

Index

About the Author

Linda Baas, PhD, MSN, RN, ACNP, FAHA, has a joint position as Professor at the University of Cincinnati and Director of Nursing Research at The Christ Hospital in Cincinnati, Ohio. In her current role, she guides staff nurses in the evaluation of evidence for practice change, assists in the design of performance improvement projects and research studies, and guides staff in publications. Prior to this position, she was the Director of the Acute Care Nurse Practitioner Program at the University of Cincinnati and she worked part-time for 10 years as an ACNP in a heart failure and transplant program. Other past experiences include staff nurse in CCU, cardiac CNS, and director of a cardiac rehabilitation program.

Over her career, she has conducted research related to self-care resources, quality of life, and technology use in cardiac patients. She also has published in various journals and has published numerous chapters in books. Linda is certified as a Cardiovascular Nurse and an ACNP from the American Nurses Credentialing Center and as a CCNS from the American Association of Critical Care Nurses (AACN). She is a Fellow in the American Heart Association Council of Cardiovascular Nursing and a member of the AACN Circle of Excellence.

Linda has been active in many organizations over the years and is currently on the Board of the American Association of Heart Failure Nurses (AAHFN) and the Board of the Society for the Advancement of Modeling and Role-Modeling, and has committee appointments with AHA and the Heart Failure Society of America and the local chapters of PCNA and Ohio Nurses Association.

She has been a speaker at AAHFN and the AACN NTI meetings, presenting on research, assessment, and exercise topics. She has presented research findings at numerous national and international meetings. For 5 years she has been a regular speaker for the ANCC, conducting the cardiovascular review seminars.

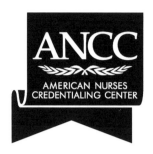

NURSING REVIEW AND RESOURCE MANUAL

Cardiac–Vascular Nursing Addendum

Published by American Nurses Credentialing Center

Author: Barbara "Bobbi" Leeper, MN, RN-BC, CNS M-S, CCRN, FAHA

NURSING CERTIFICATION REVIEW MANUAL
CLINICAL PRACTICE RESOURCE

ADDENDUM TO THE 3RD EDITION

The American Nurses Credentialing Center (ANCC), a subsidiary of the American Nurses Association (ANA), provides individuals and organizations throughout the nursing profession with the resources they need to achieve practice excellence. ANCC's internationally renowned credentialing programs certify nurses in specialty practice areas; recognize healthcare organizations for promoting safe, positive work environments through the Magnet Recognition Program® and the Pathway to Excellence® Program; and accredit providers of continuing nursing education. ANCC's Institute for Credentialing Innovation provides leading-edge information, education services, and products to support its core credentialing programs.

Contents

Introduction to the
Cardiac–Vascular Nursing
Review & Resource Manual Addendum

The management of patients with cardiovascular disease continues to evolve. Changes regarding management affects the practice of nurses caring for these patients. The American Nurses Credentialing Center recognizes the importance of staying abreast of these changes. This addendum includes the information from the revised test content outline to ensure that the *Cardiac Vascular Nursing Review and Resource Manual* is up-to-date. The revision to the test content outline includes the addition of information on complementary therapies, and there is a greater focus on the use of the nursing process for developing and modifying the patient's plan of care.

The information in this addendum serves as bridge material that will assist you with successful completion of the certification examination. It also serves as a guideline for your practice. This addendum is meant to highlight the subject matter and is not meant to be all-inclusive. For more detailed information, we encourage you to further explore the topics via other research-based references or Web sites. We hope that you will find this material useful as both a study guide and a source of information.

If you have any questions about this addendum or the review manual, please send an e-mail to revmanuals@ana.org.

—Barbara "Bobbi" Leeper, MN, RN-BC, CNS M-S, CCRN, FAHA

Complementary Therapies for Patients With Cardiovascular Disease

Many patients with cardiovascular disease (CVD) seek alternative medical therapies as a supplement to their standard of care. They may do so to address adverse effects or perceived limitations of standard therapy. Generally, when these therapies are used in addition to traditional medical practices, they are called complementary therapies, and when they are used in place of traditional medical practices they are called alternative therapies. These practices and products are often used by patients with known cardiovascular disease or by patients with risk factors for cardiovascular disease such as hypertension or elevated lipid levels. The most commonly used interventions are natural products and mind–body practices. More than half of Americans who use herbal remedies do not report their use to their provider. Of concern are the potentially dangerous interactions that may occur with prescribed medications; the more herbs a patient takes, the more likely a drug–drug interaction will occur.

Complementary and alternative medicine (CAM) is the name given to these diverse therapies and products that are not considered part of conventional medical interventions. Interest in CAM therapies for cardiovascular health has increased in recent years. The use of CAM modalities by patients with or at risk for CVD is common and more prevalent than in those without CVD.

Studies have shown that patients turn to CAM modalities to improve their health and health-related quality of life and to prevent further illness. Others are attracted to the idea of taking a holistic approach to health and wellness through CAM. Patients often want to take an active role and have a sense of control in their treatment regimen, and they may believe that natural therapies have fewer adverse effects than conventional medications. Lastly, cost may be a factor. Limited insurance coverage, the increased cost of prescriptions and services, or both may contribute to the appeal of CAM because they are less expensive.

CAM modalities include:
- Alternative medical systems: Homeopathy, naturopathic medicine, ayurveda, and traditional Chinese medicine
- Mind–body intervention: Prayer, deep breathing, meditation, yoga, biofeedback, tai chi, and guided imagery
- Manipulative and body-based therapies: Chiropractic, osteopathic manipulation, massage, reflexology, and Rolfing
- Energy therapies: Veritable and putative energy field treatments, therapeutic touch, healing touch, Reiki, magnet therapy, and sound and light therapy
- Biological therapies: These therapies may include the use of substances found in nature, including herbs, vitamins, and foods; materials such as elk horn and shark cartilage; and diets such as Atkins, macrobiotic, Ornish, Pritikin, Zone, and all types of vegetarianism. Chelation and folk medicine also are considered biological therapy.

HERBALS/SUPPLEMENTS

The most popular therapy is the use of herbals, often referred to as botanicals. Herbals are considered dietary supplements by the U.S. Food and Drug Administration (FDA), and, as a result, they do not require FDA approval. The CAM industry is quite popular with older adults, because these supplements promise to rejuvenate, eliminate ailments, and prevent further aging. Unfortunately, much of this advertising is not reliable or truthful, and the labels for herbals and other supplements often do not warn about possible drug–drug interactions (see Table 1).

Table 1. Common Herbs/Supplements With Side Effects and Precautions

Supplement	Botanical or Chemical Name(s)	Use	Mechanism of Action	Side Effects
Chondroitin, glucosamine, (e.g., Osteo Bi-flex)		Symptomatic and functional benefits for patients with osteoarthritis of knees or hips; may slow disease progression	Glucosamine is an amino sugar that is a substrate for production of glycosaminoglycans and proteoglycans (building blocks of connective tissue); chondroitin is a glycosaminoglycan that may inhibit enzymatic destruction of synovial tissue and have an antiinflammatory role (in addition to its role in cartilage formation)	Considered safe; dose is 500/400 mg, respectively, t.i.d.; may take 8 weeks before treatment response is seen
Coenzyme Q10	Ubiquinone, Ubiquinol, Ubidecarenone	Cardiac conditions; suggested to prevent statin-induced myotoxicity	Substance produced by the body that is structurally similar to vitamins E and K; considered to be an antioxidant and plays a role in mitochondrial oxidative phosphorylation	Considered safe; used in high doses (> 1,000 mg/day) in Parkinson's disease; will decrease the effect of warfarin when given concurrently; cardiac dose is 50–200 mg/day
Echinacea	Echinacea purpurea, Echinacea angustifolia, Echinacea pallida	Colds; analgesic effects	Protects the integrity of hyaluronic acid matrix by stimulating an alternative complement pathway in the immune system; promotes nonspecific T-cell activation by binding to T-cells and increasing interferon production	Skin rash; gastrointestinal upset; diarrhea
Fish oil/ Omega-3 fatty acids		Treating bipolar disorder, hypertension, lowering triglycerides, decreasing blood clotting	Interacts with warfarin, increases anticoagulant effect	Individuals cautioned to stop use before surgery

cont.

Table 1. Common Herbs/Supplements With Side Effects and Precautions (cont.)

Supplement	Botanical or Chemical Name(s)	Use	Mechanism of Action	Side Effects
Flaxseed oil	Aceite de Linaza, Acide Alpha-Linolénique, Acide Gras Omega 3	Treat high cholesterol levels, osteoarthritis, anxiety, benign prostatic hypertrophy, atherosclerosis, hypertension, heart disease, diabetes	High in omega-3 fatty acids and a source of polyunsaturated fatty acids, such as alpha-linolenic acid, which are antiinflammatory	
Garlic	*Allium sativum*	Natural cholesterol-lowering agent; effective only short-term	Sulfur-containing substances in garlic may inhibit 3-hydroxy-3-methylglutaryl coenzyme-A reductase; decreases platelet aggregation	Generally considered safe; can cause gastrointestinal distress and gas
Ginkgo	*Ginkgo biloba*	Improving memory; treating dementia, peripheral vascular disease, and tinnitus	Increases blood flow; inhibits platelet-activating factors; alters neuronal metabolism; works as an antioxidant	Rare; can cause gastrointestinal complaints or headache; case reports of spontaneous bleeding
Ginseng		Improving memory	Increases heart, blood pressure	Increased effect of blood thinners; should not be taken if hyptertensive
Grapeseed extract		Antihypertensive	Contains bioflavonoids, which have anti-inflammatory and antioxidant effects; prevents premature aging, improves skin, anti-arthritic	
Hawthorn		Treating heart failure	May improve ejection fraction, exercise tolerance and reduce subjective symptoms	

St. John's Wort	*Hypericum perforatum*	Wound healing; depression	Serotonin reuptake is primary mechanism, perhaps MAOI and catechol-O-methyltransferase activity, along with modulation of melatonin and norepinephrine uptake	Photosensitivity; possible serotonin syndrome if used with SSRIs

Note. MAOI = monoamine oxidase inhibitor; SSRI = selective serotonin reuptake inhibitors

---

Herbals are manufactured in several forms—capsules, extracts, oils, pills, salves, teas, and tinctures. Their efficacy varies depending on the form of the herb used. Herbal teas appeal to consumers, and millions of dollars are spent annually on this form of botanical. Because there are few reports of untoward effects of teas, consumers believe they are harmless. They may, in fact, be safe if they are consumed in moderation (or minimally). However, liver disease has been reported with comfrey, causing it to be removed from the market in 2002. Table 1 contains a list of common supplements whose use is reported by patients with CVD, along with side effects and precautions.

Fish Oil/Omega-3 Fatty Acids

Omega-3 fatty acids are polyunsaturated fatty acids with known health benefits. Unfortunately, the body cannot produce them. Therefore, dietary intake of omega-3 fatty acids is essential. They play an important role in:
- Cognitive function (memory and performance) and behavioral development
- Normal growth and development
- Control of inflammation

Clinical evidence is strong for a therapeutic role in:
- Reduction of risk for CVD
- Hypertension
- Diabetes (to lower triglyceride levels)
- Rheumatoid arthritis/systemic lupus erythematosis

Dietary sources include coldwater fish, such as salmon, tuna, and halibut. They are also found in flaxseed, soybeans, pumpkin seeds, and other types of seed and nuts.

Omega-3 fatty acids interact with the following drugs:
- Warfarin (Coumadin), clopidogrel (Plavix), or aspirin: Associated with increased risk of bleeding
- Diabetes medications (oral and insulin): May increase fasting blood sugar levels

Coenzyme Q10

One of the most frequently used supplements is coenzyme Q10 (CoQ10). This enzyme has a structure similar to vitamin K. It supports three biologic functions:
- Enhances mitochondrial adenosine triphosphate (ATP) energy production
- Potentiates antioxidant effects—removes oxygen radicals
- Enhances cell membrane stabilization

The body's production of CoQ10 decreases with age. Studies have shown that patients with CVD have a CoQ10 deficiency in their myocardial tissues. There is evidence supporting the therapeutic value of CoQ10 as an adjunct to standard medical therapy for the management of heart failure.

CoQ10 has been found to:
- Increase myocardial contractility
- Improve oxygen use at the cellular level
- Enhance systolic function in chronic heart failure

CoQ10 interacts with the following drugs:
- Statins: Therapy may reduce blood levels of CoQ10
- Warfarin: CoQ10 reduces coagulation effect; caution should be exercised if warfarin and CoQ10 are used together
- Insulin: Potential hypoglycemic effects; use caution with the combination
- Vasodilators: Potential hypotensive effects; use caution with the combination

EVIDENCE-BASED MIND–BODY THERAPIES

The use of mind–body therapies for stress reduction has been shown to reduce cardiovascular mortality. Studies demonstrated a 29% reduction in myocardial infarction recurrence and a 34% reduction in mortality attributable to CVD. In many cases, patients are able to practice these techniques independently.
- Acupressure/acupuncture
- Aromatherapy
- Biofeedback
- Guided imagery
- Massage
- Meditation/yoga
- Progressive muscle relaxation
- Reflexology
- Tai chi

Acupressure/Acupuncture
- Modalities that are thought to produce effects by regulating the nervous system and aiding the activity of endorphins and immune cells at different sites in the body
- Also thought to alter brain chemistry by changing the release of neurohormones and neurotransmitters
- Have been shown to lower blood pressure

Aromatherapy
- Use of plants or oils to obtain many therapeutic effects, such as analgesic, psychological, and antimicrobial effects

Biofeedback
- A process that provides a person with visual or auditory information about autonomic physiologic functions of his or her body, such as blood pressure, muscle tension, and brain wave activity.
- Through attention and practice, the person can learn to influence these functions.
- Used to control or manage a person's response to conditions as varied as:
  - Stress-related symptoms (e.g., anxiety)
  - Blood pressure and heart rate variability
  - Pain
  - Insomnia
  - Raynaud's disease
  - Urinary incontinence
  - Neuromuscular problems such as migraines, muscular tension, and tension headaches
- Said to enhance healing of injuries and improve athletic and work performance
- Desired outcomes include:
  - Positive change in baseline measures
  - Demonstrated skill at self-regulation
  - Improvement in symptoms
  - Use of skills in daily life
  - Reduction of muscle bracing
  - Increased sense of self-efficacy

Massage
- Modality believed to increase blood circulation, improve lymph flow, improve musculoskeletal tone, and have a tranquilizing effect on the mind

Meditation
- The practice of consciously directing one's attention to alter one's state of mind
- Produces physiological effects such as decreased heart rate, blood pressure, and respiratory rate; decreased anxiety; and increased alpha brain waves
- Has been shown to improve blood pressure and insulin resistance
- Associated with lower cardiovascular morbidity and mortality

Reflexology
- Based on Traditional Chinese Medicine (TCM) and a Western technique called zone therapy
  - TCM: The feet are seen as a microcosm of the body, that is, all the organs, glands, and other body parts are mirrored on the soles of the feet. All organs are interconnected with each other by a number of energy pathways. The goal is to keep the energies in balance.
  - Zone Therapy: Similar concept as TCM, with the body and its organs represented in a certain configuration on the feet. Pressure in different areas of the feet produces distinct effects in the body. Massaging the hands and ears has been shown to have similar effects.

- Reported uses include:
  – Decrease pain: Back pain, migraines
  – Decrease anxiety
  – Reduce physiologic stress
  – Reduce symptoms of multiple sclerosis
  – Promote relaxation
  – Improve sleep
  – Improve quality of life in cancer patients

Guided Imagery

- A technique that has been shown to reduce anxiety and pain associated with cardiac surgery
- Hypnosis-like guided imagery has been successful in:
  – Reducing anxiety and blood pressure
  – Affecting heart rate variability, with effects on autonomic nervous system

Tai Chi

- A Chinese movement discipline that involves coordination of different breathing patterns with different body postures and motions
- Heart failure patients have shown significant increases on quality of life scores, 6-minute walk distances, and serum brain natriuretic peptide levels

Nursing Diagnosis

A *nursing diagnosis* is a label used to identify key problems that caused the patient's change in health status. The use of this label assists the nurse in developing the patient's plan of care. The nursing diagnosis may be pathophysiologic (biological or psychosocial), treatment-related, situational (environmental or personal in nature), or maturational. Table 2 provides examples of each category.

Table 2. Nursing Diagnoses Categories

Nursing Diagnosis Category	Example
Pathophysiologic	Inadequate peripheral circulation Low cardiac output
Treatment-related	Incisional pain (following surgery) Hypotension (vasodilators)
Situational	Change in role status Loss of job
Family	Retirement

Some nursing diagnoses are considered high risk. A nurse may make a clinical judgment indicating the patient, family, or both are more vulnerable to developing a problem than other people in the same situation. For example, consider a patient who has a job requiring lifting heavy equipment who has undergone emergency coronary artery bypass surgery following a myocardial infarction. The surgeon used a median sternotomy approach. Following surgery, the surgeon tells the patient that he will not be able to return to work for at least 3 months to make sure the sternum has healed completely. This is worrisome for the patient, because he does not have enough sick leave to cover the extended time off and he is the family's sole wage earner. This situation is a major source of worry and anxiety for the patient, and can contribute to loss of sleep and impaired healing, as well as contribute to noncompliance during the recovery phase.

Formulating a Nursing Diagnosis

Today, a nursing diagnosis can be written in a variety of ways. The traditional approach recommended by the North American Nursing Diagnosis Association (NANDA) has been to have a two- or three-part statement. A three-part statement would include the diagnostic label (problem) related to the contributing factors (etiology) as evidenced by signs and symptoms (symptoms). A two-part statement would include the diagnostic label related to the contributing factors. More recently, a one-part statement—the problem statement—has become more common.

The problem can be stated in a variety of ways. One approach is to state, "Impaired skin integrity." Another is simply stating what the problem is, such as "dysphagia." The problem statement should not be a medical diagnosis such as "diabetes" or a treatment such as "chest tube." Nursing diagnoses are primarily resolved by nursing interventions. Nurses are accountable for treatment outcomes related to the interventions.

Prioritizing the Nursing Diagnoses

The list of nursing diagnoses—that is, patient problems—should be prioritized, starting with the highest-risk problem associated with preventing death. The second level would be diagnoses related to preventing disability. The final priority would be diagnoses addressing the prevention of pain and discomfort. Actual problems should always take precedence over potential problems. The problem list will aid development of the patient's plan of care and nursing interventions to be implemented while caring for the patient.

Table 3 contains a list of nursing diagnoses/patient problems that may be considered for patients with cardiovascular disease.

Table 3. Potential Nursing Diagnoses for Patients With Cardiovascular Disease

Cardiovascular Problem	Nursing Diagnosis
Hypertension	• Chest pain related to increased afterload • Decreased cardiac output • Decreased urine output • Alteration in pulmonary function • Sleep apnea – Pulmonary edema related to worsening heart failure • Alteration in neurologic status • Impaired peripheral perfusion • Noncompliance related to medications

Angina, stable	• Knowledge deficit if new onset
	  – Risk factor identification and modification
	  – Medications
	• Potential for ineffective coping
	• Risk for activity intolerance

Acute coronary syndrome • Unstable angina • Non-ST-segment MI • ST-segment MI	• Cardiac output, decreased • Gas exchange, impaired • Mobility, impaired physical • Peripheral tissue perfusion, altered • High risk for fluid volume disturbance • Family process, altered • Role performance, altered • Coping, compromised
Valvular heart disease	• Activity intolerance • Fatigue • Impaired gas exchange • Decreased cardiac output • Altered tissue perfusion • Decisional conflict related to medical and surgical management • Knowledge deficit
Peripheral vascular disease	• Activity intolerance • Altered tissue perfusion • Pain, acute or chronic • Impaired skin integrity • Impaired tissue integrity • Noncompliance related to tobacco use
Stroke	• Unilateral neglect • Impaired physical mobility • Disturbed sensory perception • Impaired verbal communication • Ineffective protection • Knowledge deficit (specify) • Ineffective coping; compromised family coping

In summary, there is no consensus on the focus of the nursing diagnosis. It is driven by the model of nursing used to guide the nursing process in a given environment. It may focus on self-care deficits, ineffective adaptations, human response patterns, patient needs, or dysfunctional health patterns. It is important to remember that the problem statement is drawn from the nurse's assessment of the patient, family, or both, and is used to develop the plan of care.

References

Anderson, J. G., & Taylor A.G. (2011). Use of complimentary therapies by individuals with or at risk for cardiovascular disease. *Journal of Cardiovascular Nursing, 27*(2), 96–102.

Carpenito, L. J. (2006). *Nursing diagnosis: Application to clinical practice* (11th ed.). Philadelphia: Lippincott Williams & Wilkins.

Gordon, M. (2010). *Manual of nursing diagnoses.* Sudbury, MA: Jones & Bartlett.

Guarneri, M., Mercado, N., & Suhar, C. (2009). Integrative approaches for cardiovascular disease. *Nutrition in Clinical Practice, 24*(6), 701–708.

Rainforth, M. V., Schneider, R. H., Nidich, S. I., Gaylord-King, C., Salerno, S. I., & Anderson, J. W. (2007). Stress reduction programs in patients with elevated blood pressure: A systematic review and meta-analysis. *Current Hypertension Reports, 9,* 520–528.

Sander, S., Coleman, C. I., Patel, A. A., Kluger, J., & White, C. M. (2006) The impact of coenzyme Q10 on systolic function in patients with chronic heart failure. *Journal of Cardiac Failure, 12*(6), 464–472.

Singh, U., Devaraj, S., & Jialal, I. (2007). Coenzyme Q10 supplementation and heart failure. *Nutrition Reviews, 65*(6), 286–293.

Skidmore-Roth, K. (2010). *Mosby's handbook of herbs and natural supplements* (4th ed.). Philadelphia: Elsevier Mosby.

Snyder, M., & Lindquist, R. (Eds.). (2010). *Complementary & alternative therapies in nursing* (6th ed.). New York: Springer.

Yeh, G. Y., Davis, R. B., & Phillips R. S. (2006). Use of complementary therapies in patients with cardiovascular disease. *American Journal of Cardiology, 98,* 673–680.